Applied Mathematical Sciences
Volume 167

Applied Mathematical Sciences
Volume 162

Editors
S.S. Antman J.E. Marsden L. Sirovich

Otmar Scherzer

Harald Grossauer

Frank Lenzen

Markus Grasmair

Markus Haltmeier

Variational Methods in Imaging

With 72 Figures

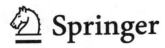 Springer

Otmar Scherzer
otmar.scherzer@uibk.ac.at

Markus Grasmair
markus.grasmair@uibk.ac.at

Harald Grossauer
harald.grossauer@uibk.ac.at

Markus Haltmeier
markus.haltmeier@uibk.ac.at

Frank Lenzen
frank.lenzen@uibk.ac.at

All affiliated with:
Department of Mathematics
University of Innsbruck
Techniker Str. 21a/2
6020 Insbruck
Austria

Editors

S.S. Antman
Department of Mathematics
and
Institute for Physical Science
  and Technology
University of Maryland
College Park, MD 20742-4015
USA
ssa@math.umd.edu

J.E. Marsden
Control and Dynamical
  Systems, 107-81
California Institute of
  Technology
Pasadena, CA 91125
USA
marsden@cds.caltech.edu

L. Sirovich
Laboratory of Applied
  Mathematics
Department of
  Biomathematical
  Sciences
Mount Sinai School
  of Medicine
New York, NY 10029-6574
USA
chico@camelot.mssm.edu

ISBN: 978-1-4419-2166-6   e-ISBN: 978-0-387-69277-7
DOI: 10.1007/978-0-387-69277-7

Mathematics Subject Classification (2000): 68U10

Printed on acid-free paper

springer.com

This book is dedicated to *Zuhair Nashed* on the occasion of his 70th birthday. Zuhair has collaborated with Heinz Engl, University of Linz, Austria. Heinz Engl in turn has supervised Otmar Scherzer, who was also supervised afterwards by Zuhair during several long- and-short term visits in the USA. Finally, Markus Grasmair was supervised by Otmar Scherzer during his PhD studies, and the thesis was also evaluated by Zuhair. Three generations of mathematicians in Austria congratulate Zuhair and his family on his 70th birthday.

Otmar Scherzer also dedicates this book to his family: Roswitha, Anna, Simon, Heide, Kurt, Therese, Franz, Paula, and Josef. Markus Haltmeier dedicates this book to his family. Frank Lenzen dedicates this book to Bettina, Gisela, Dieter, and Ulli.

Preface

Imaging is an interdisciplinary research area with profound applications in many areas of science, engineering, technology, and medicine. The most primitive form of *imaging* is *visual inspection*, which has dominated the area before the technical and computer revolution era. Today, computer imaging covers various aspects of *data filtering, pattern recognition, feature extraction, computer aided inspection,* and *medical diagnosis.* The above mentioned areas are treated in different scientific communities such as *Imaging, Inverse Problems, Computer Vision, Signal* and *Image Processing,* ..., but all share the common thread of recovery of an object or one of its properties.

Nowadays, a core technology for solving imaging problems is *regularization.* The foundations of these approximation methods were laid by Tikhonov in 1943, when he generalized the classical definition of *well-posedness* (this generalization is now commonly referred to as *conditional well-posedness*). The heart of this definition is to specify a *set of correctness* on which it is known *a priori* that the considered problem has a unique solution. In 1963, Tikhonov [371, 372] suggested what is nowadays commonly referred to as Tikhonov (or sometimes also Tikhonov–Phillips) regularization. The abstract setting of regularization methods presented there already contains all of the variational methods that are popular nowadays in imaging. Morozov's book [277], which is the English translation of the Russian edition from 1974, is now considered the first standard reference on Tikhonov regularization.

In the early days of regularization methods, they were analyzed mostly theoretically (see, for instance, [191, 277, 278, 371–373]), whereas later on numerics, efficient solutions (see, for instance, the monographs [111, 204, 207, 378]), and applications of regularization methods became important (see, for instance, [49, 112–114]).

Particular applications (such as, for instance, segmentation) led to the development of specific variational methods. Probably the most prominent among them is the Mumford–Shah model [276, 284], which had an enormous impact on the analysis of regularization methods and revealed challenges for the efficient numerical solution (see, e.g., [86, 88]). However, it is notable that the Mumford–Shah method also reveals the common features of the abstract form of Tikhonov regularization. In 1992, Rudin, Osher, and Fatemi published *total variation regularization* [339]. This paper had an enormous impact on theoretical mathematics and applied sciences. From an analytical point of view, properties of the solution of regularization functionals have been analyzed (see, for instance, [22]), and efficient numerical algorithms (see [90, 133, 304]) have been developed.

Another stimulus for regularization methods has come from the development of non-linear parabolic partial differential equations for *image denoising* and *image analysis*. Here we are interested in two types of evolution equations: *parabolic subdifferential inclusion* equations and *morphological* equations (see [8, 9, 194]). Subdifferential inclusion equations can be associated in a natural way with Tikhonov regularization functionals. This for instance applies to *anisotropic diffusion filtering* (see the monograph by Weickert [385]). As we show in this book, we can associate *non-convex* regularization functionals with morphological equations.

Originally, Tikhonov type regularization methods were developed with the emphasis on the stable solution of *inverse problems*, such as tomographical problems. These inverse problems are quite challenging to analyze and to solve numerically in an efficient way. In this area, mainly simple (quadratic) Tikhonov type regularization models have been used for a long time. In contrast, the underlying physical model in image analysis is simple (for instance, in denoising, the identity operator is inverted), but sophisticated regularization techniques are used. This discrepancy between the different scientific areas led to a split.

The abstract formulation of Tikhonov regularization can be considered in *finite dimensional* space setting as well as in *infinite dimensional function space* setting, or in a combined *finite-infinite* dimensional space setting. The latter is frequently used in spline and wavelet theory. Moreover, we mention that Tikhonov regularization can be considered in a *deterministic* setting as well as in a *stochastic* setting (see, for instance, [85, 231]).

This book attempts to bridge the gap between the two research areas of image analysis and imaging problems in inverse problems and to find a common language. However, we also emphasize that our research is biased toward *deterministic* regularization and, although we use statistics to motivate regularization methods, we do not make the attempt to give a stochastic analysis.

For applications of imaging, we have chosen examples from our own research experience, which are *denoising, telescope imaging, thermoacoustic imaging,* and *schlieren tomography*. We do not claim that these applications are most representative for imaging. Certainly, there are many other active research areas and applications that are not touched in this book.

Of course, this book is not the only one in the field of *Mathematical Imaging*. We refer for instance to [26, 98]. Imaging from an inverse problems point of view is treated in [49]. There exists also a vast number of proceedings and edited volumes that are concerned with mathematical imaging; we do not provide detailed references on these volumes. Another branch of imaging is mathematical methods in tomography, where also a vast amount of literature exists. We mention exemplarily the books [232, 288, 289].

The objective of this book certainly is to bridge the gap between regularization theory in image analysis and in inverse problems, noting that both areas have developed relatively independently for some time.

Acknowledgments

The authors are grateful for the support of the Austrian Science Foundation (FWF), which supported the authors during writing of the book. The relevant supporting grants are Y-123 INF, FSP 92030, 92070, P18172-N02, S10505.

Moreover, Otmar Scherzer is grateful to the Radon Institute in Linz and the available research possibilities there.

The authors thank the Infmath group in Innsbruck and the Imaging group in Linz for their proofreading. We are grateful to many researchers that stimulated our research and spared much time for discussion.

Otmar Scherzer acknowledges the possibility to teach preliminary parts of the book in summer schools in Vancouver (thanks to Ian Frigaard), in Jyväskylä (thanks to Kirsi Majava), and at CMLA, Paris (thanks to Mila Nikolova).

The authors are grateful to GE Medical Systems Kretz Ultrasound AG for providing the ultrasound data frequently used in the book as test data. Moreover, the authors thank Vaishali Damle and Marcia Bunda of Springer New York for their constant support during the preparation of the book.

Innsbruck,   *Markus Grasmair, Harald Grossauer, Markus Haltmeier,*
2008   *Frank Lenzen, Otmar Scherzer*

Contents

Part III Mathematical Foundations

Part I

Fundamentals of Imaging

1

Case Examples of Imaging

In this chapter, we study several imaging examples from our own research experience. The first example concerns the problem of *denoising*. The other examples are related to *inverse problems*, which in general are defined as problems of recovering the cause for an observed effect (see [152]).

1.1 Denoising

One of the most important problems in digital image processing is *denoising*. Noise is usually considered as undesired perturbation in an image. However, it appears during every data acquisition process, for instance during recording with CCD sensors (see [359]).

Denoising is the process of reducing spurious noise in an image. It is either used to make images look "nicer" or as a preprocessing step for *image analysis* and *feature extraction*.

In order to highlight the importance of denoising for image analysis, we apply a *segmentation* and an *edge detection* algorithm to the ultrasound data shown in Fig. 1.1. It can be seen from Figs. 1.2 and 1.3 that after filtering in a preprocessing step, the implementation of these algorithms yields clearly better results.

- The task of segmentation is to retrieve all pixels belonging to an object of interest in a given image.

  As an example, we consider segmentation of the vein in the ultrasound image Fig. 1.1, which is the circular, dark domain in the center. To that end we use the following *region-growing algorithm* based on *intensity thresholding* (see [336]): Given an intensity threshold c and a *seed pixel* p with an intensity less than or equal to c, we start with the initial region $R^0 := \{p\}$ and iteratively obtain regions R^{i+1} from R^i by adding pixels that are *neighboring* R^i and whose intensities are less than or equal to c. The

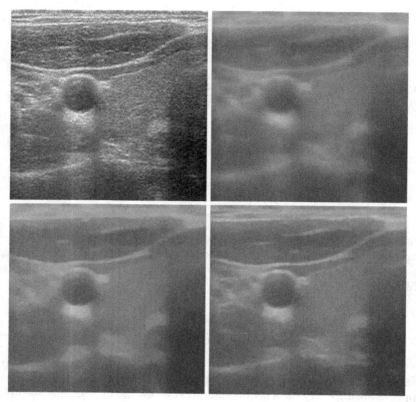

Fig. 1.1. Results of different variational regularization techniques for denoising ultrasound data (*top left*), which are described in Chapter 4.

region growing stops if no more pixels satisfying these two conditions can be found. Figure 1.2 shows the result of the region-growing algorithm applied to the original and filtered data in Fig. 1.1. The results imply that the segmentation is unsatisfactory if the algorithm is applied to unfiltered data.

- Another example that reveals the importance of denoising as preprocessing step in image analysis is edge detection. Here the goal is to extract the boundaries of objects or regions in the image.

One widely used method for edge detection is the *Sobel operator*: Let

$$G_x = \begin{pmatrix} -1 & 0 & 1 \\ -2 & 0 & 2 \\ -1 & 0 & 1 \end{pmatrix}, \quad G_y = \begin{pmatrix} -1 & -2 & -1 \\ 0 & 0 & 0 \\ 1 & 2 & 1 \end{pmatrix}.$$

We denote the discrete convolution (see [184, Sect. 3.4]) of an image $\mathbf{u}$, interpreted as real-valued matrix, with the masks G_x and G_y by $G_x * \mathbf{u}$ and $G_y * \mathbf{u}$, respectively. The Sobel operator is given by

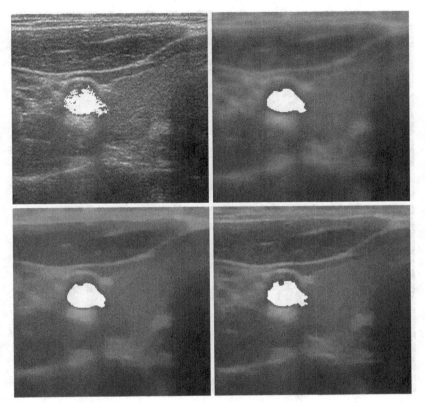

Fig. 1.2. Segmentation of the vein in the ultrasound image Fig. 1.1. The white regions indicate the results of a region-growing algorithm applied to the original data (*top left*) and the different smoothed images. Segmentation of the original data provides a region with fuzzy boundary. When the algorithm is applied to filtered data, the results show a more regular shape that better reflects the vein's true boundary.

$$G : \mathbf{u} \mapsto \sqrt{(G_x * \mathbf{u})^2 + (G_y * \mathbf{u})^2} \; .$$

The value $(G\mathbf{u})_{ij}$ is large near edges and small in homogeneous regions of the image. As can be seen from Fig. 1.3, the edge detector gives significantly better results for the filtered than for the unfiltered data, where spurious edges appear.

Among the variety of denoising techniques, two classes are of importance for this book: *variational methods*, which are discussed in Chapter 4, and *evolutionary partial differential equations*, which are discussed in Chapter 6.

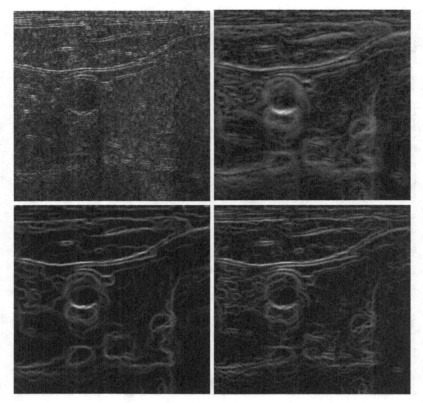

Fig. 1.3. Edge detection with the Sobel operator. The images show the value of the Sobel operator applied to the original (*top left*) and filtered data. Using filtered data improves the quality of detection, as spurious edges created by noise are suppressed.

1.2 Chopping and Nodding

Chopping and nodding (see [51, 148, 230, 252, 333]) is a common approach for the removal of background noise in infrared observations of the sky with ground-based telescopes.

The basic assumption is that the background noise can be decomposed into two components, the first of which mainly depends on the time of acquisition of the image, whereas the second, *residual noise*, varies in time at a slower rate and mainly depends on the optical path of light through the telescope.

We denote by $\mathbf{x} \in S^2$ the position in the sky the telescope, located at $0 \in \mathbb{R}^3$, is originally pointing to. Here S^2 denotes the unit sphere in $\mathbb{R}^3$. From this position $\mathbf{x}$, a signal u_1 is recorded.

Then a *chopping* procedure is performed, which consists in tilting the secondary mirror of the telescope by a certain angle (see Fig. 1.4). After tilting, the telescope points to a position $\mathbf{y} \in S^2$, and a signal u_2 is recorded. The

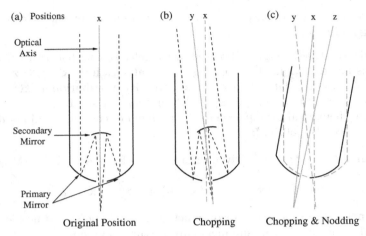

Fig. 1.4. The procedure of chopping and nodding. (**a**) Original position of the telescope pointing toward position **x** in the sky. (**b**) *Chopping*: tilting the secondary mirror provides a signal from position **y**. (**c**) After *nodding*, the telescope points toward **z**. A second chopping procedure is performed, after which the telescope points at position **x**, where the signal is recorded again.

shift $\mathbf{x} - \mathbf{y}$ is called *chopping throw*, its size $|\mathbf{y} - \mathbf{x}|$ the *chopping amplitude*. Chopping is performed at a high rate to cope with the time-varying background noise. Thus it can be assumed that the difference signal $u_1 - u_2$ is little affected by background noise. After chopping, the secondary mirror is moved back to its original position.

For reduction of the residual noise, the whole telescope is tilted to point at a position that is chosen in a way that $|\mathbf{z} - \mathbf{x}| = |\mathbf{y} - \mathbf{x}|$ and the points $\mathbf{x}, \mathbf{y}, \mathbf{z}$, and 0 are coplanar. A signal u_3 then is acquired. In the literature, the tilting is referred to as *nodding*. Because u_1 and u_3 are recorded with the same optical path through the telescope, they contain similar residual noise, which can be removed by taking the difference of u_1 and u_3.

While the telescope is in tilted position, a second chopping procedure is performed, after which the telescope again points toward position **x**. From this position the signal $\tilde{u}_1$ is recorded. Note that also the difference $\tilde{u}_1 - u_3$ shows little background noise, while the difference $\tilde{u}_1 - u_2$ shows little residual noise, as the signals $\tilde{u}_1$ and u_2 are recorded with the same optical path.

Finally the signals are fused as follows:

$$v = u_1 - u_2 - u_3 + \tilde{u}_1 .$$

The motivation for the chopping and nodding procedure is that the collected data v contain little background and residual noise, as v consists of the differences $u_1 - u_2$ and $\tilde{u}_1 - u_3$, as well as the differences $u_1 - u_3$ and $\tilde{u}_1 - u_2$. Therefore, the difficult modeling of the background noise can be avoided.

Figure 1.4 schematically illustrates the movement of the telescope for chopping and nodding.

We identify the sky region observed by the telescope with a subset Ω of $\mathbb{R}^2$. After this identification, the chopping throw satisfies $\mathbf{h} := \mathbf{x} - \mathbf{y} = \mathbf{z} - \mathbf{x}$. In the case of noise-free data, there exists an intensity distribution $u : \mathbb{R}^2 \to \mathbb{R}_{\geq 0}$ such that $u_1 = \tilde{u}_1 = u(\mathbf{x})$, $u_2 = u(\mathbf{x} - \mathbf{h})$, and $u_3 = u(\mathbf{x} + \mathbf{h})$.

The mathematical formulation of the problem of chopping and nodding is as follows (see also [50, 52]):

Problem 1.1. Let $\Omega \subset \mathbb{R}^2$. Given data $v : \Omega \to \mathbb{R}$, find $u : \mathbb{R}^2 \to \mathbb{R}_{\geq 0}$ such that

$$2u(\mathbf{x}) - u(\mathbf{x} - \mathbf{h}) - u(\mathbf{x} + \mathbf{h}) = v(\mathbf{x}), \quad \mathbf{x} \in \Omega \,.$$

In general, the problem of reconstruction from chopped and nodded data is more difficult, as the measurements are perturbed by noise.

For simulations, we use corresponding chopped and nodded data from an artificial test image (see Fig. 1.5). Variational methods for solving Problem 1.1 are presented in Section 3.4.

1.3 Image Inpainting

The process of filling in artificial image data into a missing or occluded image region is referred to as *image inpainting*. The processed region is called the *inpainting domain*. The task is to insert new image data that fit nicely into the

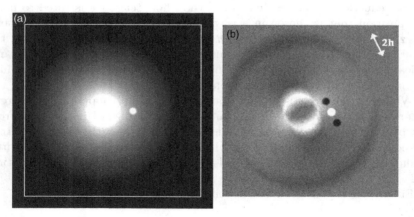

Fig. 1.5. Artificial test image. (a) The white square marks the domain where chopped and nodded data are acquired. (b) Simulated chopped and nodded data, which additionally are perturbed by Gaussian noise. The white arrow indicates the double chopping throw 2**h**. The data v are represented as a function defined on Ω, the boundary of which is indicated by the white rectangle on the left-hand side.

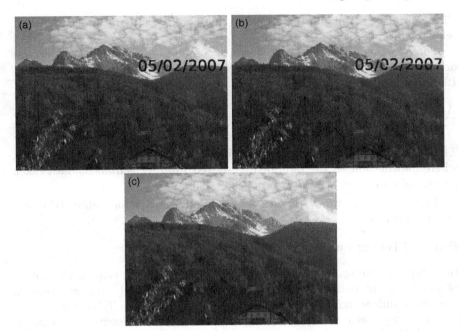

Fig. 1.6. Image inpainting. (**a**) The original image with superimposed text, which should be inpainted. (**b**) The most prominent edges have been completed across the text. (**c**) The remaining superimposed text parts have been filled with texture from the surroundings.

surrounding data, such that a hasty observer does not notice the manipulation. Practical applications are, for example, restoration of old photographs whose color coating peels off, or the removal of overlaid pieces of text (date/time information included in images taken with digital cameras).

The underlying *inpainting model* has to meet the following specifications (see Fig. 1.6):

1. Salient image structures, such as for instance edges, have to be continued smoothly into and across the inpainting domain (*geometry inpainting*).
2. The remaining empty space must be filled up with a pattern that fits into its surroundings (*texture inpainting*).

Typically, *geometry inpainting* is performed with variational methods and partial differential equations. Variational methods for inpainting are presented in Chapter 3.

The most important approach in *texture inpainting* is to model images as the output of a stochastic process. The characteristic of the stochastic process is estimated from the available texture. Missing image regions are then filled by texture that is synthesized from samples of the same stochastic process.

This approach is outside the scope of this book. For more information, we refer to [141, 208, 384].

Some further algorithms have been proposed that are more or less variants or combinations of geometry and texture inpainting, see for example [120, 138, 193, 224].

1.4 X-ray–Based Computerized Tomography

The term *tomography* is used for various *non-invasive imaging techniques*, where information on the interior is retrieved from measurement data taken outside of an object, see for instance [289, 360].

In this section, we focus on X-ray computerized tomography (CT) for medical purposes.

Physical Background

In X-ray CT, the spatially varying *attenuation coefficient*, that is, the ability of the tissue to reduce the X-ray intensity, is visualized. The attenuation coefficient differs significantly within the human body (see Table 1.2).

Electromagnetic radiation is characterized by its wavelength λ or, equivalently, by its frequency $\nu = c/\lambda$, where c is the speed of light. Electromagnetic radiation of frequency ν consists of photons, each carrying energy $E = h\nu$, where h is Planck's constant (see Table 1.1). The wavelength of X-rays used in medical applications is relatively small, varying between 0.01 nm and 0.1 nm. Radiation with small wavelength (high frequency) is *ionizing*.

X-rays are hardly scattered in tissue. Therefore, in contrast with *non-ionizing radiation* such as visible light and microwaves, X-rays propagate mainly along a line (see Fig. 1.7).

Mathematical Modeling

In the sequel, we derive the basic mathematical model for X-ray CT. As illustrated in Fig. 1.7, an X-ray beam is initialized at $\mathbf{x}_{\mathrm{init}}$ with intensity I_{init}

Table 1.1. Physical variables used to describe the X-radiation (*top*) and interactions between radiation and tissue (*bottom*).

Physical quantity	Symbol	Order of magnitude
Speed of light	c	300,000 km/s
Frequency of X-rays	ν	10^{19} /s
Wavelength of X-rays	λ	0.05 nm
Planck's constant	h	4×10^{-15} eV s
Energy of X-rays	$E = h\nu$	100 keV
Intensity of X-ray	$I(\mathbf{x})$	W/m^2
Attenuation coefficient	$u(\mathbf{x})$	See Table 1.2

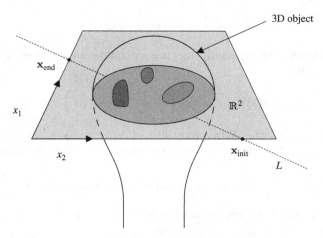

Fig. 1.7. Basic setup of computerized tomography.

and propagates along the line L through a slice of the tissue (modeled as the plane $\mathbb{R}^2$).

We describe the line L by its initialization point $\mathbf{x}_{\text{init}}$ and the normalized direction $\mathbf{a}$ (that is, $|\mathbf{a}| = 1$). Therefore, each point $\mathbf{x}(s)$ on L has the unique representation

$$\mathbf{x}(s) = \mathbf{x}_{\text{init}} + s\mathbf{a}, \qquad s \in \mathbb{R}.$$

We denote by $I(\mathbf{x}(s))$ the intensity of the X-ray beam at $\mathbf{x}(s)$ and set $I_{\text{init}} = I(\mathbf{x}(0))$. Due to absorption and scattering, the intensity is a non-increasing function in s. It is common to model the losses in intensity due to absorption and scattering by the *law of attenuation*

Table 1.2. Average attenuation coefficient of X-rays for different photon energies. Note the significant difference between soft tissue and bone and the small difference between various soft tissues.

Photon energy (keV)	30	60	90	120
Material/tissue	Attenuation coefficient (1/cm)			
Lead	344.13	56.988	83.172	46.932
Air	0.0004	0.0002	0.0002	0.0002
Water	0.3756	0.2059	0.1772	0.1626
Breast	0.3471	0.2046	0.1783	0.1642
Lung	0.4006	0.2156	0.1849	0.1695
Brain	0.3963	0.2140	0.1837	0.1685
Muscle	0.3972	0.2150	0.1846	0.1693
Blood	0.4083	0.2180	0.1867	0.1711
Bone	0.5555	0.6044	0.3921	0.3274

$$\frac{\mathrm{d}I(\mathbf{x}(s))}{\mathrm{d}s} = -u(\mathbf{x}(s))\, I(\mathbf{x}(s))\,, \tag{1.1}$$

where $u(\mathbf{x})$ denotes the spatially varying attenuation coefficient. Integration of (1.1) shows that

$$I(\mathbf{x}(s)) = I_{\mathrm{init}} \exp\left(-\int_0^s u(\mathbf{x}(\tau))\,\mathrm{d}\tau\right)\,.$$

Measurements of the X-ray intensity at $\mathbf{x}_{\mathrm{end}} := \mathbf{x}(s_{\mathrm{end}})$ provide data $I_{\mathrm{end}} := I(\mathbf{x}_{\mathrm{end}})$. Assuming that $u(\mathbf{x}(s))$ vanishes outside $[0, s_{\mathrm{end}}]$, we find that

$$-\log\left(I_{\mathrm{end}}/I_{\mathrm{init}}\right) = \int_{\mathbb{R}} u(\mathbf{x}(\tau))\,\mathrm{d}\tau =: (\mathrm{R}_{\mathrm{line}}\, u)(\mathbf{n}, r)\,.$$

Here $\mathbf{n} \in S^1$ denotes the unit vector normal to L such that $(\mathbf{a}, \mathbf{n})$ is a positively oriented basis (that is, $\det(\mathbf{a}, \mathbf{n}) > 0$), and

$$r := \mathbf{x}_{\mathrm{init}} \cdot \mathbf{n}$$

denotes the signed distance of L from the origin.

For fixed $\mathbf{n}$, the one-dimensional function $(\mathrm{R}_{\mathrm{line}}\, u)(\mathbf{n}, \cdot)$ is called *linear projection* of u in direction orthogonal to $\mathbf{n}$. Figure 1.8 shows a function and its projections for two different directions. The transformation that maps u to $\mathrm{R}_{\mathrm{line}}\, u$ is called linear Radon transform. See Fig. 1.9 for an example of an intensity function and its linear Radon transform.

To summarize, two-dimensional X-ray CT can be formulated in mathematical terms as follows:

Problem 1.2 (Reconstruction of a function from its linear projections). Let $\emptyset \neq \Gamma \subset S^1$. Given one-dimensional functions

$$v(\mathbf{n}, \cdot): \mathbb{R} \to \mathbb{R}\,, \qquad \mathbf{n} \in \Gamma\,,$$

find $u: \mathbb{R}^2 \to \mathbb{R}$ such that

$$(\mathrm{R}_{\mathrm{line}}\, u)(\mathbf{n}, \cdot) = v(\mathbf{n}, \cdot)\,, \qquad \mathbf{n} \in \Gamma\,.$$

Problem 1.2 with $\Gamma = S^1$ was considered first by Radon [324]; The original paper is reprinted in [209, pp. 177–192]. In [324] it is proven that the function u is uniquely determined by the Radon transform $\mathrm{R}_{\mathrm{line}}\, u$, and an analytic formula for the reconstruction of u from $v(\mathbf{n}, \cdot)$ is given.

In 1963, Cormack [117] was the first to point out the possible application of Problem 1.2 for medical diagnostics. He also made important mathematical contributions, for example he derived an inversion formula using harmonic decompositions of u and $\mathrm{R}_{\mathrm{line}}\, u$. The first commercially available CT system was constructed by Hounsfield [218], and the first patient brain-scan in a hospital was made in 1972. Cormack and Hounsfield shared the Nobel Prize in medicine in 1979 for the development of computer-assisted tomography.

1.5 Thermoacoustic Computerized Tomography

Thermoacoustic CT (also called *optoacoustic* or *photoacoustic* CT) is a hybrid imaging technique that is used to visualize the electromagnetic absorption coefficient at low frequencies, that is, the capability of a medium to absorb non-ionizing radiation. It has demonstrated great promise for important medical applications, including functional brain imaging of animals [244,381,399], soft-tissue characterization and early cancer diagnostics [16,246,248,382], and imaging of vasculature [213,242,404].

Physical Background

In photoacoustic CT, a body is illuminated with short pulses of electromagnetic radiation, absorbs a fraction of the energy thereof, heats up, and reacts with an expansion. This consequently induces acoustic waves, which are recorded at the boundary of the object. The recorded acoustical data are used to reconstruct the electromagnetic absorption coefficient.

X-ray CT has the drawback of low contrast in soft tissue (compare Table 1.2). However, different soft biological tissues have significantly varying

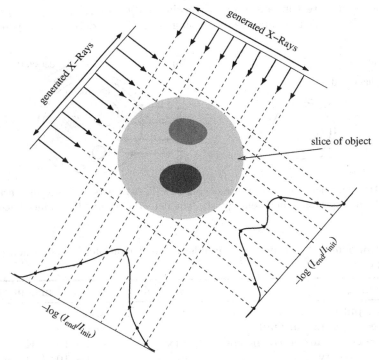

Fig. 1.8. The basics of an X-ray CT scanner. Each detector array pointing in direction $\mathbf{n}$ collects a one-dimensional linear projection $(\mathrm{R}_{\text{line}}\, u)(\mathbf{n}, \cdot)$.

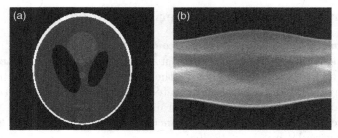

Fig. 1.9. Example of Radon transformed data. (**a**) Shepp–Logan phantom that is often used for testing of reconstruction algorithms in CT. (**b**) Radon transform (sinogram) of Shepp–Logan phantom. Each column represents a linear projection $(R_{line} u)(\mathbf{n}, \cdot)$.

absorption coefficients at certain low frequencies in the electromagnetic spectrum. Exemplarily, for radiation in the near infrared domain, as for instance produced by a Nd:YAG laser, the absorption coefficient in human soft tissues varies in the range of 0.1/cm to 0.5/cm (see [107]).

The first clinical prototype for breast cancer diagnosis with a thermoacoustic CT scanner was constructed by Kruger in 1998 (see [247]). It uses small acoustic detectors and offers a spatial resolution in the mm range (see [17, 395]). Existing imaging systems using optical line detectors in principle

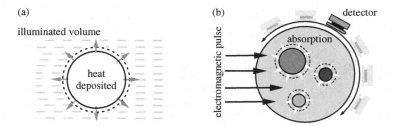

Fig. 1.10. Data acquisition in thermoacoustic CT. (**a**) Parts of a specimen are illuminated with electromagnetic energy. (**b**) The detector records the induced acoustic pressure.

Table 1.3. Some relevant physical variables in the derivation of the thermoacoustic wave equation.

Meaning	Symbol	Order of magnitude
Laser pulse duration	τ_{em}	$<$ ns
Speed of sound (in fluid)	v_s	$\sim 1500 \,\mathrm{m/s}$
Thermal expansion coefficient	$\beta(\mathbf{x})$	$\sim 4 \times 10^{-4}/\mathrm{K}$
Heat capacity	$c_p(\mathbf{x})$	$\sim 4 \times 10^3 \,\mathrm{J/(K\,kg)}$
Absorption coefficient	$\mu_{abs}(\mathbf{x})$	$\sim 0.5/\mathrm{cm}$

allow a resolution in the range of $100\,\mu\mathrm{m}$ (see, for example, [68, 317]). For practical aspects of thermoacoustic computerized tomography, like safety and applications in medicine, we refer to [397].

Mathematical Modeling

In the sequel, we derive the wave equation that models the physical principle of thermoacoustic CT.

Relevant physical quantities are depicted in Table 1.3. We assume that the object to be investigated is an inviscid fluid, which is homogeneous and isotropic with respect to acoustic wave propagation. First we derive a relation between the *mass density* ϱ and the *acoustic pressure* p.

- The *linearized continuity equation* (see, for instance, [161, (49.2)])

$$\frac{\partial \varrho}{\partial \hat{t}}(\mathbf{x}, \hat{t}) = -\varrho_0 \, \nabla \cdot \mathbf{v}(\mathbf{x}, \hat{t}) \tag{1.2}$$

  is derived from the principle of *conservation of mass*, if the *velocity* $\mathbf{v}(\mathbf{x}, \hat{t})$ is small and the total mass density $\varrho_{\mathrm{tot}}(\mathbf{x}, \hat{t}) = \varrho_0 + \varrho(\mathbf{x}, \hat{t})$ is just slightly varying, that is, $|\varrho(\mathbf{x}, \hat{t})| \ll \varrho_0$.
- The *linearized Euler equation* (see, for instance, [161, (49.3)])

$$\varrho_0 \frac{\partial \mathbf{v}}{\partial \hat{t}}(\mathbf{x}, \hat{t}) = -\nabla p(\mathbf{x}, \hat{t}) \tag{1.3}$$

  is derived from the principle of *conservation of momentum* for an *inviscid, non-turbulent* flow in the absence of external forces and just slightly varying total pressure $p_{\mathrm{tot}}(\mathbf{x}, \hat{t}) = p_0 + p(\mathbf{x}, \hat{t})$, that is, $|p(\mathbf{x}, \hat{t})| \ll p_0$.

Taking the first derivative with respect to time in (1.2) and applying the divergence to both sides of (1.3), the velocity $\mathbf{v}$ can be eliminated and the equation of motion that relates the acoustic pressure to the mass density follows:

$$\frac{\partial^2 \varrho}{\partial \hat{t}^2}(\mathbf{x}, \hat{t}) = \Delta p(\mathbf{x}, \hat{t}) \,. \tag{1.4}$$

The assumption that the object is illuminated with a short electromagnetic pulse implies that the intensity of the electromagnetic radiation is given by

$$I_{\mathrm{em}}(\mathbf{x}, \hat{t}) = J(\mathbf{x}) j(\hat{t}) \,, \tag{1.5}$$

where j denotes the temporal and J the spatial intensity distribution. Equation (1.5) takes into account that, due to the high magnitude of speed of light, the time delay between illumination of different parts of tissue (see the right picture in Fig. 1.10) can be neglected. For laser illumination, the function j typically has small support $[0, \tau_{\mathrm{em}}]$ with pulse duration τ_{em} in the range of some ps (picoseconds). The *absorbed electromagnetic power* is given by

$$r(\mathbf{x}, \hat{t}) = I_{\mathrm{em}}(\mathbf{x}, \hat{t})\, \mu_{\mathrm{abs}}(\mathbf{x})\,,$$

where $\mu_{\mathrm{abs}}(\mathbf{x})$ is the absorption coefficient. Absorption of electromagnetic power causes thermal *heating*.

In thermoacoustic CT the pulse duration τ_{em} is very short, and effects of thermal conduction can be neglected (see [369]). Therefore, the variation of temperature per time unit $(\partial T / \partial \hat{t})(\mathbf{x}, \hat{t})$ is proportional to the absorbed power, that is,

$$\frac{\partial T}{\partial \hat{t}}(\mathbf{x}, \hat{t}) = \frac{r(\mathbf{x}, \hat{t})}{c_p(\mathbf{x})}\,. \tag{1.6}$$

Here $c_p(\mathbf{x})$ denotes the *specific heat capacity*, which specifies how much energy is needed to increase the temperature of a substance.

Heating causes thermal *expansion* (decrease of density) and an increase of pressure. Taking (1.6) into account, the relation between heating, expansion, and pressure is expressed by the *linearized expansion equation* [200, 369] that reads as follows:

$$\frac{\beta(\mathbf{x}) r(\mathbf{x}, \hat{t})}{c_p(\mathbf{x})} = \frac{1}{v_s^2} \frac{\partial p}{\partial \hat{t}}(\mathbf{x}, \hat{t}) - \frac{\partial \varrho}{\partial \hat{t}}(\mathbf{x}, \hat{t})\,. \tag{1.7}$$

Here v_s is the speed of sound and $\beta(\mathbf{x})$ the thermal expansion coefficient, which specifies the increase of volume if the temperature increases by one Kelvin. We adopt the common assumption that the speed of sound v_s is constant in the investigated sample.

By taking the time derivative in (1.7) and inserting (1.4), we find that

$$\frac{1}{v_s^2} \frac{\partial^2 p}{\partial \hat{t}^2}(\mathbf{x}, \hat{t}) - \Delta p(\mathbf{x}, \hat{t}) = \frac{\mathrm{d}j}{\mathrm{d}\hat{t}}(\hat{t}) \left(\frac{\mu_{\mathrm{abs}}(\mathbf{x}) \beta(\mathbf{x}) J(\mathbf{x})}{c_p(\mathbf{x})} \right)\,. \tag{1.8}$$

The assumption that there is no acoustic pressure before the object is illuminated at time $\hat{t} = 0$ is expressed by

$$p(\mathbf{x}, \hat{t}) = 0\,, \qquad \hat{t} < 0\,. \tag{1.9}$$

In experiments with laser illumination (compare Fig. 1.12), the duration τ_{em} of the laser pulse is about 20 ps and the speed of sound v_s in tissue is $1500\,\mathrm{m/s} = 1.5\,\mathrm{nm/ps}$. Consequently, the function j can be replaced by a δ-distribution, at least as long as we are not interested in a spatial resolution below $20 \times 1.5\,\mathrm{nm} = 30\,\mathrm{nm}$.

With this approximation and by using the time scaling $t := v_s \hat{t}$, (1.8), and (1.9), it follows that p satisfies (principle of Duhamel [156, p. 81])

$$
\frac{\partial^2 p}{\partial t^2}(\mathbf{x}, t) - \Delta p(\mathbf{x}, t) = 0, \qquad (\mathbf{x}, t) \in \mathbb{R}^3 \times (0, \infty),
$$

$$
p(\mathbf{x}, 0) = u(\mathbf{x}) := \frac{\mu_{\mathrm{abs}}(\mathbf{x})\beta(\mathbf{x})J(\mathbf{x})v_s^2}{c_p(\mathbf{x})}, \qquad \mathbf{x} \in \mathbb{R}^3, \tag{1.10}
$$

$$
\frac{\partial p}{\partial t}(\mathbf{x}, 0) = 0, \qquad \mathbf{x} \in \mathbb{R}^3.
$$

The initial value problem (1.10) characterizes the forward model in thermo-acoustic CT. The actual imaging problem consists in reconstruction of the initial pressure distribution $u(\mathbf{x})$ from pressure data measured at the boundary of the sample. Different experimental setups have been proposed in the literature, leading to different mathematical problems (see [165, 197, 249]). They can be classified into three main categories as described in the following.

Small Detectors: Spherical Projections

The standard approach in thermoacoustic CT is to record acoustic data with small piezoelectric detectors used to simulate point detectors. In mathematical terms, a point detector records the solution of (1.10) pointwise on a surface outside the object of interest.

The unique solution of (1.10) can be written as (see [156, p. 72])

$$
p(\mathbf{x}, t) = \frac{\partial}{\partial t}\left[\frac{(\mathrm{R}_{\mathrm{sph}}\, u)(\mathbf{x}, t)}{4\pi t}\right], \tag{1.11}
$$

where

$$
(\mathrm{R}_{\mathrm{sph}}\, u)(\mathbf{x}, t) := \int_{\partial B_t(\mathbf{x})} u(\mathbf{y})\, \mathrm{d}\mathcal{H}^2(\mathbf{y}), \qquad (\mathbf{x}, t) \in \mathbb{R}^3 \times [0, \infty),
$$

denotes the integration of u over a sphere with center $\mathbf{x}$ and radius t. The time-dependent function $(\mathrm{R}_{\mathrm{sph}}\, u)(\mathbf{x}, \cdot)$ is called *spherical projection* of u at center $\mathbf{x}$.

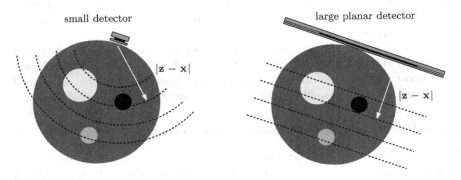

Fig. 1.11. Small area versus large area detector.

After integrating (1.11) with respect to (scaled) time, we find that, at the position $\mathbf{x}$ of a transducer outside the support of u,

$$(\mathrm{R}_{\mathrm{sph}}\, u)(\mathbf{x}, t) = 4\pi t \int_0^t p(\mathbf{x}, s)\, \mathrm{d}s \,.$$

For data acquisition, detectors are placed on a surface enclosing the support of the initially generated pressure u (see (1.10)).

The image reconstruction problem in thermoacoustic CT with point-detector measurement data can be stated as follows:

Problem 1.3 (Reconstruction of a function from its spherical projections). Let $\emptyset \neq \Omega \subset \mathbb{R}^3$ be a domain with boundary $\partial\Omega$ and let $\emptyset \neq \Gamma \subset \partial\Omega$. Given time-dependent functions

$$v(\mathbf{z}, \cdot) : (0, \infty) \to \mathbb{R}\,, \qquad \mathbf{z} \in \Gamma\,,$$

find $u : \mathbb{R}^3 \to \mathbb{R}$ with $\mathrm{supp}(u) \subset \Omega$ satisfying

$$(\mathrm{R}_{\mathrm{sph}}\, u)(\mathbf{z}, \cdot) = v(\mathbf{z}, \cdot)\,, \qquad \mathbf{z} \in \Gamma\,.$$

If $\Gamma = \partial\Omega$, then $(\mathrm{R}_{\mathrm{sph}}\, u)(\mathbf{z}, \cdot)$, $\mathbf{z} \in \Gamma$, is called the *complete set of spherical projections*. The integral transform that maps the function u to the complete set of spherical projections is called *spherical Radon transform*.

The reconstruction of a function from spherical integrals has been studied by many authors. See [226] for early work in this subject; for more recent development we refer to [165, 166, 249, 289, 314]. Despite the long history of the problem, analytical reconstruction formulas are quite rare and have been discovered only recently. In the case when Ω is a half space, such formulas have been derived in [15, 158], motivated by applications of Problem 1.3 in SAR (synthetic aperture radar) [297] and SONAR (sound navigation and ranging) [256]. In the case when Ω is either a ball or a cylinder, formulas have been discovered in [300]. For the case that Ω is a ball, exact formulas of the so-called back-projection type have been derived in [164]. Later, a formula of the back-projection type has been discovered that is exact for balls and cylinders [396, 397]. Approximate reconstruction formulas of the back-projection type are derived in [69, 245, 300, 394, 398].

Due to practical constraints, the transducer locations $\mathbf{z}$ may be restricted to a proper subset $\Gamma \neq \partial\Omega$. A typical example is breast imaging, where Γ covers at most a hemisphere. In such a limited data situation, however, analytical inversion formulas are only known when Γ is part of a plane (see [15]).

Large Planar Detectors: Planar Projections

In practice, every acoustic detector has a finite size, and therefore algorithms that are based on the assumption of point measurement data give blurred reconstructions (see [395, 397]).

In order to overcome this resolution limit for thermoacoustic CT, in [199] it is suggested to use *sufficiently large planar* detectors and measure the total acoustic pressure therewith. For the sake of simplicity, we assume that the initial pressure distribution u is supported in the open ball $B_R(0) \subset \mathbb{R}^3$ with radius R centered at the origin. Let $p(\mathbf{x}, t)$ be the solution of the three-dimensional wave equation (1.10). Moreover, we denote by $E(\mathbf{n}, d) := \{\mathbf{x} \in \mathbb{R}^3 : \mathbf{x} \cdot \mathbf{n} = d\}$ the plane with normal vector $\mathbf{n} \in S^2$ and distance d to the origin.

A *planar detector*, placed tangentially to $\partial B_R(0)$, records the total acoustic pressure

$$P(\mathbf{n}, t) := \int_{E(\mathbf{n}, R)} p(\mathbf{x}, t)\, \mathrm{d}\mathcal{H}^2(\mathbf{x})\,, \qquad t \in [0, \infty)\,. \qquad (1.12)$$

For large planar detectors, the following relationship between the measured data P and the initial pressure distribution u holds (see [199, 397]):

$$\boxed{(\mathrm{R}_{\mathrm{plane}}\, u)(\mathbf{n}, R - t) := \int_{E(\mathbf{n}, R-t)} u(\mathbf{y})\, \mathrm{d}\mathcal{H}^2(\mathbf{y}) = \frac{P(\mathbf{n}, t)}{2}\,.} \qquad (1.13)$$

As illustrated in Fig. 1.11, a planar detector provides integrals of u over planes parallel to $E(\mathbf{n}, R)$. The factor $1/2$ in (1.13) indicates that the planar detector records only one of two counter-propagating plane waves.

For fixed $\mathbf{n}$, the one-dimensional function $(\mathrm{R}_{\mathrm{plane}}\, u)(\mathbf{n}, \cdot)$ is called *planar projection* and the mapping of a function u onto the complete set of planar projections $(\mathrm{R}_{\mathrm{plane}}\, u)(\mathbf{n}, \cdot)$, $\mathbf{n} \in S^2$, is called *planar Radon transform*. The planar projection $(\mathrm{R}_{\mathrm{plane}}\, u)(\mathbf{n}, \cdot)$ vanishes outside $[-R, R]$, and in order to measure the planar projection we can choose $2R$ as the final recording time. For three-dimensional imaging, the large planar detector is rotated around S^2 in order to obtain information from various directions. According to (1.13), this setup for thermoacoustic CT leads to the following mathematical problem:

Problem 1.4 (Reconstruction of a function from its planar projections). Let $\emptyset \neq \Gamma \subset S^2$. Given one-dimensional functions

$$v(\mathbf{n}, \cdot) : \mathbb{R} \to \mathbb{R}\,, \qquad \mathbf{n} \in \Gamma\,,$$

find $u : \mathbb{R}^3 \to \mathbb{R}$ with $\mathrm{supp}(u) \subset B_R(0)$, such that

$$(\mathrm{R}_{\mathrm{plane}}\, u)(\mathbf{n}, \cdot) = v(\mathbf{n}, \cdot)\,, \qquad \mathbf{n} \in \Gamma\,.$$

In 1917, Radon [324] proved that the function u is uniquely determined by $\mathrm{R}_{\mathrm{plane}}\, u$. Moreover, he gave an explicit formula for its reconstruction.

In practical experiments, a large planar detector can be realized with a thin film made of piezoelectric PVDF (polyvinylidene fluoride) mounted on a

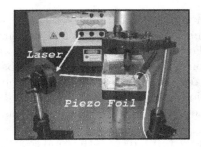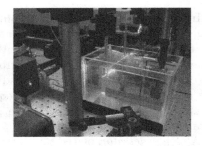

Fig. 1.12. Experimental realization of large planar detector and single line detector.

rigid baffle (see Fig. 1.12). We emphasize that the large detector size does not limit the spatial resolution of thermoacoustic CT, as the shape of the detector is explicitly included in the reconstruction method (see [68, 199]).

Line Detectors: Circular Projections

Three-dimensional imaging with a large planar detector requires complicated scanning motions. To simplify the setup for three-dimensional imaging, in [68, 317] it is proposed to measure the acoustic signals with an array of parallel line detectors that are rotated around a single axis (see Fig. 1.13). In such a situation, three-dimensional imaging involves the inversion of the classical linear Radon transform (see Problem 1.2) and the inversion of the *circular Radon transform* as outlined in the following.

Let $p(\mathbf{x}, t)$ denote the unique solution of (1.10). For simplicity of presentation, we assume that the line detectors point into direction $\mathbf{e}_1 := (1, 0, 0)$. Moreover, write $\mathbf{x} = (x_1, \mathbf{x}')$, $x_1 \in \mathbb{R}$, $\mathbf{x}' \in \mathbb{R}^2$, and let

$$\bar{u}(\mathbf{x}') := \int_{\mathbb{R}} u(x_1, \mathbf{x}') \, dx_1 \,, \qquad \mathbf{x}' \in \mathbb{R}^2 \,,$$

$$\bar{p}(\mathbf{x}', t) := \int_{\mathbb{R}} p(x_1, \mathbf{x}', t) \, dx_1 \,, \qquad (\mathbf{x}', t) \in \mathbb{R}^2 \times [0, \infty) \,, \qquad (1.14)$$

denote the linear projections of u and p in direction $\mathbf{e}_1$. We assume that $\bar{u}$ has support in Ω, where Ω is a domain in $\mathbb{R}^2$. Then the array of line detectors measures $\bar{p}$ on a subset of $\partial\Omega$.

Using the commutation relation between the wave equation and the two-dimensional linear Radon transform (see [209, 288]), it follows that $\bar{p}$ satisfies the *two-dimensional* wave equation (see [67, 197]):

$$\boxed{\begin{aligned} \frac{\partial^2 \bar{p}}{\partial t^2}(\mathbf{x}', t) - \Delta \bar{p}(\mathbf{x}', t) &= 0 \,, & (\mathbf{x}', t) \in \mathbb{R}^2 \times (0, \infty) \,, \\ \bar{p}(\mathbf{x}', 0) &= \bar{u}(\mathbf{x}') \,, & \mathbf{x}' \in \mathbb{R}^2 \,, \\ \frac{\partial \bar{p}}{\partial t}(\mathbf{x}', 0) &= 0 \,, & \mathbf{x}' \in \mathbb{R}^2 \,. \end{aligned}} \qquad (1.15)$$

The unique solution of (1.15) can be written as (see [227, (1.24a)])

$$\bar{p}(\mathbf{x}',t) = \frac{1}{2\pi} \frac{\partial}{\partial t} \int_0^t \frac{(\mathrm{R}_{\mathrm{circ}}\,\bar{u})(\mathbf{x}',s)}{\sqrt{t^2 - s^2}}\,\mathrm{d}s\,, \qquad (1.16)$$

where

$$(\mathrm{R}_{\mathrm{circ}}\,\bar{u})(\mathbf{x}',t) := \int_{\partial B_t(\mathbf{x}')} \bar{u}(\mathbf{y}')\,\mathrm{d}\mathcal{H}^1(\mathbf{y}')$$

denotes the integration of $\bar{u}$ over the circle $\partial B_t(\mathbf{x}') \subset \mathbb{R}^2$ with center $\mathbf{x}'$ and radius t.

Equation (1.16) can be solved for $\mathrm{R}_{\mathrm{circ}}\,\bar{u}$ using standard methods for solving Abel type equations (see [185, 288]). The result is

$$\boxed{(\mathrm{R}_{\mathrm{circ}}\,\bar{u})(\mathbf{x}',t) = 4t \int_0^t \frac{\bar{p}(\mathbf{x}',s)}{\sqrt{t^2 - s^2}}\,\mathrm{d}s\,.} \qquad (1.17)$$

The one-dimensional function $(\mathrm{R}_{\mathrm{circ}}\,\bar{u})(\mathbf{x}',\cdot)$ is called *circular projection* of $\bar{u}$. The integral transform $\mathrm{R}_{\mathrm{circ}}$ that maps $\bar{u}$ onto the complete set of circular projections

$$(\mathrm{R}_{\mathrm{circ}}\,\bar{u})(\mathbf{x}',\cdot)\,, \qquad \mathbf{x}' \in \partial\Omega\,,$$

is called *circular Radon transform*.

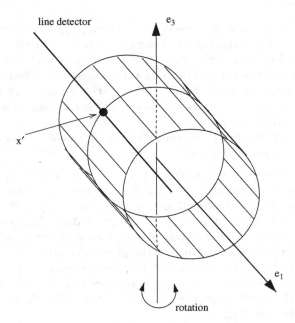

Fig. 1.13. The complete array of line detectors records the acoustic field while rotating around the sample.

Solving (1.17) for $\bar{u}$, we are able to obtain the line integrals of u along lines parallel to $\mathbf{e}_1$ from the measured data $\bar{p}$. Rotating the measurement device around the $\mathbf{e}_3$-axis, we can collect the complete set of linear projections in each plane normal to $\mathbf{e}_3$. Consequently, the reconstruction of u is reduced to a consecutive inversion of the circular and the linear Radon transform.

As the linear Radon transform has been treated already in the previous section, we concentrate here on the inversion of the circular Radon transform. We write u instead of $\bar{u}$ in order to be consistent with the notation in Section 3.4, where we study the solution of the following problem by means of variational methods.

Problem 1.5 (Reconstruction of a function from circular projections). Let $\emptyset \neq \Omega \subset \mathbb{R}^2$ be a domain with boundary $\partial\Omega$ and let $\emptyset \neq \Gamma \subset \partial\Omega$. Given time-dependent functions

$$v(\mathbf{z}, \cdot) : (0, \infty) \to \mathbb{R}, \quad \mathbf{z} \in \Gamma,$$

find $u : \mathbb{R}^2 \to \mathbb{R}$ with $\operatorname{supp}(u) \subset \Omega$ such that

$$(R_{\mathrm{circ}}\, u)(\mathbf{z}, \cdot) = v(\mathbf{z}, \cdot), \quad \mathbf{z} \in \Gamma.$$

Recovering a function from its integrals over circles is the two-dimensional analogue of Problem 1.3. Analytical reconstruction formulas exist for $\Gamma = \partial\Omega$ in the cases where Ω is either a disk (see [163, 198, 251, 299]) or a half plane (see [15, 44, 158, 313]).

Remark 1.6 (Minimal size of integrating detector). In practice, every integrating detector has a finite size (area or length). It may appear that the assumption of infinite size in the definitions of $P(\mathbf{n}, t)$ (see (1.12)) and $\bar{p}(\mathbf{x}', t)$ (see (1.14)), which cannot be fulfilled in applications, negatively affects the imaging resolution. However, as shown below, there exists a criterion for the minimal size of a real detector such that it provides the same data as a detector of infinite size (see [199, 316]).

For the sake of simplicity, we consider the case where a planar detector is used to record the acoustic data:

1. The initial data $u(\mathbf{x}) = p(\mathbf{x}, 0)$ in (1.10) are supported in $B_R(0)$. Therefore, the planar projections $(R_{\mathrm{plane}}\, u)(\mathbf{n}, \cdot)$ are supported in $(-R, R)$. According to (1.13), the function $P(\mathbf{n}, t) = 2(R_{\mathrm{plane}}\, u)(\mathbf{n}, R - t)$ vanishes for $t \geq 2R$. Therefore, it is sufficient to collect data $P(\mathbf{n}, t)$ up to a time $2R$, which is given by the arrival time of a wave initiated at the point in $B_R(0)$ with the largest distance to the planar detector.
2. From the finite speed of sound and the assumption $\operatorname{supp}(u) \subset B_R(0)$, it follows that $p(\cdot, t)$, $0 \leq t < 2R$, is supported in $B_{3R}(0)$. Thus, $p(\cdot, t)$, $0 \leq t \leq 2R$, vanishes outside $D(\mathbf{n}, R) := E(\mathbf{n}, R) \cap B_{3R}(0)$, which is a disk of radius (see Fig. 1.14)

$$\sqrt{(3R)^2 - R^2} = \sqrt{8}R.$$

3. From the consideration in Items 1 and 2, it follows that in (1.12) (which is the definition of $P(\mathbf{n}, R)$), the infinite plane $E(\mathbf{n}, R)$ can be replaced by an area that contains $D(\mathbf{n}, R)$, because all parts of the detector outside of this region do not contribute to the integrated signal. In such a situation, the finite detector size introduces no approximation errors in (1.13).

Similar considerations lead to a criterion for the length of a real line detector. For example, if u is supported in $B_R(0)$ and the line detector is tangential to $B_R(0)$, then it must contain a line segment of length $2R\sqrt{8}$ (compare again with Fig. 1.14). $\Diamond$

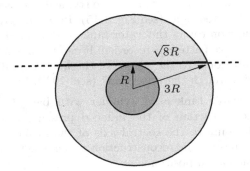

Fig. 1.14. The initial source $p(\cdot, 0)$ is supported in $B_R(0)$. Therefore, $p(\cdot, t)$, $0 \le t \le 2R$, is supported in $B_{3R}(0)$ and vanishes outside the disk $D(\mathbf{n}, R)$.

Remark 1.7. Tomographic problems can be considered a special instance of a *deblurring problem*. These problems can be written as solving the operator equation

$$Ku = v, \tag{1.18}$$

where the operator K has the following form,

$$Ku(\mathbf{x}) = \int_\Omega k(\mathbf{x}, \hat{\mathbf{x}})\, u(\hat{\mathbf{x}})\, \mathrm{d}\hat{\mathbf{x}},$$

and is called *blurring operator*. The problem of solving (1.18) is then called *deblurring*.

A special instance of deblurring is *deconvolution*, where the operator

$$Ku(\mathbf{x}) = \int_\Omega k(|\mathbf{x} - \hat{\mathbf{x}}|)\, u(\hat{\mathbf{x}})\, \mathrm{d}\hat{\mathbf{x}} =: (k * u)(\mathbf{x})$$

is called *convolution operator*; the function k is called *convolution kernel*. The problem of solving $k * u = v$ is called *deconvolution*. Several deconvolution and deblurring problems and their efficient numerical solution can be found for instance in [36, 49].

Blind deconvolution is concerned with the simultaneous identification of the kernel k and the function u (see, for example, [48, 66, 78, 101, 102, 229], which are concerned with variational methods for deconvolution). $\Diamond$

1.6 Schlieren Tomography

Schlieren tomography is used for the visualization of pressure waves in a fluid (see Fig. 1.15). One important application of schlieren imaging is testing of ultrasonic transducers, in particular to measure the focal spot size, beam symmetry, and the general geometry and intensity of side-lobes. Schlieren tomography utilizes the fact that pressure waves in fluids cause density variations, which in turn cause transmitted light to be diffracted (see [58, 104, 203, 322, 402]).

A measurement device for schlieren tomography consists of an optical system that contains a water tank, a light source (typically a laser), and a screen for recording the diffracted light (see Fig. 1.15). In a tomographic setup, the ultrasound transducer on top of the water tank is rotated, and for each angle of rotation the diffractive pattern is recorded. It can be shown that the diffractive pattern is proportional to the square of the line integral of the pressure along the light path through the water tank (see [203]).

We model the water tank as a cylinder with base $B_1(0) \subset \mathbb{R}^2$ (see Fig. 1.15). The reconstruction of the induced pressure is similar for each planar section orthogonal to the central axis of the cylinder. Therefore, the three-dimensional tomographic reconstruction reduces to two-dimensional reconstructions for each axial position.

Let $u : B_1(0) \to \mathbb{R}$ denote the induced pressure at a certain height in the water tank. For fixed angular position $\mathbf{n} \in S^1$ of the ultrasound transducer, the recorded data are modeled by

$$v(\mathbf{n}, r) = \left(\int_{\mathbb{R}} u(r\mathbf{n} + s\mathbf{a}) \, ds \right)^2, \qquad r \in (-1, 1),$$

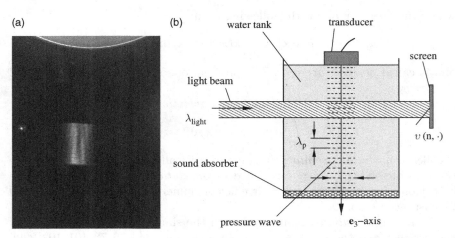

Fig. 1.15. Schlieren imaging. **(a)** Schlieren image provided by *GE Medical Systems Kretz Ultrasound*; **(b)** Schematic illustration of taking a schlieren image.

where $\mathbf{a}$ is orthogonal to $\mathbf{n}$, and r corresponds to the signed distance of the line $r\mathbf{n} + \mathbb{R}\mathbf{a}$ to the origin. The function $v(\mathbf{n}, \cdot)$ is the square of the linear projection $(\mathrm{R}_{\mathrm{line}}\, u)(\mathbf{n}, \cdot)$ considered in Section 1.4. Schlieren tomography then can be formulated as reconstructing u from data $v(\mathbf{n}, \cdot)$, $\mathbf{n} \in S^1$.

To summarize, the mathematical formulation of the problem of schlieren tomography is as follows:

Problem 1.8 (Schlieren tomography). Given $v(\mathbf{n}, \cdot)$, $\mathbf{n} \in S^1$, find $u : \mathbb{R}^2 \to \mathbb{R}$ supported in $B_1(0)$ such that

$$(\mathrm{R}_{\mathrm{line}}\, u)^2(\mathbf{n}, \cdot) = v(\mathbf{n}, \cdot)\,, \qquad \mathbf{n} \in S^1\,. \tag{1.19}$$

In Problem 1.8, the functions u and $(\mathrm{R}_{\mathrm{line}}\, u)(\mathbf{n}, \cdot)$ may attain negative values. Therefore, (1.19) cannot be reduced to a linear system of equations for u, given the linear projections $(\mathrm{R}_{\mathrm{line}}\, u)(\mathbf{n}, \cdot)$, $\mathbf{n} \in S^1$.

2

Image and Noise Models

Maximum a posteriori (MAP) estimation is a statistical method for denoising of data, which takes into account statistical prior information on the clean data and on the noise process. The maximum a posteriori estimate is the most likely data under the assumption of priors for the data and the noise.

Typically, noise is assumed to be Gaussian, Laplacian, or Poisson distributed. Prior distributions of images are derived from histograms of training data. Under such assumptions, MAP estimation reduces to a discrete variational regularization problem.

In this chapter, we first review basic statistical concepts. Applying these concepts to discrete, digital images, we discuss several noise models and derive priors for image data from histograms of "comparable" image data. Finally, we show how this information can be used for MAP estimation.

2.1 Basic Concepts of Statistics

A *random experiment* is a "process, whose outcome is not known in advance with certainty" (see [129, p. 5]). The set of possible outcomes is referred to as the *sampling space* of the process. A *probability distribution* or *probability measure* P on a sampling space Ω is a measure that satisfies $P(\Omega) = 1$.

Let Ω be a sampling space with probability distribution P. A measurable function $\Delta : \Omega \to \mathbb{R}$ is called *random variable*. By $\mathrm{Ran}(\Delta) := \{\Delta(\omega) : \omega \in \Omega\}$ we denote the *range* of Δ. The random variable Δ induces a measure P_Δ on $\mathbb{R}$ by

$$P_\Delta(A) := P(\Delta^{-1}A), \qquad A \subset \mathbb{R} \text{ measurable} .$$

An element $x \in \mathrm{Ran}(\Delta)$ is called *realization* of Δ, and a P_Δ-measurable subset of $\mathbb{R}$ is called an *event*. For simplicity we write $P_\Delta(x) := P_\Delta(\{x\})$.

If $\mathrm{Ran}(\Delta)$ is discrete, then P_Δ is called *discrete* probability distribution. In this case, the probability distribution is uniquely determined by the values $P_\Delta(x)$, $x \in \mathrm{Ran}(\Delta)$.

O. Scherzer et al., *Variational Methods in Imaging*,
© Springer Science+Business Media, LLC 2009

If there exists a non-negative Borel function $p_\Delta : \mathbb{R} \to \mathbb{R}_{\geq 0}$ such that

$$P_\Delta(A) = \int_A p_\Delta \,, \qquad A \subset \mathbb{R} \text{ measurable} \,,$$

then P_Δ is called a *(absolutely) continuous* probability distribution. In this case, the function p_Δ is called the *probability density* of Δ.

Assume that Ω is a sampling space with probability distribution P. An n-dimensional *random vector* $\boldsymbol{\Delta} = (\Delta_1, \ldots, \Delta_n)$ is a measurable function $\boldsymbol{\Delta} : \Omega \to \mathbb{R}^n$. The *joint probability* $P_{\boldsymbol{\Delta}}$ of $\boldsymbol{\Delta}$ is the measure on $\mathbb{R}^n$ defined by

$$P_{\boldsymbol{\Delta}}(A) := P\big(\boldsymbol{\Delta}^{-1}(A)\big) \,, \qquad A \subset \mathbb{R}^n \text{ measurable} \,.$$

The probability density of a random vector $\boldsymbol{\Delta}$ is defined analogously to the probability density of a random variable.

If $\boldsymbol{\Delta}$ is an n-dimensional random vector on Ω, then its components Δ_i, $1 \leq i \leq n$, are themselves random variables on Ω. We say that the random vector $\boldsymbol{\Delta}$ consists of *independent* random variables Δ_i, if

$$P_{\boldsymbol{\Delta}}(A_1 \times \cdots \times A_n) = P_{\Delta_1}(A_1) \cdots P_{\Delta_n}(A_n) \,, \qquad A_1, \ldots, A_n \subset \mathbb{R} \text{ measurable} \,,$$

where P_{Δ_i} are the probability distributions of Δ_i, $1 \leq i \leq n$. If additionally $P_{\Delta_i} = P_{\Delta_j}$ for all $1 \leq i,j \leq n$, then $\boldsymbol{\Delta}$ consists of *independent and identically distributed*, in short i.i.d., random variables.

The probability density of a random vector of independent continuous random variables can be determined by the following result:

Theorem 2.1. *Let $\boldsymbol{\Delta}$ be a random vector consisting of independent random variables Δ_i, $1 \leq i \leq n$, with continuous probability distributions P_{Δ_i} and corresponding densities p_{Δ_i}. Then $P_{\boldsymbol{\Delta}}$ is continuous, and its probability density $p_{\boldsymbol{\Delta}}$ is given by*

$$p_{\boldsymbol{\Delta}} = \prod_{i=1}^n p_{\Delta_i} \,.$$

Proof. See, e.g., [321, Thm. I.3.2.]. □

Definition 2.2. *Assume that $\boldsymbol{\Delta}$ is an n-dimensional random vector with probability distribution $P_{\boldsymbol{\Delta}}$, and that $f : \mathbb{R}^n \to \mathbb{R}^m$, $1 \leq m \leq n$, is continuous. The* push forward $f^\# \boldsymbol{\Delta}$ *of $\boldsymbol{\Delta}$ is the m-dimensional random vector defined by the probability distribution*

$$P_{f^\# \boldsymbol{\Delta}}(A) := P_{\boldsymbol{\Delta}}(f^{-1}A) \,, \qquad A \subset \mathbb{R}^m \text{ measurable} \,.$$

For a Lipschitz function $f : \mathbb{R}^n \to \mathbb{R}^m$, $1 \leq m \leq n$, the Jacobian is defined as

$$J_f := \sqrt{\det(\nabla f \, \nabla f^T)} \,. \tag{2.1}$$

If f is Lipschitz and has a non-vanishing Jacobian almost everywhere and Δ has a continuous probability distribution, then also $P_{f\#\Delta}$ is a continuous probability distribution. In this case, its density can be determined by means of the following lemma.

Lemma 2.3. *Let* Δ *be an* n-*dimensional continuous random vector with probability distribution* P_Δ *and density* p_Δ. *Assume that* $f : \mathbb{R}^n \to \mathbb{R}^m$, $1 \le m \le n$, *is locally Lipschitz such that its Jacobian satisfies* $J_f \ne 0$ *almost everywhere in* $\mathbb{R}^n$. *Then*

$$p_{f\#\Delta}(\mathbf{y}) = \int_{f^{-1}(\mathbf{y})} \frac{p_\Delta(\mathbf{x})}{J_f(\mathbf{x})} \, d\mathcal{H}^{n-m}, \qquad \mathbf{y} \in \mathbb{R}^m,$$

where $\mathcal{H}^{n-m}$ *denotes the* $(n-m)$-*dimensional Hausdorff measure (see* (9.1)).

Proof. By definition, we have for every measurable set $A \subset \mathbb{R}^m$ that

$$\int_A p_{f\#\Delta}(\mathbf{y}) = P_{f\#\Delta}(A) = P_\Delta(f^{-1}(A)) = \int_{f^{-1}(A)} p_\Delta(\mathbf{x}) \,. \qquad (2.2)$$

Using the coarea formula (see [159, Thm. 3.2.12], where as function g there we use $g = (p_\Delta/J_f)\chi_{f^{-1}(A)}$), we find that

$$\int_{f^{-1}(A)} p_\Delta(\mathbf{x}) = \int_A \int_{f^{-1}(\mathbf{y})} \frac{p_\Delta(\mathbf{x})}{J_f(\mathbf{x})} \, d\mathcal{H}^{n-m}\,. \qquad (2.3)$$

Combining (2.2) and (2.3), it follows that

$$\int_A p_{f\#\Delta}(\mathbf{y}) = \int_A \int_{f^{-1}(\mathbf{y})} \frac{p_\Delta(\mathbf{x})}{J_f(\mathbf{x})} \, d\mathcal{H}^{n-m}, \qquad A \subset \mathbb{R}^m \text{ measurable }.$$

This shows the assertion. $\qquad\qquad\qquad\qquad\qquad\qquad\qquad\qquad\qquad\qquad\quad\square$

Definition 2.4 (Mean and variance). *Let* Δ *be a random variable with probability distribution* P_Δ. *We define the* mean *(or expectation)* $\mathrm{E}(\Delta)$ *and the* variance $\mathrm{Var}(\Delta)$ *by*

$$\mathrm{E}(\Delta) := \int_\mathbb{R} x \, dP_\Delta, \qquad \mathrm{Var}(\Delta) := \int_\mathbb{R} (x - E(\Delta))^2 \, dP_\Delta,$$

provided the integrals exist. If the distribution P_Δ *is continuous with density* p_Δ, *then we have*

$$\mathrm{E}(\Delta) := \int_\mathbb{R} p_\Delta(x)\, x, \qquad \mathrm{Var}(\Delta) := \int_\mathbb{R} p_\Delta(x)\big(x - E(\Delta)\big)^2\,.$$

We call $\sqrt{\mathrm{Var}(\Delta)}$ *the* standard deviation *of* Δ.

Remark 2.5. Repeating a random experiment, we obtain a finite number of realizations (a *sample*) of a random variable. Based on this sample, we can define a discrete probability distribution on $\mathbb{R}$:

Let $\delta_1, \ldots, \delta_n$ denote n realizations of a random variable Δ. Then the vector $\boldsymbol{\delta} = (\delta_1, \ldots, \delta_n)$ defines a probability distribution on $\mathbb{R}$ by

$$P_{\boldsymbol{\delta}}(x) := \frac{1}{n} \left| \{ i \in \{1, \ldots, n\} : \delta_i = x \} \right| . \tag{2.4}$$

We refer to $P_{\boldsymbol{\delta}}(x)$ as the *empirical* probability distribution of $\boldsymbol{\delta}$. We denote

$$\mathrm{E}(\boldsymbol{\delta}) := \frac{1}{n} \sum_{i=1}^{n} \delta_i$$

the *sample mean* and

$$\mathrm{Var}(\boldsymbol{\delta}) := \frac{1}{n} \sum_{i=1}^{n} \left(\delta_i - E(\delta) \right)^2$$

the *sample variance* of $\boldsymbol{\delta}$, i.e., $\mathrm{E}(\boldsymbol{\delta})$ and $\mathrm{Var}(\boldsymbol{\delta})$ are the mean and variance of the probability density $P_{\boldsymbol{\delta}}(x)$ defined in (2.4), respectively.

In particular, $\mathrm{E}(\boldsymbol{\delta})$ and $\mathrm{Var}(\boldsymbol{\delta})$ are the mean and variance, respectively, of the empirical probability distribution of $\boldsymbol{\delta}$. $\diamond$

Remark 2.6. Let Δ be a random variable. Assume that $\mathrm{Var}(\Delta)$ and $\mathrm{E}(\Delta)$ exist. Then

$$\mathrm{Var}(\Delta) = \mathrm{E}(\Delta^2) - \mathrm{E}(\Delta)^2 ,$$

where Δ^2 is the push-forward of Δ by the function $f(x) = x^2$ (see, e.g., [129, Thm. 4.3.3]). $\diamond$

Example 2.7. We recall some important distributions on $\mathbb{R}$ and $\mathbb{R}^n$, which are required below for the definitions of image noise models. Details and motivations for these distributions can be found in [129].

1. The *Poisson distribution* is a discrete distribution P with range $\mathrm{Ran}(P) = \mathbb{N} \cup \{0\}$. It is given by

$$P(k) = \frac{\lambda^k}{k!} \exp(-\lambda), \qquad k \in \mathbb{N} \cup \{0\}, \tag{2.5}$$

   where the parameter $\lambda \geq 0$ is at the same time the mean and the variance of P.

2. Let $I \subset \mathbb{R}$ be measurable with $0 < \mathcal{L}^1(I) < \infty$. The *uniform distribution* on I is given by the probability density

$$p(x) = \begin{cases} \mathcal{L}^1(I)^{-1}, & \text{if } x \in I , \\ 0, & \text{if } x \notin I . \end{cases}$$

3. The *Laplacian distribution* on $\mathbb{R}$ with mean $\bar{x} \in \mathbb{R}$ and $\sigma_1 > 0$ is given by the probability density

$$p(x) = \frac{1}{2\sigma_1} \exp\left(-\frac{|x - \bar{x}|}{\sigma_1}\right), \qquad x \in \mathbb{R}. \qquad (2.6)$$

4. The *Gaussian distribution* on $\mathbb{R}$, also called *normal distribution*, with mean $\bar{x}$ and standard deviation $\sigma_2 > 0$ is given by the probability density

$$p(x) = \frac{1}{\sigma_2 \sqrt{2\pi}} \exp\left(-\frac{|x - \bar{x}|^2}{2\sigma_2^2}\right). \qquad (2.7)$$

5. If $\boldsymbol{\Delta}$ is a random vector consisting of i.i.d. random variables, then the probability density of $\boldsymbol{\Delta}$ is given as the product of the probability densities of Δ_i (cf. Theorem 2.1). For example, for i.i.d. Gaussian random variables we have

$$p(\mathbf{x}) = \frac{1}{(\sigma_2 \sqrt{2\pi})^n} \exp\left(-\frac{|\mathbf{x} - \bar{\mathbf{x}}|^2}{2\sigma_2^2}\right),$$

where $\bar{\mathbf{x}} = (\bar{x}, \ldots, \bar{x})^T \in \mathbb{R}^n$ (compare with the more general definition of *multivariate* (or *vectorial*) Gaussian distribution in the literature, see for example [321, Sect. VIII.4]). Note that here $|\mathbf{x} - \bar{\mathbf{x}}|$ denotes the Euclidean norm on $\mathbb{R}^n$. $\diamondsuit$

2.2 Digitized (Discrete) Images

In this section, we give the basic model of discrete and continuous images as used in the sequel.

Let $h > 0$ and $n_x, n_y \in \mathbb{N}$. *Discrete images* of size $n_x \times n_y$ are given as matrices $\mathbf{u} = (u_{ij})_{(i,j) \in \mathcal{I}_1}$, where

$$\boxed{u_{ij} \in \mathbb{R}, \qquad (i,j) \in \mathcal{I}_1 := \{1, \ldots, n_x\} \times \{1, \ldots, n_y\},}$$

describe the intensity values of a digital image at the nodal points

$$\boxed{x_{ij} = (ih, jh), \qquad (i,j) \in \mathcal{I}_1,}$$

of a regular rectangular *pixel grid* $\mathbf{x} = (x_{ij})$. The parameter h controls the resolution of the image, that is, the horizontal and vertical distance of the pixels x_{ij} (see Fig. 2.1). Note that in the literature, sometimes pixels are defined as rectangles with midpoints x_{ij}.

In contrast with digital photography, where intensities are assumed to be integers in a certain range (for instance, between 0 and 255), we allow for arbitrary real values in the consideration below.

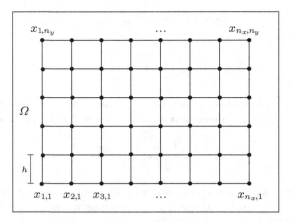

Fig. 2.1. Pixel grid with nodes $x_{ij} = (ih, jh)$.

A *continuous image* is given by its *intensity function* $u : \Omega \to \mathbb{R}$, where

$$\Omega := \big(0, (n_x + 1)h\big) \times \big(0, (n_y + 1)h\big) .$$

Note that Ω is chosen in such a way that the pixel grid $\mathbf{x}$ is contained in the *interior* of Ω.

To every pair (i, j) in the set

$$\mathcal{I}_2 := \{1, \ldots, n_x - 1\} \times \{1, \ldots, n_y - 1\}$$

we assign the discrete gradient v_{ij} of u at x_{ij} setting

$$v_{ij} := \frac{1}{h} \begin{pmatrix} u_{i+1,j} - u_{ij} \\ u_{i,j+1} - u_{ij} \end{pmatrix} . \qquad (2.8)$$

The resulting mapping $\mathbf{v} : \mathcal{I}_2 \to \mathbb{R}^2$ is called the *discrete gradients matrix*. Note that this matrix is not an ordinary matrix of scalars, but its entries are actually vectors. Moreover, we denote the matrix of norms of the discrete gradients $|v_{ij}|$ by $|\mathbf{v}|$.

We distinguish discrete gradients $\mathbf{v}$ of a *discrete image* from one-sided discrete gradients $\nabla_h u$ of a *continuous image* u, which are defined by

$$\nabla_h u(x_{ij}) := \frac{1}{h} \begin{pmatrix} u(x_{i+1,j}) - u(x_{ij}) \\ u(x_{i,j+1}) - u(x_{ij}) \end{pmatrix} , \qquad (i, j) \in \mathcal{I}_2 .$$

In the special case that the discrete image $\mathbf{u}$ is given as pointwise discretization of a continuous image u, that is, $u_{ij} = u(x_{ij})$, we obtain the equality of gradients $v_{ij} = \nabla_h u(x_{ij})$. It is, however, convenient in certain applications to also allow more general discretizations with respect to which the equality does not necessarily hold.

2.3 Noise Models

In this section, we discuss noise models corresponding to different distortions in image recording. We concentrate first on intensity errors, which are realizations of independent random variables, acting on each pixel location separately, and then on sampling errors, where the observed error depends on surrounding pixels as well.

Intensity Errors

The simplest model for intensity errors is *additive noise*. Let $\mathbf{u}$ be a discrete image and $\boldsymbol{\delta} = (\delta_{ij})_{ij}$ be an $n_x \times n_y$ matrix of realizations of i.i.d. random variables. If the recorded data are

$$\boxed{\mathbf{u}^\delta = \mathbf{u} + \boldsymbol{\delta}\,,}$$

(2.9)

then we speak of *additive intensity errors* in the image data. If each random variable is Gaussian distributed, we speak of *Gaussian intensity errors*. Other commonly used noise models assume a Laplacian, uniform, or Poisson distribution (with constant parameter) of the random variables. Variational approaches for removing additive Gaussian intensity errors are discussed in the subsequent sections.

A model of *multiplicative noise* is given by

$$\boxed{\mathbf{u}^\delta = \mathbf{u} \cdot \boldsymbol{\delta}\,,}$$

where, again, $\boldsymbol{\delta} = (\delta_{ij})_{ij}$ is a matrix of realizations of (non-negative) i.i.d. random variables, and the multiplication is understood pointwise, that is, $u_{ij}^\delta = u_{ij}\delta_{ij}$. We then speak of *multiplicative intensity errors*. A variational denoising approach taking into account such a noise model has been studied in [337, 346, 347]. Aubert & Aujol [25] have considered multiplicative *Gamma noise* and developed an adequate variational denoising approach.

Poisson noise and *Salt-and-Pepper noise* are prominent noise models with a functional dependency of the noise $\boldsymbol{\delta}$ on $\mathbf{u}$, which is neither multiplicative nor additive, that is,

$$\boxed{\mathbf{u}^\delta = \boldsymbol{\delta}(\mathbf{u})\,.}$$

Photon counting errors produced by CCD sensors are typically modeled by Poisson noise [40, 223, 359]. Let us consider a camera with a two-dimensional array of CCD sensors, each sensor (i, j) corresponding to a position x_{ij} of the sensor. During exposure, each sensor counts the number of incoming photons at x_{ij}. Because this number is non-negative, the vector $\mathbf{u}$ has non-negative entries.

The number of photons $\delta_{ij}(\mathbf{u})$ detected by the CCD sensor can be modeled as a realization of a Poisson distributed random variable with mean u_{ij}. Then the probability for measuring the value $k \in \mathbb{N} \cup \{0\}$ at the pixel position x_{ij} is given by the probability distribution $P_{\Delta_{ij}} =: P_{ij}$ defined by (cf. (2.5))

$$P_{ij}(k) = \frac{u_{ij}^k}{k!} \exp(-u_{ij}), \qquad k \in \mathbb{N} \cup \{0\} .$$

In the case of Salt-and-Pepper noise, it is assumed that uniform bounds $c_{\min} \leq u_{ij} \leq c_{\max}$ of the data $\mathbf{u}$ are given. On each pixel x_{ij}, the noise process either sets the intensity u_{ij} to $c_{\min}$ or $c_{\max}$, or leaves the intensity unchanged. This can be modeled by considering $\delta_{ij}(\mathbf{u})$ a realization of the random variable P_{ij} with range $\{c_{\min}, u_{ij}, c_{\max}\}$ given by

$$P_{ij}(c_{\min}) = \lambda_1 , \qquad P_{ij}(u_{ij}) = \lambda_2 , \qquad P_{ij}(c_{\max}) = \lambda_3 ,$$

where $\lambda_i \geq 0$ satisfy $\lambda_1 + \lambda_2 + \lambda_3 = 1$. One application is the modeling of corrupt sensors that are either in an "always on" or "always off" state. In this case, $c_{\min} = 0$ represents black (off) pixels and $c_{\max} = 1$ white (on) pixels. For more details, we refer to [184, p. 316] or [92].

Sampling Errors

We consider the noise model

$$\boxed{\mathbf{u}^\delta = \mathbf{u} + \boldsymbol{\delta} \, |\mathbf{v}| ,} \qquad (2.10)$$

where $|\mathbf{v}|$ is the matrix of the norms of the discrete gradients defined in (2.8) and $\boldsymbol{\delta}$ is an $(n_x - 1) \times (n_y - 1)$ matrix of realizations of i.i.d. Gaussian random variables Δ_{ij}. We assume that each Δ_{ij} has zero mean and standard deviation $\sigma_{\Delta_{ij}} := \sigma_\Delta > 0$. As in the case of multiplicative intensity errors, all operations in (2.10) are understood pointwise. For the sake of simplicity of presentation, we do not notationally distinguish between the $n_x \times n_y$ matrices $\mathbf{u}$ and $\mathbf{u}^\delta$ on the one hand and the sub-matrices consisting of the first $(n_x - 1)$ columns and first $(n_y - 1)$ rows on the other hand.

The relevance of this noise model becomes evident from the following considerations: Let us assume that u_{ij}, $(i,j) \in \mathcal{I}_2$, are obtained by sampling a function $u \in C_0^2(\Omega)$ at sampling points $x_{ij} \in \Omega$, $(i,j) \in \mathcal{I}_2$. The following results state that the error model defined in (2.10) approximates an error model, where each sampling point is randomly shifted in direction of $\nabla u(x_{ij})$.

Theorem 2.8. *Let $h > 0$ fixed. Assume that $u \in C_0^2(\mathbb{R}^2)$ satisfies*

$$u_{ij} = u(x_{ij}), \qquad (i,j) \in \mathcal{I}_2 .$$

Moreover, let

$$x_{ij}^\delta := x_{ij} + \delta_{ij} n_{ij} , \qquad n_{ij} := \begin{cases} \dfrac{\nabla u(x_{ij})}{|\nabla u(x_{ij})|}, & \text{if } \nabla u(x_{ij}) \neq 0 , \\ 0, & \text{else} , \end{cases}$$

that is, n_{ij} is orthogonal to the level line $\partial\, \mathrm{level}_{u_{ij}}(u)$ at x_{ij}. Then there exists a constant C only depending on u, such that

$$\frac{1}{|\mathcal{I}_2|} \sum_{(i,j)\in\mathcal{I}_2} |u(x_{ij}^{\delta}) - u_{ij}^{\delta}| \leq \frac{C}{|\mathcal{I}_2|} \Big(h \sum_{(i,j)\in\mathcal{I}_2} |\delta_{ij}| + \sum_{(i,j)\in\mathcal{I}_2} \delta_{ij}^2 \Big) . \qquad (2.11)$$

Proof. Because $u(x_{ij}) = u_{ij}$, it follows that also $\nabla_h u(x_{ij}) = v_{ij}$. Because by assumption $u \in C_0^2(\mathbb{R}^2)$, Taylor's theorem shows that there exists $C_1 > 0$ only depending on $\left\| \nabla^2 u \right\|_{\infty}$, such that

$$\left| u(x_{ij} + \delta_{ij} n_{ij}) - u(x_{ij}) - \delta_{ij} \nabla u(x_{ij}) \cdot n_{ij} \right| \leq C_1 \delta_{ij}^2 , \qquad (i,j) \in \mathcal{I}_2 . \quad (2.12)$$

Using (2.12) shows that

$$\begin{aligned}
\left| u(x_{ij}^{\delta}) - u_{ij}^{\delta} \right| &= \left| u(x_{ij} + \delta_{ij} n_{ij}) - u(x_{ij}) - \delta_{ij} |\nabla_h u(x_{ij})| \right| \\
&\leq \left| \delta_{ij} \nabla u(x_{ij}) \cdot n_{ij} - \delta_{ij} |\nabla_h u(x_{ij})| \right| + C_1 \delta_{ij}^2 .
\end{aligned} \qquad (2.13)$$

Because $\nabla u(x_{ij}) \cdot n_{ij} = |\nabla u(x_{ij})|$, it follows from (2.13) that

$$\begin{aligned}
\left| u(x_{ij}^{\delta}) - u_{ij}^{\delta} \right| &\leq |\delta_{ij}| \, \big| |\nabla u(x_{ij})| - |\nabla_h u(x_{ij})| \big| + C_1 \delta_{ij}^2 \\
&\leq |\delta_{ij}| \, \big| \nabla u(x_{ij}) - \nabla_h u(x_{ij}) \big| + C_1 \delta_{ij}^2 .
\end{aligned} \qquad (2.14)$$

Moreover, there exists $C_2 > 0$, again only depending on $\left\| \nabla^2 u \right\|_{\infty}$, such that

$$\left| \nabla u(x_{ij}) - \nabla_h u(x_{ij}) \right| \leq C_2 h , \qquad (i,j) \in \mathcal{I}_2 . \qquad (2.15)$$

Inserting (2.15) in (2.14), we derive

$$\frac{1}{|\mathcal{I}_2|} \sum_{(i,j)\in\mathcal{I}_2} |u(x_{ij}^{\delta}) - u_{ij}^{\delta}| \leq \frac{C_2 \, h}{|\mathcal{I}_2|} \sum_{(i,j)\in\mathcal{I}_2} |\delta_{ij}| + \frac{C_1}{|\mathcal{I}_2|} \sum_{(i,j)\in\mathcal{I}_2} \delta_{ij}^2 ,$$

which proves the assertion. $\qquad \square$

Remark 2.9. We now study the influence of the mesh size h on the above defined sampling errors. To that end, we indicate the parameter h by a superscript in all occurring variables and sets.

Recall that the sample means of δ^h and $|\delta^h|$ and the sample variance of δ^h are defined as (see Definition 2.4 and Remark 2.6)

$$\mathrm{E}(\delta^h) = \frac{1}{|\mathcal{I}_2^h|} \sum_{(i,j)\in\mathcal{I}_2^h} \delta_{ij}^h , \qquad \mathrm{E}(|\delta^h|) = \frac{1}{|\mathcal{I}_2^h|} \sum_{(i,j)\in\mathcal{I}_2^h} |\delta_{ij}^h| ,$$

$$\mathrm{Var}(\delta^h) = \frac{1}{|\mathcal{I}_2^h|} \sum_{(i,j)\in\mathcal{I}_2^h} \left(\delta_{ij}^h - \mathrm{E}(\delta^h) \right)^2 = \frac{1}{|\mathcal{I}_2^h|} \sum_{(i,j)\in\mathcal{I}_2^h} (\delta_{ij}^h)^2 - \mathrm{E}(\delta^h)^2 .$$

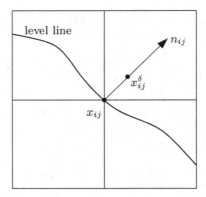

Fig. 2.2. Distortion of a sampling point in 2D. The shift is assumed to be orthogonal to the level line.

Inserting these definitions in the right-hand side of (2.11) yields

$$\frac{1}{|\mathcal{I}_2^h|} \sum_{(i,j)\in\mathcal{I}_2^h} \left| u(x_{ij}^{h,\delta}) - u_{ij}^{h,\delta} \right| \le C\big(h\, \mathrm{E}(|\boldsymbol{\delta}^h|) + \mathrm{E}(\boldsymbol{\delta}^h)^2 + \mathrm{Var}(\boldsymbol{\delta}^h) \big)\,.$$

For $h > 0$, denote by $P_{\boldsymbol{\Delta}^h}$ the distribution of the random vector $\boldsymbol{\Delta}^h$. The law of large numbers (see, e.g., [160, VII.7, Thm. 1]) implies that $\mathrm{E}(\boldsymbol{\delta}^h) \to 0$ in probability, that is,

$$\lim_{h\to 0} P_{\boldsymbol{\Delta}^h}\big(\{ |\mathrm{E}(\boldsymbol{\delta}^h)| > \varepsilon \}\big) = 0\,, \qquad \varepsilon > 0\,.$$

Similarly, the law of large numbers implies that $\mathrm{E}(|\boldsymbol{\delta}^h|)$ converges in probability to a finite number, which implies that $h\, \mathrm{E}(|\boldsymbol{\delta}^h|) \to 0$. As a consequence, it follows from Theorem 2.8 that

$$\limsup_{h\to 0} \frac{1}{|\mathcal{I}_2^h|} \sum_{(i,j)\in\mathcal{I}_2^h} \left| u(x_{ij}^{h,\delta}) - u_{ij}^{h,\delta} \right| \le C\, \mathrm{Var}(\boldsymbol{\delta}^h) \quad \text{in probability}\,, \quad (2.16)$$

that is,

$$\lim_{h\to 0} P_{\boldsymbol{\Delta}^h}\left(\left\{ \frac{1}{|\mathcal{I}_2^h|} \sum_{(i,j)\in\mathcal{I}_2^h} \left| u(x_{ij}^{h,\delta}) - u_{ij}^{h,\delta} \right| > C\, \mathrm{Var}(\boldsymbol{\delta}^h) + \varepsilon \right\}\right) = 0\,, \qquad \varepsilon > 0\,.$$

Using (2.16), it follows that the error model (2.10) for small variances approximately describes displacement errors of the sampling points in direction orthogonal to the level lines (compare Fig. 2.2).   ◇

2.4 Priors for Images

In the following, we show how images themselves can be modeled as realizations of a random vector, the distribution of which is called *prior distribution* or *prior* (see [129, 231]). The method of MAP estimation, to be introduced in

Section 2.5, then provides a statistical motivation for variational methods for denoising. We attempt to use as simple as possible priors, and assume that either the intensities of the image or the discrete gradients are i.i.d. Below we show with three test examples that this assumption, though extremely simplifying, still provides enough information to be used in MAP estimation for efficient denoising.

In this book, we consider three digitized test images shown in Figs. 2.3, 2.5, and 2.7:

- a digital photo, which we refer to as the *mountain* image,
- a synthetic image, which we refer to as the *cards* image, and
- ultrasound data.

As additional test data, we use noisy variants of the mountain and cards images. We have artificially distorted the images by adding either *Gaussian intensity errors* or by simulating *sampling errors*.

The test data with Gaussian intensity errors are plotted in Figs. 2.9 and 2.11. The test data with sampling errors are shown in Figs. 2.10 and 2.12.

Histograms of the Intensities

Histograms are important for motivating variational regularization techniques. The *histogram* of an image is determined by partitioning $\mathbb{R}$ into congruent half-open sub-intervals of length $\Delta I > 0$,

$$I_k := \left[k\,\Delta I, (k+1)\Delta I\right), \qquad k \in \mathbb{Z},$$

and counting the occurrences of $\mathbf{u}$ in the sub-intervals, that is,

$$c_k := |\{(i,j) \in \mathcal{I}_1 : u_{ij} \in I_k\}| \ .$$

The histogram is represented as a probability density p on $\mathbb{R}$ that is constant on each interval I_k and there attains the value

$$\boxed{p|_{I_k} := \frac{c_k}{\Delta I \, |\mathcal{I}_1|}, \qquad k \in \mathbb{Z}.}$$

Comparing the histograms of the intensities of the test images with the corresponding histograms of the distorted images reveals that, by adding Gaussian noise to an image, the histogram of the intensities becomes smoother (compare the histograms of Figs. 2.4 and 2.6).

The ultrasound image in Fig. 2.7 contains speckle noise. Because no noise-free version is available, we compare the original data with a filtered version of the image (see Fig. 2.8). For filtering, the total variation regularization method discussed in Chapter 4 is used. Again, the histogram of the noisy data is smoother than that of the filtered image.

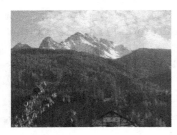

Fig. 2.3. Mountain image.

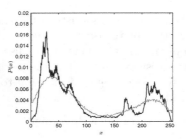

Fig. 2.4. Histogram of mountain image (*black line*) and histogram of the image distorted with Gaussian noise (*gray line*).

Fig. 2.5. Cards image.

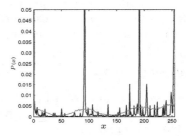

Fig. 2.6. Histogram of cards image (*black line*) and histogram of the image distorted with Gaussian noise (*gray line*).

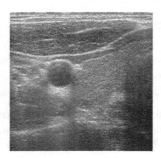

Fig. 2.7. Ultrasound data.

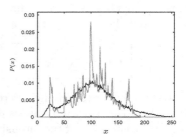

Fig. 2.8. Histogram of original ultrasound data (*black line*) and of filtered data (*gray line*).

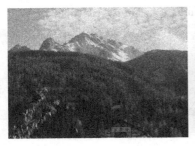

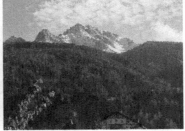

Fig. 2.9. Mountain image distorted by additive Gaussian noise.

Fig. 2.10. Mountain image distorted by sampling point errors.

Fig. 2.11. Cards image distorted by additive Gaussian noise.

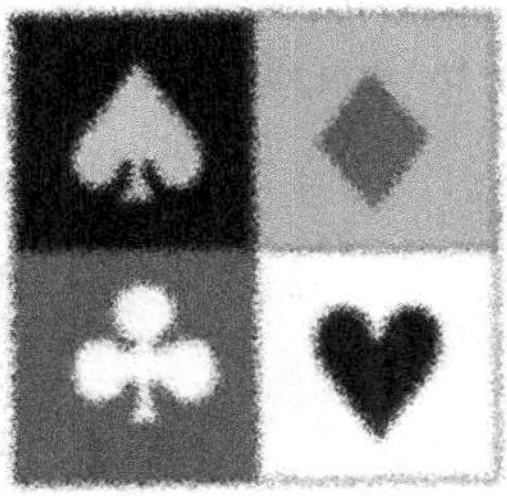

Fig. 2.12. Cards image distorted by sampling point errors.

The above examples show that the intensity histograms of images strongly depend on the image content. Therefore it is difficult to provide an *a priori* probability density $p(\mathbf{u})$ that approximates the histograms of a variety of different images.

Histograms of the Discrete Gradients

In image processing, commonly the histograms of *norms of the discrete gradients* of intensities are preferred to intensity histograms. Figures 2.14, 2.16, and 2.18 show the histograms of $|\mathbf{v}|$ for our test images. It can be recognized that the histograms are pronounced at around 0 and look very similar to the probability distributions considered above. In Figs. 2.13, 2.15, and 2.17, the histograms for the distorted and the original test images are compared to highlight the differences.

For both the card and the mountain image without distortions, the histograms of the discrete gradients are concentrated around zero, indicating that the images have dominant flat regions. For the data distorted with Gaussian noise, the histogram is significantly flatter. Distortions of sampling points strongly change the histogram in the mountain image but not in the cards image. This is due to the fact that the cards image consists of piecewise constant parts, in which sampling errors have no effect.

Distribution of |**v**| and fitted Gaussian and Laplacian distribution

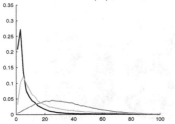

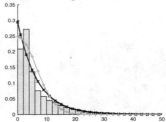

Fig. 2.13. Empirical distribution of the discrete gradient: mountain image (*black line*), distorted by Gaussian noise (*dark gray line*) and distorted by sampling errors (*light gray line*).

Fig. 2.14. Histogram of |**v**| (*bar plot*) for the mountain image and fitted Laplacian (*black line*) and Gaussian (*gray line*) distribution.

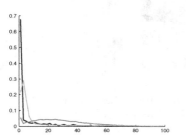

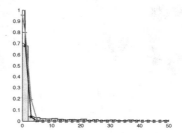

Fig. 2.15. Empirical density of |**v**| for the cards image (*black line*), distorted by Gaussian noise (*dark gray line*) and distorted by sampling errors (*light gray line*).

Fig. 2.16. Histogram of |**v**| (*bar plot*) for the cards image and fitted Laplacian (*black line*) and Gaussian (*gray line*) distribution.

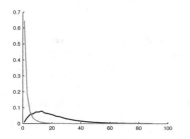

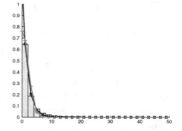

Fig. 2.17. Histogram of |**v**| for the ultrasound (*black line*) and filtered ultrasound data (*gray line*).

Fig. 2.18. Histogram of |**v**| for the filtered ultrasound data and fitted Laplacian (*black line*) and Gaussian (*gray line*) distribution.

Table 2.1. Optimal approximation (w.r.t. l^2-error) by Gaussian and Laplacian probability densities to the histograms of the absolute value of discrete gradients of the images.

Test image	l^2-error – Gauss	l^2-error – Laplace
Mountain	3.13×10^{-3}	2.61×10^{-3}
Cards	10.25×10^{-3}	1.14×10^{-3}

In order to derive image priors, we compare the histograms of $|\mathbf{v}|$ with an appropriate subset of well-established continuous probability density functions supported in $[0, \infty)$. For a continuous density function $\tilde{p}$ we use the approximation

$$\tilde{P}|_{I_k} := \frac{1}{|I_k|} \int_{I_k} \tilde{p}(s) \approx \tilde{p}(k), \qquad k \in \mathbb{Z},$$

and minimize the l^2-error between the histogram and the vector $(\tilde{p}(k))$.

In the following, we denote by $\mathbf{U}$ a random vector and by $p_{\mathbf{U}}$ the probability density of $\mathbf{U}$. The image $\mathbf{u}$ is considered as a realization of $\mathbf{U}$.

We now assume that the probability density $p_{\mathbf{U}}(\mathbf{u})$ only depends on the matrix $|\mathbf{v}|$ of the norms of the discrete gradients $\mathbf{v}$ of $\mathbf{u}$. Additionally, we assume that the norms of the discrete gradients are i.i.d. In this case, the probability density of $\mathbf{U}$ is the product of the densities of $|v_{ij}|$.

A typical assumption on the absolute values of the discrete gradients is that they are Gaussian distributed, in which case the prior is

$$p_{\mathbf{U}}(\mathbf{u}) := C \exp\left(-\frac{1}{2\sigma_2^2} \sum_{(i,j) \in \mathcal{I}_2} |v_{ij}|^2 \right), \tag{2.17}$$

or that they are Laplacian distributed (see [39]), in which case the prior is

$$p_{\mathbf{U}}(\mathbf{u}) := C \exp\left(-\frac{1}{\sigma_1} \sum_{(i,j) \in \mathcal{I}_2} |v_{ij}| \right).$$

We refer to these priors as the *Gaussian prior* and the *Laplacian prior*, respectively.

Example 2.10. We determine the best approximation of discrete gradients of the cards and mountain histogram, respectively, within the set of Laplacian and Gaussian densities. To that end, we have to determine the parameters $\sigma_q > 0$, $q \in \{1, 2\}$, in such a way that the density p as introduced in (2.6) and

(2.7), respectively, optimally fits the histogram. In Figs. 2.14 and 2.16, we have plotted the optimal Laplacian density ($q = 1$) and the optimal Gaussian density ($q = 2$). Table 2.1 shows that the histogram can be better approximated within the set of Laplacian distributions than within the set of Gaussian distributions. $\diamond$

In the case of the mountain image, one can see that the histogram of the discrete gradients attains its maximum away from zero (see Fig. 2.14). The reason is that natural images often include regions containing texture, where small oscillations cause a non-vanishing discrete gradient. The Gaussian and Laplacian prior, however, both attain their maximum at zero. In order to mirror this situation, we introduce a new density, in the following referred to as *log-prior* (see Fig. 2.19),

$$p_{\mathbf{U}}(\mathbf{u}) := C \exp \left(\sum_{(i,j)\in\mathcal{I}_2} -\frac{|v_{ij}|^q}{q\,\sigma_3^q} + \log|v_{ij}| \right) ,$$

where $C > 0$ is a normalizing constant, and $q = 1$ or $q = 2$.

We motivate the log-prior as follows: Let $v \in \mathbb{R}^2$ be a realization of a two-dimensional random vector V, which is Gaussian or Laplacian distributed, that is, it has a probability density of the form

$$p_V(v) = C \exp \left(-\frac{|v|^q}{q\,\sigma_3^q} \right) ,$$

where $\sigma_3 > 0$, $q \in \{1,2\}$, and $C := \left(\int_{\mathbb{R}^2} \exp\left(-|\tilde{v}|^q/q\sigma_3^q\right) \right)^{-1}$. We are interested in the distribution of $|V|$, and therefore we consider its probability density $p_{|V|}$. Using Lemma 2.3 with $f(v) = |v|$, which implies that the Jacobian of f (see (2.1)) satisfies $J_f = 1$ almost everywhere, we find that

$$p_{|V|}(s) = C \int_{|\tilde{v}|=s} \exp \left(-\frac{|\tilde{v}|^q}{q\sigma_3^q} \right) \, \mathrm{d}\mathcal{H}^1 , \qquad s \geq 0, \qquad (2.18)$$

where $\mathcal{H}^1$ is the one-dimensional Hausdorff measure (see (9.1)). Because the integrand in (2.18) is constant on $\{|\tilde{v}| = s\}$, it follows from the fact that $\mathcal{H}^1(\{|\tilde{v}| = s\}) = 2\pi s$ that

$$p_{|V|}(s) = 2\pi s\, C \exp \left(-\frac{s^q}{q\sigma_3^q} \right) , \qquad s \geq 0, \qquad (2.19)$$

the maximum of which is attained for $s = \sigma_3$. Figure 2.19 shows the graphs of the probability density (2.19) for $q = 1$ and $q = 2$. For $q = 2$, the function $p_{|V|}$ is the density of the *Rayleigh distribution* (see, for example, [388]).

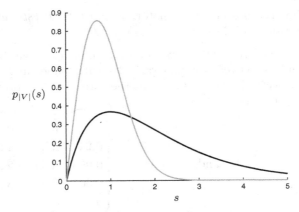

Fig. 2.19. Probability density $p_{|V|}(s) = Cs\exp(-s^q/q\sigma_3^q)$ with $\sigma_3 = 1$, $C = \left(\int_0^\infty s\exp(-s^q/q\sigma_3^q)\right)^{-1}$ for $q = 1$ (*black line*) and $q = 2$ (*gray line*).

2.5 Maximum A Posteriori Estimation

We consider the following situation:

Let $\tilde{\mathbf{U}} = (\mathbf{U}, \mathbf{U}^\delta)$ be an $(n + m)$-dimensional random vector. The probability distribution of $\tilde{\mathbf{U}}$ is just the joint probability distribution of $\mathbf{U}$ and $\mathbf{U}^\delta$, denoted by $P_{\mathbf{U},\mathbf{U}^\delta}$.

Moreover, let $\mathbf{u}^\delta$ be a realization of the m-dimensional random vector $\mathbf{U}^\delta$. We want to find a realization $\mathbf{u}^0$ of $\mathbf{U}$ that makes the pair $(\mathbf{u}, \mathbf{u}^\delta)$ most likely. Typically, $\mathbf{u}^\delta$ is interpreted as noisy data, which are formed from the clean data by means of a known noise process.

If $\mathbf{U}$ is a discrete random vector, the task of reconstructing $\mathbf{u}^0$ is comparatively easy. The most likely realization $\mathbf{u}^0$ is the one that, for fixed $\mathbf{u}^\delta$, maximizes the joint probability $P_{\mathbf{U},\mathbf{U}^\delta}(\cdot, \mathbf{u}^\delta)$. In order to make the definition suited for generalization to the non-discrete case, we define maximum a posteriori estimation for discrete random vectors by means of conditional probabilities:

Definition 2.11. *Let* $\mathbf{U}$ *and* $\mathbf{U}^\delta$ *be discrete random vectors. The* conditional probability *of* $\mathbf{u}$ *for given realization* $\mathbf{u}^\delta$ *of* $\mathbf{U}^\delta$ *is defined by*

$$P_{\mathbf{U}|\mathbf{U}^\delta}(\mathbf{u}|\mathbf{u}^\delta) := \begin{cases} \dfrac{P_{\mathbf{U},\mathbf{U}^\delta}(\mathbf{u}, \mathbf{u}^\delta)}{P_{\mathbf{U}^\delta}(\mathbf{u}^\delta)}, & \text{if } P_{\mathbf{U}^\delta}(\mathbf{u}^\delta) > 0, \\ 0, & \text{if } P_{\mathbf{U}^\delta}(\mathbf{u}^\delta) = 0. \end{cases} \tag{2.20}$$

The mapping

$$\mathbf{u}^\delta \mapsto \mathbf{u}^0 := \arg\max_{\mathbf{u}} P_{\mathbf{U}|\mathbf{U}^\delta}(\mathbf{u}|\mathbf{u}^\delta)$$

is called maximum a posteriori estimator, *in short MAP estimator, and the function* $\mathbf{u}^0$ *is called* MAP estimate *(see [383, 391])*.

Example 2.12. We apply MAP estimation to a simple example: Let U and Δ be two independent discrete random variables with values in $I_1 := \{1,2,3\}$ and $I_2 := \mathbb{Z}$, respectively. We assume that the corresponding probability distributions are defined by

$$P_U(u) = \frac{1}{3} \quad \text{and} \quad P_\Delta(\delta) = \begin{cases} 0.4 & \text{if } \delta = 0, \\ 0.24 & \text{if } |\delta| = 1, \\ 0.055 & \text{if } |\delta| = 2, \\ 0.005 & \text{if } |\delta| = 3, \\ 0 & \text{else}. \end{cases}$$

Let $U^\delta = U + \Delta$. Then

$$P_{U^\delta}(u^\delta) = \sum_{u \in I_1} P_{U,\Delta}(u, u^\delta - u) = \sum_{u \in I_1} P_U(u)\, P_\Delta(u^\delta - u)$$

$$= \frac{1}{3} \sum_{u \in I_1} P_\Delta(u^\delta - u) = \begin{cases} 0.002 & \text{if } u^\delta = -2 \text{ or } 6, \\ 0.02 & \text{if } u^\delta = -1 \text{ or } 5, \\ 0.1 & \text{if } u^\delta = 0 \text{ or } 4, \\ 0.232 & \text{if } u^\delta = 1 \text{ or } 3, \\ 0.293 & \text{if } u^\delta = 2, \\ 0 & \text{else}. \end{cases}$$

For $u^\delta \in \{-2,\ldots,6\}$, the probabilities $P_{U,U^\delta}(u, u^\delta)$ and $P_{U|U^\delta}(u|u^\delta)$ can be read from the following tables, for $u^\delta \notin \{-2,\ldots 6\}$ we have $P_{U,U^\delta}(u, u^\delta) = P_{U|U^\delta}(u|u^\delta) = 0$ for every u.

					u^δ				
P_{U,U^δ}	-2	-1	0	1	2	3	4	5	6
u=1	0.002	0.018	0.080	0.133	0.080	0.018	0.002	0.000	0.000
u=2	0.000	0.002	0.018	0.080	0.133	0.080	0.018	0.002	0.000
u=3	0.000	0.000	0.002	0.018	0.080	0.133	0.080	0.018	0.002

$P_{U|U^\delta}$	-2	-1	0	1	2	3	4	5	6
u=1	1.0	0.917	0.800	0.576	0.273	0.079	0.017	0.000	0.0
u=2	0.0	0.083	0.183	0.345	0.455	0.345	0.183	0.083	0.0
u=3	0.0	0.000	0.017	0.079	0.273	0.576	0.800	0.917	1.0

(Note that these values have been rounded.)

For given u^δ, we can determine from $P_{U|U^\delta}$ the most probable value $u \in \{1,2,3\}$. For example, the probability $P_{U|U^\delta}$ for the value of $U^\delta = 0$ attains the maximum at $U = 1$. $\diamond$

In the following, we study the problem of MAP estimation for absolutely continuous distributions. The argumentation follows [321, pp. 98–99]. We assume that the random vectors $\mathbf{U}$, $\mathbf{U}^\delta$, and $\tilde{\mathbf{U}} = (\mathbf{U}, \mathbf{U}^\delta)$ have absolutely continuous probability distributions $P_{\mathbf{U}}$, $P_{\mathbf{U}^\delta}$, and $P_{\mathbf{U},\mathbf{U}^\delta}$ with according densities $p_{\mathbf{U}}$, $p_{\mathbf{U}^\delta}$, and $p_{\mathbf{U},\mathbf{U}^\delta}$.

Analogously to (2.20), we define the conditional probability of a measurable set $A \subset \mathbb{R}^n$ for given measurable $B \subset \mathbb{R}^m$ by

$$P_{\mathbf{U}|\mathbf{U}^\delta}(A|B) := \begin{cases} \dfrac{P_{\mathbf{U},\mathbf{U}^\delta}(A, B)}{P_{\mathbf{U}^\delta}(B)}, & \text{if } P_{\mathbf{U}^\delta}(B) > 0, \\ 0, & \text{if } P_{\mathbf{U}^\delta}(B) = 0. \end{cases}$$

Now let $\mathbf{u}^\delta$ be a realization of $\mathbf{U}^\delta$. We define the *conditional density* $p_{\mathbf{U}|\mathbf{U}^\delta}$ of $\mathbf{u} \in \mathbb{R}^n$ given $\mathbf{u}^\delta$ by

$$p_{\mathbf{U}|\mathbf{U}^\delta}(\mathbf{u}|\mathbf{u}^\delta) := \begin{cases} \dfrac{p_{\mathbf{U},\mathbf{U}^\delta}(\mathbf{u}, \mathbf{u}^\delta)}{p_{\mathbf{U}^\delta}(\mathbf{u}^\delta)}, & \text{if } p_{\mathbf{U}^\delta}(\mathbf{u}^\delta) > 0, \\ 0, & \text{if } p_{\mathbf{U}^\delta}(\mathbf{u}^\delta) = 0. \end{cases} \tag{2.21}$$

The next result reveals the connection between conditional density and conditional probability:

Theorem 2.13. *Let $\mathbf{u}$ and $\mathbf{u}^\delta$ be realizations of the random vectors $\mathbf{U}$ and $\mathbf{U}^\delta$, respectively. Assume that the densities $p_{\mathbf{U}^\delta}$ and $p_{\mathbf{U},\mathbf{U}^\delta}$ are continuous, and $p_{\mathbf{U}^\delta}(\mathbf{u}^\delta) > 0$.*

For $\rho > 0$, let $\mathcal{U}_\rho(\mathbf{u})$ and $\mathcal{U}_\rho(\mathbf{u}^\delta)$ denote the open cubes with side length 2ρ around $\mathbf{u}$ and $\mathbf{u}^\delta$,

$$\mathcal{U}_\rho(\mathbf{u}) := (u_1 - \rho, u_1 + \rho) \times \cdots \times (u_n - \rho, u_n + \rho),$$
$$\mathcal{U}_\rho(\mathbf{u}^\delta) := (u_1^\delta - \rho, u_1^\delta + \rho) \times \cdots \times (u_m^\delta - \rho, u_m^\delta + \rho).$$

Then

$$p_{\mathbf{U}|\mathbf{U}^\delta}(\mathbf{u}|\mathbf{u}^\delta) = \lim_{\rho \to 0} 2^{-n} \rho^{-n} P_{\mathbf{U}|\mathbf{U}^\delta}\big(\mathcal{U}_\rho(\mathbf{u})|\mathcal{U}_\rho(\mathbf{u}^\delta)\big).$$

Proof. Because the probability densities $p_{\mathbf{U}^\delta}$ and $p_{\mathbf{U},\mathbf{U}^\delta}$ are continuous, it follows from the mean value theorem for integration that

$$p_{\mathbf{U}^\delta}(\mathbf{u}^\delta) = \lim_{\rho \to 0} \frac{1}{2^m \rho^m} \int_{\mathcal{U}_\rho(\mathbf{u}^\delta)} p_{\mathbf{U}^\delta}(\mathbf{u}^\delta) = \lim_{\rho \to 0} \frac{P_{\mathbf{U}^\delta}\big(\mathcal{U}_\rho(\mathbf{u}^\delta)\big)}{2^m \rho^m}, \tag{2.22}$$

$$p_{\mathbf{U},\mathbf{U}^\delta}(\mathbf{u}, \mathbf{u}^\delta) = \lim_{\rho \to 0} \frac{P_{\mathbf{U},\mathbf{U}^\delta}\big(\mathcal{U}_\rho(\mathbf{u}) \times \mathcal{U}_\rho(\mathbf{u}^\delta)\big)}{2^{n+m} \rho^{n+m}}. \tag{2.23}$$

Thus the assertion follows from the definitions of conditional probability in (2.20) and conditional density in (2.21). □

Note that (2.22) and (2.23) are simple versions of the Lebesgue–Besicovitch differentiation theorem (see, e.g., [157, Sect. 1.7] for a formulation with balls instead of cubes), which also applies to discontinuous densities, in which case (2.22) and (2.23) only hold almost everywhere.

As a consequence of Theorem 2.13, maximization of $p_{\mathbf{U}|\mathbf{U}^\delta}(\cdot|\mathbf{u}^\delta)$ can be considered as continuous analogue to discrete MAP estimation.

In many applications, the vector $\mathbf{u}^\delta$ is considered a noisy perturbation of some unknown data $\mathbf{u}$. The noise process that generates $\mathbf{u}^\delta$ is described by the conditional density $p_{\mathbf{U}^\delta|\mathbf{U}}(\mathbf{u}^\delta|\mathbf{u})$ of $\mathbf{u}^\delta$ given $\mathbf{u}$. Thus we have to find a way that links the two conditional densities $p_{\mathbf{U}|\mathbf{U}^\delta}(\mathbf{u}|\mathbf{u}^\delta)$ and $p_{\mathbf{U}^\delta|\mathbf{U}}(\mathbf{u}^\delta|\mathbf{u})$. This is achieved by means of the *formula of Bayes* (see, for instance, [129]),

$$
p_{\mathbf{U}|\mathbf{U}^\delta}(\mathbf{u}|\mathbf{u}^\delta) = \begin{cases} \dfrac{p_{\mathbf{U}^\delta|\mathbf{U}}(\mathbf{u}^\delta|\mathbf{u})\,p_{\mathbf{U}}(\mathbf{u})}{p_{\mathbf{U}^\delta}(\mathbf{u}^\delta)}\,, & \text{if } p_{\mathbf{U}^\delta}(\mathbf{u}^\delta) > 0\,, \\ 0\,, & \text{if } p_{\mathbf{U}^\delta}(\mathbf{u}^\delta) = 0\,. \end{cases}
$$

Therefore, we call *continuous MAP estimation* the problem of maximizing the functional

$$
\mathcal{T}^{\mathrm{MAP}}(\mathbf{u}) = \frac{p_{\mathbf{U}^\delta|\mathbf{U}}(\mathbf{u}^\delta|\mathbf{u})\,p_{\mathbf{U}}(\mathbf{u})}{p_{\mathbf{U}^\delta}(\mathbf{u}^\delta)}\,. \tag{2.24}
$$

Note that in (2.24), the constant factor $p_{\mathbf{U}^\delta}(\mathbf{u}^\delta)$ can be omitted without affecting the maximization problem. A maximizer of (2.24) is called *MAP estimate*.

To simplify the maximization, the logarithmic MAP estimator

$$
\mathcal{T}^{\mathrm{logMAP}}(\mathbf{u}) := -\log p_{\mathbf{U}^\delta|\mathbf{U}}(\mathbf{u}^\delta|\mathbf{u}) - \log p_{\mathbf{U}}(\mathbf{u}) \tag{2.25}
$$

is often used in applications. Because the logarithm is a strictly increasing function, the transformation does not change the extrema. The problem of minimization of $\mathcal{T}^{\mathrm{logMAP}}$ is referred to as log MAP estimation.

2.6 MAP Estimation for Noisy Images

We now show how the method of MAP estimation can be applied to image denoising and analysis.

We always assume that we are given a noisy image $\mathbf{u}^\delta$ that is a distortion of the clean image by one of the noise processes introduced in Section 2.3. Moreover, we denote by $\mathbf{U}$ a random variable associated with one of the image priors introduced in Section 2.4. In addition, $\mathbf{u}$ denotes a realization of $\mathbf{U}$.

Intensity Errors

We first assume additive Gaussian intensity errors on the image. In this case, the data $\mathbf{u}^\delta$ are given as (see (2.9))

$$\mathbf{u}^\delta = \mathbf{u} + \boldsymbol{\delta} \,,$$

where $\boldsymbol{\delta}$ is a realization of the random vector $\boldsymbol{\Delta} = (\Delta_{ij})$, $(i,j) \in \mathcal{I}_2$, where Δ_{ij} are i.i.d. Gaussian random variables with zero mean and variance σ^2. For fixed $\mathbf{u}$, the random vector $\mathbf{U}^\delta$ is given by

$$\mathbf{U}^\delta = \mathbf{u} + \boldsymbol{\Delta} \,.$$

We immediately see that U_{ij}^δ for given $\mathbf{u}$ are independently Gaussian distributed with mean u_{ij} and variance σ^2. Thus the conditional probability density $p(\mathbf{u}^\delta|\mathbf{u}) := p_{\mathbf{U}^\delta|\mathbf{U}}(\mathbf{u}^\delta|\mathbf{u})$ is given by

$$p(\mathbf{u}^\delta|\mathbf{u}) = \left(\frac{1}{\sigma\sqrt{2\pi}}\right)^{|\mathcal{I}_2|} \prod_{(i,j)\in\mathcal{I}_2} \exp\left(-\frac{(u_{ij}^\delta - u_{ij})^2}{2\sigma^2}\right) \,. \tag{2.26}$$

For simplicity of presentation, we now omit the subscripts of the probability densities $p_{\mathbf{U}^\delta|\mathbf{U}}(\mathbf{u}^\delta|\mathbf{u})$ and $p_{\mathbf{U}}(\mathbf{u})$, which can always be identified from the context. From (2.26), it follows that

$$-\log p(\mathbf{u}^\delta|\mathbf{u}) = |\mathcal{I}_2| \log(\sigma\sqrt{2\pi}) + \sum_{(i,j)\in\mathcal{I}_2} \frac{(u_{ij}^\delta - u_{ij})^2}{2\sigma^2} \,.$$

The goal of maximum a posteriori estimators (see also (2.24)) is to determine $\mathbf{u}$ by maximizing the product of the conditional probability density $p(\mathbf{u}^\delta|\mathbf{u})$ and the probability density of $\mathbf{u}$, which is given by its image prior $p(\mathbf{u})$. Maximizing the conditional probability density is equivalent to minimization of the negative logarithm of the conditional probability density.

Assuming a Gaussian prior (2.17), the second term in (2.25) reads as

$$-\log p(\mathbf{u}) = \sum_{(i,j)\in\mathcal{I}_2} \frac{1}{2\sigma_2^2} |v_{ij}|^2 + C \,.$$

Thus, the *log MAP estimator* for denoising images with intensity errors and Gaussian prior consists in minimization of the functional

$$\boxed{\arg\min_{\mathbf{u}\in\mathbb{R}^{\mathcal{I}_1}} \sum_{(i,j)\in\mathcal{I}_2} \left((u_{ij} - u_{ij}^\delta)^2 + \alpha\,|v_{ij}|^2\right),}$$

where $\alpha := \sigma^2/\sigma_2^2 > 0$.

Sampling Errors

As above, we now determine MAP estimators for the model of sampling errors, where the noise model is given by (2.10).

Again we assume that $\boldsymbol{\delta}$ is a realization of a random vector $\boldsymbol{\Delta} = (\Delta_{ij})$, $(i,j) \in \mathcal{I}_2$, consisting of i.i.d. Gaussian random variables Δ_{ij} all having zero mean and variance σ^2. Let $\mathbf{u}$ be fixed (and therefore also $\mathbf{v}$), then it follows that the random variables

$$U_{ij}^{\delta} = u_{ij} + |v_{ij}| \, \Delta_{ij} \,, \qquad (i,j) \in \mathcal{I}_2 \,, \tag{2.27}$$

are independent.

Assuming that $|v_{ij}| > 0$ for all $(i,j) \in \mathcal{I}_2$, it follows from (2.27) by using Lemma 2.3 with $f(x) = u_{ij} + |v_{ij}| \, x$ (and therefore $J_f = |v_{ij}|$) that

$$\begin{aligned}
p(u_{ij}^{\delta}|\mathbf{u}) &= \int_{\left\{\delta_{ij} = \frac{u_{ij}^{\delta} - u_{ij}}{|v_{ij}|}\right\}} \frac{1}{|v_{ij}|} \, p_{\Delta_{ij}}(\delta_{ij}) \, \mathrm{d}\mathcal{H}^0 \\
&= \left(\frac{1}{\sigma\sqrt{2\pi}}\right) \frac{1}{|v_{ij}|} \exp\left(-\frac{(u_{ij} - u_{ij}^{\delta})^2}{2\sigma^2 \, |v_{ij}|^2}\right) \,.
\end{aligned} \tag{2.28}$$

Because U_{ij}^{δ}, $(i,j) \in \mathcal{I}_2$, are independent, we have that

$$p(\mathbf{u}^{\delta}|\mathbf{u}) = \prod_{(i,j) \in \mathcal{I}_2} p(u_{ij}^{\delta}|\mathbf{u}) \,. \tag{2.29}$$

Inserting (2.28) into (2.29), it follows that

$$p(\mathbf{u}^{\delta}|\mathbf{u}) = \left(\frac{1}{\sigma\sqrt{2\pi}}\right)^{|\mathcal{I}_2|} \prod_{(i,j) \in \mathcal{I}_2} \frac{1}{|v_{ij}|} \exp\left(-\frac{(u_{ij} - u_{ij}^{\delta})^2}{2\sigma^2 \, |v_{ij}|^2}\right) \,. \tag{2.30}$$

As an example, the log MAP estimator, defined in (2.25), according to the conditional probability density (2.30) and the log-prior (2.19) is given by

$$\underset{\mathbf{u} \in \mathbb{R}^{\mathcal{I}_1}}{\arg\min} \sum_{(i,j) \in \mathcal{I}_2} \left(\frac{1}{2} \frac{(u_{ij} - u_{ij}^{\delta})^2}{|v_{ij}|^2} + \frac{\alpha}{q} |v_{ij}|^q\right) \,, \qquad q = 1, 2 \,. \tag{2.31}$$

Here $\alpha := \sigma^2/\sigma_3^q > 0$.

It is convenient for this book to study (2.31) in a more general setting. We consider

$$\underset{\mathbf{u} \in \mathbb{R}^{\mathcal{I}_1}}{\arg\min} \sum_{(i,j) \in \mathcal{I}_2} \left(\frac{1}{p} \frac{(u_{ij} - u_{ij}^{\delta})^p}{|v_{ij}|^q} + \frac{\alpha}{r} |v_{ij}|^r\right) \tag{2.32}$$

with $p > 1$ and $r \geq 1$, and $q \geq 0$. In Chapters 4 and 5, we investigate continuous formulations

$$\boxed{\underset{u \in X}{\arg\min} \left(\frac{1}{p} \int_{\Omega} \frac{(u - u^{\delta})^p}{|\nabla u|^q} + \frac{\alpha}{r} \int_{\Omega} |\nabla u|^r\right)} \tag{2.33}$$

of the discrete variational problem defined in (2.32), where X is an appropriate space of functions $u : \Omega \to \mathbb{R}$.

Further Reading

Background on statistical modeling of MAP estimators can be found for instance in [129, 321].

The standard reference for statistical approaches in inverse problems is [231]. Computational methods for statistical inverse problems are discussed in [378].

The relation between variational methods and MAP estimation is discussed in [39, 79, 186, 201, 202, 296]. An early reference on the topic on MAP estimators in imaging is [179].

Part II

Regularization

3

Variational Regularization Methods for the Solution of Inverse Problems

In this chapter, we review variational methods for the solution of *inverse problems*. It is common to consider inverse problems to be *ill-posed* in the sense that the solution (provided it exists) is unstable with respect to data perturbations. Typical examples of inverse problems are *differentiation* or *inversion of the Radon transform (computerized tomography)*. See Chapter 1 for some case examples of inverse and ill-posed problems.

For the stable approximation of a solution of the operator equation

$$F(u) = v \,, \tag{3.1}$$

where we assume that only noisy data v^δ of the exact data v are available, Tikhonov proposed to minimize the functional

$$\boxed{\mathcal{T}_{\alpha,v^\delta}(u) := \rho(F(u), v^\delta) + \alpha \mathcal{R}(u) \,,}$$

only assuming that ρ is a functional measuring the error between $F(u)$ and v^δ, $\alpha > 0$, and $\mathcal{R}$ is a non-negative functional, see for instance [277]. The number α is called the *regularization parameter*.

Iterative variants consist in iteratively calculating

$$\boxed{\begin{aligned} u_\alpha^{(k+1)} &:= \arg\min \mathcal{T}_{\alpha,v^\delta}^{(k)}(u) \,, \\ \mathcal{T}_{\alpha,v^\delta}^{(k)}(u) &:= \rho\big(F(u), v^\delta\big) + \alpha_k D(u, u_\alpha^{(k)}) \,, \qquad k = 0, 1, \dots \,. \end{aligned}}$$

Here $D(u,v)$ denotes an appropriate distance measure between u and v, like for instance a squared Hilbert space norm or the Bregman distance (see Definition 3.15). Moreover, $u_\alpha^{(0)}$ is an *a priori* guess of the solution of (3.1). We stress that for $D(u, u_\alpha^{(0)}) = \mathcal{R}(u)$, we have that $u_\alpha^{(1)} = u_\alpha$ minimizes $\mathcal{T}_{\alpha,v^\delta}$.

In most applications of Tikhonov regularization for the solution of inverse problems, a Sobolev space setting has been used with

O. Scherzer et al., *Variational Methods in Imaging*,
© Springer Science+Business Media, LLC 2009

$$\rho\big(F(u), v^\delta\big) = \int_{\tilde{\Omega}} \big(F(u) - v^\delta\big)^2 \qquad \text{and} \qquad \mathcal{R}(u) = \|u - u_0\|^2_{W^{l,2}(\Omega)}$$

for some $l \in \mathbb{N}$. Note that for inverse problems, the desired reconstruction and the measurement data can be functions defined on different domains Ω and $\tilde{\Omega}$. In recent years, regularization with convex functionals $\mathcal{R}$ in Banach spaces has been of growing interest.

We now clarify some notation used throughout this chapter: We assume that $F : \mathcal{D}(F) \subset U \to V$ is a mapping between linear spaces U and V, and that $v^\delta \in V$. Moreover, $u_0 \in U$ is considered a guess of a solution of (3.1). We denote by u_α^δ a minimizer of the functional $\mathcal{T}_{\alpha,v^\delta}$. If instead of v^δ the *noise free* (unperturbed by measurement errors) data v are used (that is, the case when $\delta = 0$), then a minimizer of $\mathcal{T}_{\alpha,v}$ is denoted by u_α. The subscript α describes the amount of regularization; the superscript δ in u_α^δ indicates that only erroneous data with $\rho(v, v^\delta) \leq \delta$ are given.

As we show below, a very important piece of information in the analysis of variational regularization methods is the distance $\rho(v, v^\delta)$ between unperturbed and noisy data, which is considered the amount of noise in the data v.

3.1 Quadratic Tikhonov Regularization in Hilbert Spaces

Quadratic Tikhonov regularization in a Hilbert space setting consists in minimizing the functional

$$\boxed{\mathcal{T}_{\alpha,v^\delta}(u) := \left\|F(u) - v^\delta\right\|^2_V + \alpha \left\|u - u_0\right\|^2_U}$$

over the Hilbert space U. The precise understanding is that we set $\mathcal{T}_{\alpha,v^\delta}(u) = \infty$ if $u \notin \mathcal{D}(F)$, thus minimization actually happens over $\mathcal{D}(F)$.

The norms on the Hilbert spaces U and V are denoted by $\|\cdot\|_U$, $\|\cdot\|_V$, respectively. Moreover, the inner products on U and V are denoted by $\langle \cdot, \cdot \rangle_U$ and $\langle \cdot, \cdot \rangle_V$. In the Hilbert space context, $\rho(v, v^\delta) = \left\|v^\delta - v\right\|^2$, and we assume the information on the noisy data v^δ that $\left\|v^\delta - v\right\|_V \leq \delta$. The amount of regularization (that is, the value of the regularization parameter α) has to correlate with the amount of noise, when stability and approximation properties of the regularizer are desired.

We review some analytical results collected from [152, 153, 277, 354, 373] for quadratic Tikhonov regularization for the solution of non-linear operator equations. Of course, these results also apply to linear ill-posed problems. However, in the linear case, the according results can be motivated more easily and derived with several different mathematical techniques. An excellent survey for quadratic variational regularization methods for linear ill-posed problems is [191].

For variational regularization methods, typically five results are of most interest:

- *Existence:* For fixed regularization parameter $\alpha > 0$ and every $\tilde{v} \in V$, there exist minimizers of the regularization functional $\mathcal{T}_{\alpha,\tilde{v}}$.
- *Stability* is required to ensure that, for fixed α, the regularized solution u_α^δ depends continuously on v^δ.
- *Convergence* ensures that for $\alpha \to 0$ and $v^\delta \to v$, the regularized solution u_α^δ converges to a solution of (3.1).
- *Convergence rates* provide an estimate of the difference between the minimizers of the regularization functional and the solution of (3.1) (provided it exists).
- *Stability estimates* provide a bound to the difference between u_α^δ and u_α depending on the error δ.

The following assumption is central for proving existence and stability of regularization methods in Hilbert spaces.

Assumption 3.1

- *The operator $F : \mathcal{D}(F) \subset U \to V$ is acting between Hilbert spaces U and V, and $\mathcal{D}(F)$ is a non-empty set.*
- *F is sequentially closed with respect to the weak topologies on U and V (see Definition 8.5).*

Below we omit the subscripts in the norms and inner products, as the spaces and topologies can be easily identified from the context. If we feel that it is necessary to clarify the spaces, we add the subscripts.

Because in general the solution of (3.1) is not unique, we concentrate on u_0-*minimal norm solutions* $u^\dagger$, which satisfy

$$\left\| u^\dagger - u_0 \right\| = \inf \left\{ \| u - u_0 \| : u \in \mathcal{D}(F) \text{ and } F(u) = v \right\}.$$

We emphasize that a u_0-minimal norm solution need **not** exist, and even if it exists, it need not be unique. In practical applications, however, the number of feasible solutions is drastically reduced by this restriction.

Lemma 3.2. *Let F, $\mathcal{D}(F)$, U, and V satisfy Assumption 3.1. Assume that there exists a solution of (3.1) in $\mathcal{D}(F)$. Then there exists a u_0-minimal norm solution in $\mathcal{D}(F)$.*

Proof. There exists a sequence (u_k) of solutions of (3.1) in $\mathcal{D}(F)$ such that

$$\| u_k - u_0 \| \to c := \inf \left\{ \| u - u_0 \| : u \in \mathcal{D}(F),\ F(u) = v \right\}.$$

Thus (u_k) is bounded in U, and consequently has a weakly convergent subsequence (see Corollary 8.52), which we again denote by (u_k). The weak limit is denoted by $\tilde{u}$. From the weak lower semi-continuity of a norm in a Hilbert space (see Lemma 10.6), it follows that $\| \tilde{u} - u_0 \| \leq c$. Moreover, because F is weakly closed and $F(u_k) = v$ for all k, it follows that $\tilde{u} \in \mathcal{D}(F)$ and $F(\tilde{u}) = v$. This shows that $\tilde{u}$ is a u_0-minimal norm solution. $\square$

The following results are by now standard and can be found for instance in [152]. Therefore the proofs are omitted. Anyhow, the results are reproven below in Section 3.2 in a more general setting. The results in [152] are formulated with the additional assumption that F is continuous. This assumption is not required, as the inspection of the proofs shows.

In the sequel, we state well-posedness of the regularization method.

Theorem 3.3 (Existence). *Let F, $\mathcal{D}(F)$, U, and V satisfy Assumption 3.1. Assume that $\alpha > 0$, $\tilde{v} \in V$, and $u_0 \in U$. Then $\mathcal{T}_{\alpha,\tilde{v}}$ attains a minimizer.*

Note that without posing additional assumptions, $\mathcal{T}_{\alpha,\tilde{v}}$ can have multiple minimizers.

It has been shown by several authors (see, for instance, [34, 151]) that the information on the noise level

$$\left\| v^\delta - v \right\| \leq \delta \tag{3.2}$$

is essential for an analysis of regularization methods. In fact, without this information, the regularization cannot be chosen such that convergence of u_α^δ to a u_0-minimal norm solution can be guaranteed.

Theorem 3.4 (Stability). *Let F, $\mathcal{D}(F)$, U, and V satisfy Assumption 3.1. Assume that $\alpha > 0$ and $v_k \to v^\delta$. Moreover, let*

$$u_k \in \arg\min \mathcal{T}_{\alpha,v_k}, \qquad k \in \mathbb{N}.$$

Then (u_k) has a convergent subsequence. Every convergent subsequence converges to a minimizer of $\mathcal{T}_{\alpha,v^\delta}$.

The following theorem clarifies the role of the regularization parameter α. It has to be chosen in dependence of the noise level to guarantee approximation of the solution of (3.1).

Theorem 3.5 (Convergence). *Let F, $\mathcal{D}(F)$, U, and V satisfy Assumption 3.1. Assume that (3.1) has a solution in $\mathcal{D}(F)$ and that $\alpha : (0, \infty) \to (0, \infty)$ satisfies*

$$\boxed{\alpha(\delta) \to 0 \ and \ \frac{\delta^2}{\alpha(\delta)} \to 0, \ as \ \delta \to 0.}$$

Moreover, let the sequence (δ_k) of positive numbers converge to 0, and assume that the data $v_k := v^{\delta_k}$ satisfy $\|v - v_k\| \leq \delta_k$.

Let $u_k \in \arg\min \mathcal{T}_{\alpha(\delta_k),v_k}$. Then (u_k) has a convergent subsequence. The limit $u^\dagger$ is a u_0-minimal norm solution. If in addition the u_0-minimal norm solution $u^\dagger$ is unique, then $u_k \to u^\dagger$.

Remark 3.6. Under the assumptions of Theorem 3.5, there exists a minimal norm solution $u^\dagger$ of (3.1). Assume that u_0 and $u^\dagger$ satisfy $\left\| u^\dagger - u_0 \right\| < \rho$ for some fixed $\rho > 0$. Then it follows that

$$\alpha \left\| u_\alpha^\delta - u_0 \right\|^2 \leq \left\| F(u_\alpha^\delta) - v^\delta \right\|^2 + \alpha \left\| u_\alpha^\delta - u_0 \right\|^2$$

$$\leq \left\| F(u^\dagger) - v^\delta \right\|^2 + \alpha \left\| u^\dagger - u_0 \right\|^2 = \left\| v - v^\delta \right\|^2 + \alpha \left\| u^\dagger - u_0 \right\|^2 ,$$

and therefore $\left\| u_\alpha^\delta - u_0 \right\|^2 \leq \delta^2/\alpha + \left\| u^\dagger - u_0 \right\|^2$. Because $\delta^2/\alpha \to 0$ and $\left\| u^\dagger - u_0 \right\| < \rho$, the above estimate implies that $\left\| u_\alpha^\delta - u_0 \right\| < \rho$ for sufficiently small $\delta > 0$. In other words, the minimizer u_α^δ is contained in the ball $B_\rho(u_0)$. $\diamondsuit$

The following Theorem 3.12 provides an estimate of $\left\| u_\alpha^\delta - u^\dagger \right\|$. Such estimates require a source-wise representation of the solution to be recovered (see (3.4)). Here we only review the most basic convergence rates results from [153]. A convergence rate result of order $O(\delta^{2/3})$ has been proven in [290], and results of logarithmic type have been proven in [216, 345]. These results, however, require significantly stronger assumptions on the operator F and are technically difficult.

Below, we review convergence rates results, thereby requiring the following assumptions:

Assumption 3.7

1. *F, $\mathcal{D}(F)$, U, and V satisfy Assumption 3.1.*
2. *There exist $\rho > 0$ and a u_0-minimal norm solution $u^\dagger \in \mathcal{D}(F)$ such that*
   (a) $B_\rho(u_0) \subset \mathcal{D}(F)$,
   (b) $\left\| u_0 - u^\dagger \right\| < \rho$,
   (c) F is Gâteaux differentiable in $B_\rho(u_0)$ (see Definition 10.30).
3. *There exists $\gamma \geq 0$ such that for all $u \in B_\rho(u_0)$*

$$\left\| F(u) - F(u^\dagger) - F'(u^\dagger)(u - u^\dagger) \right\| \leq \frac{\gamma}{2} \left\| u - u^\dagger \right\|^2 . \qquad (3.3)$$

4. *A source-wise representation of the solution exists, that is, there exists $\omega \in V$ such that*

$$u^\dagger - u_0 = F'(u^\dagger)^* \omega \qquad and \qquad \gamma \left\| \omega \right\| < 1 . \qquad (3.4)$$

Here $F'(u^\dagger)^*$ denotes the adjoint of $F'(u^\dagger)$ (see Theorem 8.26).

Example 3.8. Let Ω be bocL. We denote by $\mathcal{W}$ either one of the spaces $W_0^{1,2}(\Omega)$ or $W_\diamond^{1,2}(\Omega)$ associated with the norm $|u|_{1,2}^2 = \int_\Omega |\nabla u|^2$ and the inner product $\langle u, v \rangle_{1,2} := \int_\Omega \nabla u \cdot \nabla v$. We consider the embedding operator

$$\mathrm{i} : \mathcal{W} \to \mathcal{L}, \qquad u \mapsto \mathrm{i}\, u := u ,$$

which is a compact mapping (see Theorem 9.39). Here $\mathcal{L}$ either denotes $L^2(\Omega)$ or $L_\diamond^2(\Omega)$ associated with standard L^2-inner product, respectively.

The adjoint i^* of i satisfies

$$\langle i\,u, v \rangle_2 = \langle u, i^*\,v \rangle_{1,2} = \langle \nabla u, \nabla i^*\,v \rangle_2 \,, \qquad u \in \mathcal{W}, \; v \in \mathcal{L} \,.$$

This is the definition of the weak solution $w = i^*\,v$ of $-\Delta w = v$, which

- for $\mathcal{W} = W_0^{1,2}(\Omega)$, satisfies homogeneous Dirichlet conditions $w = 0$ on $\partial\Omega$ (see [156, p. 296]), and
- for $\mathcal{W} = W_\diamond^{1,2}(\Omega)$, satisfies homogeneous Neumann conditions $\partial w/\partial \mathbf{n} = 0$ on $\partial\Omega$ (see [195]).

Therefore, it is instructive to write the adjoint of the embedding operator $i : \mathcal{W} \to \mathcal{L}$ as $i^* = -\Delta^{-1} : \mathcal{L} \to \mathcal{W}$. $\diamond$

Remark 3.9. Let us assume that there exists a singular value decomposition (SVD) (u_k, v_k, σ_k) for the operator $F'(u^\dagger)$ (see Definition 8.38). Then (3.4) becomes

$$u^\dagger - u_0 = F'(u^\dagger)^*\omega = \sum_k \sigma_k \, \langle \omega, v_k \rangle \, u_k$$

and $\gamma^2 \|\omega\|^2 = \gamma^2 \sum_k |\langle \omega, v_k \rangle|^2 < 1$. As a consequence of (3.4), $u^\dagger$ has to be an element of the set $\{u_0 + F'(u^\dagger)^*\omega : \gamma \|\omega\|_V < 1\}$, which in this situation is an ellipsoid with center u_0 and axes in direction of the singular values. Moreover, the axes' lengths are the absolute values of the singular values. $\diamond$

Remark 3.10. Assumption 3.1 is part of Assumption 3.7. Therefore, we can conclude the following:

- According to Lemma 3.2, the existence of a solution of (3.1) in $\mathcal{D}(F)$ implies the existence of a u_0-minimal norm solution in $\mathcal{D}(F)$. Therefore, in Assumption 3.7, it would be sufficient to require the existence of a solution instead of a u_0-minimal norm solution.
- Item 2 in Assumption 3.7 requires that $u^\dagger \in B_\rho(u_0)$. In Remark 3.6, it has been shown that if $\delta^2/\alpha \to 0$, then $u_\alpha^\delta \in B_\rho(u_0)$ for sufficiently small δ. This shows that (3.3) is applicable for $u^\dagger$, u_α, and u_α^δ, provided that Assumption 3.7 holds.
- In [152, 153], instead of (3.3) and the Gâteaux differentiability of F, it is assumed that F is Fréchet differentiable in $B_{\tilde{\rho}}(u_0)$ (with $\tilde{\rho}$ sufficiently large) and satisfies

$$\left\| F'(u) - F'(u^\dagger) \right\| \leq \gamma \left\| u - u^\dagger \right\| \,, \qquad u \in B_{\tilde{\rho}}(u_0) \,.$$

These conditions imply that (3.3) holds in a neighborhood of u_0.

                    $\diamond$

In the following, if $\alpha : (0,\infty) \to (0,\infty)$, we write $\alpha \sim \delta^s$, $s > 0$, if there exist constants $0 < c \leq C$ and $\delta_0 > 0$, such that $c\delta^s \leq \alpha(\delta) \leq C\delta^s$ for $0 < \delta < \delta_0$.

Theorem 3.11 (Convergence rates). *Let Assumption 3.7 hold. Moreover, assume that $v^\delta \in V$ satisfies (3.2). Then, for $\alpha : (0,\infty) \to (0,\infty)$ satisfying $\alpha \sim \delta$, we have*

$$\left\| u_\alpha^\delta - u^\dagger \right\|^2 = O(\delta) \quad and \quad \left\| F(u_\alpha^\delta) - v^\delta \right\| = O(\delta) \quad as \ \delta \to 0 \ .$$

Proof. The proof of the theorem is similar to [153] (see also [152, Chap. 10]) when Remark 3.10 is taken into account.   □

Next we state a qualitative stability estimate derived in [343].

Theorem 3.12 (Stability estimates). *Let Assumption 3.7 hold. Moreover, assume that $v^\delta \in V$ satisfies (3.2). Additionally, we assume that $2\gamma \|\omega\| < 1$, such that*

$$\left\| F(u) - F(\tilde{u}) - F'(\tilde{u})(u - \tilde{u}) \right\| \le \frac{\gamma}{2} \|u - \tilde{u}\|^2 \tag{3.5}$$

for all $u, \tilde{u} \in B_\rho(u_0)$. Then, for δ sufficiently small, we have

$$\left\| u_\alpha^\delta - u_\alpha \right\|^2 \le \frac{4}{1 - 2\gamma \|\omega\|} \frac{\delta^2}{\alpha} \ .$$

In particular, for $\alpha \sim \delta$, we have the stability estimate

$$\left\| F(u_\alpha^\delta) - F(u_\alpha) \right\| = O(\delta) \quad and \quad \left\| u_\alpha^\delta - u_\alpha \right\| = O(\sqrt{\delta}) \ .$$

Proof. From Remark 3.6, it follows that, for δ sufficiently small, $u_\alpha, u_\alpha^\delta \in B_\rho(u_0)$. Because u_α^δ is a minimizer of $\mathcal{T}_{\alpha,v^\delta}$, we have

$$\left\| F(u_\alpha^\delta) - v^\delta \right\|^2 + \alpha \left\| u_\alpha^\delta - u_0 \right\|^2 \le \left\| F(u_\alpha) - v^\delta \right\|^2 + \alpha \left\| u_\alpha - u_0 \right\|^2 \ .$$

The last inequality implies that

$$\begin{aligned}
\left\| F(u_\alpha^\delta) \right. & \left. - F(u_\alpha) \right\|^2 + \alpha \left\| u_\alpha^\delta - u_\alpha \right\|^2 \\
& \le \left\| F(u_\alpha^\delta) - F(u_\alpha) \right\|^2 + \left\| F(u_\alpha) - v^\delta \right\|^2 - \left\| F(u_\alpha^\delta) - v^\delta \right\|^2 \\
& \quad + \alpha \left(\left\| u_\alpha^\delta - u_\alpha \right\|^2 + \|u_\alpha - u_0\|^2 - \left\| u_\alpha^\delta - u_0 \right\|^2 \right) \\
& = 2 \left\langle F(u_\alpha) - v^\delta, F(u_\alpha) - F(u_\alpha^\delta) \right\rangle + 2\alpha \left\langle u_\alpha^\delta - u_\alpha, u_0 - u_\alpha \right\rangle \ .
\end{aligned}$$

Because F is Gâteaux differentiable, the chain rule (Theorem 10.34) implies that also $\mathcal{T}_{\alpha,v^\delta}$ is Gâteaux differentiable. Therefore, the minimizer u_α of $\mathcal{T}_{\alpha,v}$ satisfies

$$0 = \mathcal{T}_{\alpha,v}'(u_\alpha) = F'(u_\alpha)^* \big(F(u_\alpha) - v \big) + \alpha(u_\alpha - u_0) \ .$$

The last equation and the Cauchy–Schwarz inequality (9.3) show that

$$\begin{aligned}
\left\| F(u_\alpha^\delta) - F(u_\alpha) \right\|^2 + \alpha \left\| u_\alpha^\delta - u_\alpha \right\|^2 & \le 2 \left\langle F(u_\alpha) - v, F(u_\alpha) - F(u_\alpha^\delta) \right\rangle \\
& \quad + 2 \left\langle F'(u_\alpha)(u_\alpha^\delta - u_\alpha), F(u_\alpha) - v \right\rangle + 2\delta \left\| F(u_\alpha) - F(u_\alpha^\delta) \right\| \ .
\end{aligned}$$

This together with (3.5) implies that

$$\left\| F(u_\alpha^\delta) - F(u_\alpha) \right\|^2 + \alpha \left\| u_\alpha^\delta - u_\alpha \right\|^2$$
$$\leq \gamma \left\| F(u_\alpha) - v \right\| \left\| u_\alpha^\delta - u_0 \right\|^2 + 2\delta \left\| F(u_\alpha) - F(u_\alpha^\delta) \right\| .$$

Following the proof of [152, Thm. 10.4], we find that $\left\| F(u_\alpha) - v \right\| \leq 2\alpha \left\| \omega \right\|$ and thus

$$\left\| F(u_\alpha^\delta) - F(u_\alpha) \right\|^2 + \alpha(1 - 2\gamma \left\| \omega \right\|) \left\| u_\alpha^\delta - u_\alpha \right\|^2 \leq 2\delta \left\| F(u_\alpha) - F(u_\alpha^\delta) \right\| .$$
(3.6)

Because $2\gamma \left\| \omega \right\| < 1$, it follows that $\left\| F(u_\alpha^\delta) - F(u_\alpha) \right\| \leq 2\delta$ and thus the assertion follows from (3.6). □

3.2 Variational Regularization Methods in Banach Spaces

In this section, we consider a particular instance of Tikhonov type variational regularization models, consisting in minimization of

$$\boxed{\mathcal{T}_{\alpha, v^\delta}(u) := \left\| F(u) - v^\delta \right\|_V^p + \alpha \mathcal{R}(u),}$$
(3.7)

where $F : \mathcal{D}(F) \subset U \to V$ is an operator between Banach spaces U and V, and $1 \leq p < \infty$. As in the Hilbert space setting, we set $\mathcal{T}_{\alpha, v^\delta}(u) = \infty$ if $u \notin \mathcal{D}(F)$. Moreover, $\mathcal{R} : U \to [0, \infty]$ is a convex and proper functional with domain

$$\mathcal{D}(\mathcal{R}) := \left\{ u \in U : \mathcal{R}(u) \neq \infty \right\} .$$

Recall that the functional $\mathcal{R}$ is called *proper* if $\mathcal{D}(\mathcal{R}) \neq \emptyset$.

In this section, we make the following assumptions:

Assumption 3.13

1. *The Banach spaces U and V are associated with topologies τ_U and τ_V, which are weaker than the norm topologies.*
2. *The exponent p is greater or equal than 1.*
3. *The norm $\left\| \cdot \right\|_V$ is sequentially lower semi-continuous with respect to τ_V.*
4. *The functional $\mathcal{R} : U \to [0, \infty]$ is convex and sequentially lower semi-continuous with respect to τ_U.*
5. *$\mathcal{D} := \mathcal{D}(F) \cap \mathcal{D}(\mathcal{R}) \neq \emptyset$ (which, in particular, implies that $\mathcal{R}$ is proper).*
6. *For every $\alpha > 0$ and $M > 0$, the level sets (see Definition 8.4)*

$$\mathcal{M}_\alpha(M) := \text{level}_M(\mathcal{T}_{\alpha, v})$$

are sequentially pre-compact with respect to τ_U.

7. For every $\alpha > 0$ and $M > 0$, the set $\mathcal{M}_\alpha(M)$ is sequentially closed with respect to τ_U and the restriction of F to $\mathcal{M}_\alpha(M)$ is sequentially continuous with respect to the topologies τ_U and τ_V.

We stress that the sets $\mathcal{M}_\alpha(M)$ are defined based on the Tikhonov functional for unperturbed data v, and we do not *a priori* exclude the case that $\mathcal{M}_\alpha(M) = \emptyset$. Moreover, for every $M > 0$ fixed, the family $\bigl(\mathcal{M}_\alpha(M)\bigr)_{\alpha>0}$ is inversely ordered, that is, $\mathcal{M}_\alpha(M) \subset \mathcal{M}_\beta(M)$, for $0 < \beta \leq \alpha$.

Remark 3.14. Consider the case where U and V are Hilbert spaces, $p = 2$, $\mathcal{R}(u) = \|u - u_0\|_U^2$, and τ_U and τ_V the weak topologies on U and V. Then Item 3 of Assumption 3.13 is satisfied. The functional $\mathcal{R}$ is convex and sequentially lower semi-continuous with respect to τ_U, and $\mathcal{D}(\mathcal{R}) = U$. Consequently, Item 5 is equivalent to the assumption that $\mathcal{D}(F)$ is non-empty. Because $\mathcal{T}_{\alpha,v}(u) \leq \alpha \mathcal{R}(u) = \alpha \|u - u_0\|_U^2$ for every $u \in U$ and U is a Hilbert space, it follows that the level sets $\mathcal{M}_\alpha(M)$, $M > 0$, are sequentially pre-compact.

In the following, we show that Item 7 is equivalent to the assumption that F is weakly sequentially closed.

First assume that F is weakly sequentially closed. Let $(u_k) \subset \mathcal{M}_\alpha(M)$ weakly converge to $u \in U$. Then $\bigl(F(u_k)\bigr)$ is bounded in V implying the existence of a weakly convergent subsequence $\bigl(F(u_{k'})\bigr)$. The weak sequential closedness of F shows that $u \in \mathcal{D}(F)$ and $F(u_{k'}) \rightharpoonup F(u)$. Because $\|\cdot\|_V$ and $\mathcal{R}$ are weakly sequentially lower semi-continuous, it follows that $u \in \mathcal{M}_\alpha(M)$. The weak sequential continuity of F on $\mathcal{M}_\alpha(M)$ follows from a subsequence argument (cf. Lemma 8.2).

Now assume that Item 7 holds. Let $(u_k) \rightharpoonup u$ and $F(u_k) \rightharpoonup w$. Then $\bigl(\|u_k - u_0\|_U^2\bigr)$ and $\bigl(\|F(u_k) - v\|_V^2\bigr)$ are bounded sequences, and therefore for every fixed $\alpha > 0$ there exists $M > 0$ with $(u_k) \subset \mathcal{M}_\alpha(M)$. Because $\mathcal{M}_\alpha(M)$ is weakly sequentially closed and F is weakly sequentially continuous on $\mathcal{M}_\alpha(M)$, it follows that $u \in \mathcal{M}_\alpha(M)$ and $F(u) = \lim_k F(u_k) = w$. $\diamond$

In the Banach space theory of variational regularization methods, the *Bregman distance* plays an important role.

Definition 3.15. Let $\mathcal{R} : U \to \mathbb{R} \cup \{\infty\}$ be a convex and proper functional with subdifferential $\partial \mathcal{R}$. The Bregman distance of $\mathcal{R}$ at $u \in U$ and $\xi^* \in \partial \mathcal{R}(u) \subset U^*$ is defined by

$$\boxed{D_{\xi^*}(\tilde{u}, u) := \mathcal{R}(\tilde{u}) - \mathcal{R}(u) - \langle \xi^*, \tilde{u} - u \rangle_{U^*, U}\,, \quad \tilde{u} \in U\,.} \qquad (3.8)$$

The Bregman distance can be visualized as the difference between the tangent and the convex function (compare Fig. 3.1). It is only defined at a point $u \in \mathcal{D}(\mathcal{R})$ where the subdifferential is not empty. Moreover, it may attain the value ∞. The set

$$\mathcal{D}_B(\mathcal{R}) := \bigl\{u \in \mathcal{D}(\mathcal{R}) : \partial \mathcal{R}(u) \neq \emptyset\bigr\}$$

is called the *Bregman domain*.

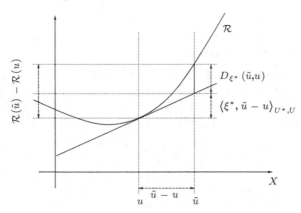

Fig. 3.1. Bregman distance.

Lemma 3.16. *The Bregman domain $\mathcal{D}_B(\mathcal{R})$ is dense in $\mathcal{D}(\mathcal{R})$. Moreover the interior of $\mathcal{D}(\mathcal{R})$ is a subset of $\mathcal{D}_B(\mathcal{R})$. In particular, if $\mathcal{D}(\mathcal{R}) = U$, then we have $\mathcal{D}_B(\mathcal{R}) = \mathcal{D}(\mathcal{R}) = U$.*

Proof. This is a standard result from convex analysis concerning the existence of the subdifferential (see, for example, [144, Chap. I, Prop. 5.2, Cor. 6.1]).

The following lemma shows that the Bregman distance can in fact be viewed as a measure of similarity of two elements of U, as it is non-negative. The proof is an immediate consequence of the definitions of the Bregman distance and the subdifferential.

Lemma 3.17. *Let $\mathcal{R} : U \to \mathbb{R} \cup \{\infty\}$ be a convex and proper functional on a Banach space U. Then, for $u \in \mathcal{D}_B(\mathcal{R})$ and $\xi^* \in \partial\mathcal{R}(u)$, the mapping $\tilde{u} \mapsto D_{\xi^*}(\tilde{u}, u)$ is convex, non-negative, and satisfies $D_{\xi^*}(u, u) = 0$.*

If, additionally, $\mathcal{R}$ is strictly convex, then $D_{\xi^*}(\tilde{u}, u) = 0$ if and only if $\tilde{u} = u$.

In the following, we compute the Bregman distance for the square of the norm on a Hilbert space.

Example 3.18. Let U be a Hilbert space and $\mathcal{R}(u) = \|u - u_0\|_U^2$. Then $\partial\mathcal{R}(u) = \{\xi^*\}$ with $\xi^* = \mathcal{J}_U\xi$, where $\xi = 2(u - u_0)$ and $\mathcal{J}_U$ is the duality mapping from U into U^*. In such a situation, $\langle\xi^*, \tilde{u}\rangle_{U^*,U} = \langle\xi, \tilde{u}\rangle_U = 2\langle u - u_0, \tilde{u}\rangle_U$ and $D_{\xi^*}(\tilde{u}, u) = \|\tilde{u} - u\|_U^2$.   ◇

Remark 3.19. For $U = L^p(\Omega)$, $1 \leq p < \infty$, we use Convention 10.17 and identify U^* with $L^{p^*}(\Omega)$. In this case, $\xi^* \in \partial\mathcal{R}(u)$ is identified with a function $\xi \in L^{p^*}(\Omega)$. The exact relation is $\xi^* = (\Im_p)^{-1}\xi$, where $\Im_p : U^* \to L^{p^*}(\Omega)$ is the isometric isomorphism defined in Lemma 9.11.   ◇

Well-posedness

We now prove existence, stability, and convergence of variational regularization methods consisting in minimization of (3.7).

Before deriving these results, we need two lemmas that are used in the proofs of the main results.

Lemma 3.20. *Let U be a normed space and $p \geq 1$. Then*

$$\|x + y\|^p \leq 2^{p-1}\big(\|x\|^p + \|y\|^p\big), \qquad x, y \in U . \tag{3.9}$$

Proof. For $p = 1$, the inequality is just the triangle inequality and thus satisfied.

For $p > 1$, we define $f : \mathbb{R} \to \mathbb{R}$,

$$f(t) := 2^{p-1}\big(|t|^p + |1 - t|^p\big) .$$

Then f is a convex function. The unique minimizer of f is $1/2$ and satisfies $f(1/2) = 1$. This shows that $f(t) \geq 1$ for all t. Now let $x, y \in U$. Without loss of generality, assume that $d := \|x\| + \|y\| \neq 0$. Then $\|y/d\| = 1 - \|x/d\|$, and thus

$$\begin{aligned}
2^{p-1}\big(\|x\|^p + \|y\|^p\big) &= 2^{p-1}\,|d|^p\,\big(\|x/d\|^p + \|y/d\|^p\big) \\
&= |d|^p\,2^{p-1}\big(\|x/d\|^p + |1 - \|x/d\|\|^p\big) \\
&= |d|^p\,f(\|x/d\|) \geq |d|^p = \big(\|x\| + \|y\|\big)^p \geq \|x + y\|^p ,
\end{aligned}$$

which shows (3.9). $\qquad\square$

Lemma 3.21. *For all $u \in \mathcal{D}$ and $v_1, v_2 \in V$, we have*

$$\mathcal{T}_{\alpha,v_1}(u) \leq 2^{p-1}\mathcal{T}_{\alpha,v_2}(u) + 2^{p-1}\|v_1 - v_2\|^p .$$

Proof. From Lemma 3.20, it follows that

$$\begin{aligned}
\mathcal{T}_{\alpha,v_1}(u) &= \|F(u) - v_1\|^p + \alpha\mathcal{R}(u) \\
&\leq 2^{p-1}\big(\|F(u) - v_2\|^p + \|v_1 - v_2\|^p\big) + \alpha\mathcal{R}(u) \\
&\leq 2^{p-1}\big(\|F(u) - v_2\|^p + \alpha\mathcal{R}(u)\big) + 2^{p-1}\|v_1 - v_2\|^p \\
&= 2^{p-1}\mathcal{T}_{\alpha,v_2} + 2^{p-1}\|v_1 - v_2\|^p .
\end{aligned}$$

$\qquad\square$

Theorem 3.22 (Existence). *Let F, $\mathcal{R}$, $\mathcal{D}$, U, and V satisfy Assumption 3.13. Assume that $\alpha > 0$ and $v^\delta \in V$. Then there exists a minimizer of $\mathcal{T}_{\alpha,v^\delta}$.*

Proof. Because $\mathcal{D} \neq \emptyset$, there exists at least one $\tilde{u} \in U$ such that $\mathcal{T}_{\alpha,v^\delta}(\tilde{u}) < \infty$. Thus there exists a sequence (u_k) in $\mathcal{D}$ such that

$$\lim_k \mathcal{T}_{\alpha,v^\delta}(u_k) = c := \inf\left\{\mathcal{T}_{\alpha,v^\delta}(u) : u \in \mathcal{D}\right\}.$$

From Lemma 3.21, we obtain that there exists $k_0 \in \mathbb{N}$ such that for $k \geq k_0$

$$M := 2^{p-1}c + 1 + 2^{p-1}\delta^p \geq 2^{p-1}\mathcal{T}_{\alpha,v^\delta}(u_k) + 2^{p-1}\left\|v - v^\delta\right\|^p \geq \mathcal{T}_{\alpha,v}(u_k).$$

Thus $u_k \in \mathcal{M}_\alpha(M)$ for $k \geq k_0$, and from Assumption 3.13 it follows that (u_k) has a τ_U-convergent subsequence, which we denote again by (u_k). The associated limit is denoted by $\tilde{u} \in U$. Because $\mathcal{R}$ is sequentially lower semi-continuous with respect to τ_U, we have

$$\mathcal{R}(\tilde{u}) \leq \liminf_k \mathcal{R}(u_k). \tag{3.10}$$

By assumption, the set $\mathcal{M}_\alpha(M)$ is sequentially closed with respect to τ_U, showing that $\tilde{u} \in \mathcal{M}_\alpha(M)$. Moreover, F is continuous on $\mathcal{M}_\alpha(M)$ with respect to the topologies τ_U and τ_V, and therefore $F(u_k)$ converges to $F(\tilde{u})$ with respect to τ_V. Because $\|\cdot\|_V$ is sequentially lower semi-continuous with respect to τ_V, it follows that

$$\left\|F(\tilde{u}) - v^\delta\right\| \leq \liminf_k \left\|F(u_k) - v^\delta\right\|. \tag{3.11}$$

Combination of (3.10) and (3.11) shows that $\tilde{u}$ minimizes $\mathcal{T}_{\alpha,v^\delta}$. $\square$

Theorem 3.23 (Stability). *Let F, $\mathcal{R}$, $\mathcal{D}$, U, and V satisfy Assumption 3.13. If (v_k) is a sequence converging to v^δ in V with respect to the norm topology, then every sequence (u_k) with*

$$u_k \in \arg\min\left\{\mathcal{T}_{\alpha,v_k}(u) : u \in \mathcal{D}\right\}$$

has a subsequence that converges with respect to τ_U. The limit of every τ_U-convergent subsequence $(u_{k'})$ of (u_k) is a minimizer $\tilde{u}$ of $\mathcal{T}_{\alpha,v^\delta}$, and $(\mathcal{R}(u_{k'}))$ converges to $\mathcal{R}(\tilde{u})$.

Proof. Because u_k is a minimizer of $\mathcal{T}_{\alpha,v_k}$, we have

$$\mathcal{T}_{\alpha,v_k}(u_k) \leq \mathcal{T}_{\alpha,v_k}(u), \quad u \in \mathcal{D}. \tag{3.12}$$

Because $\mathcal{D} \neq \emptyset$, we can select $\bar{u} \in \mathcal{D}$. By applying (3.12) to $u = \bar{u}$ and twice using Lemma 3.21, it follows that

$$\mathcal{T}_{\alpha,v}(u_k) \leq 2^{p-1}\mathcal{T}_{\alpha,v_k}(u_k) + 2^{p-1}\left\|v_k - v\right\|^p$$
$$\leq 2^{p-1}\mathcal{T}_{\alpha,v_k}(\bar{u}) + 2^{p-1}\left\|v_k - v\right\|^p \leq 4^{p-1}\mathcal{T}_{\alpha,v}(\bar{u}) + 4^p\left\|v_k - v\right\|^p.$$

It follows from the convergence of v_k to v^δ with respect to the norm topology that there exists $k_0 \in \mathbb{N}$ such that

$$M := 4^{p-1}\mathcal{T}_{\alpha,v}(\bar{u}) + 1 \geq \mathcal{T}_{\alpha,v}(u_k), \qquad k \geq k_0.$$

Thus (u_k) is contained in $\mathcal{M}_\alpha(M)$ for $k \geq k_0$ and, according to Item 6 in Assumption 3.13, has a subsequence that converges with respect to τ_U.

Now let $(u_{k'})$ denote an arbitrary subsequence of (u_k) that converges to $\tilde{u} \in \mathcal{D}$ with respect to τ_U. Because F is continuous on $\mathcal{M}_\alpha(M)$ with respect to τ_U and τ_V (see Item 7 in Assumption 3.13), it follows that $F(u_{k'})$ converges to $F(\tilde{u})$ with respect to τ_V. Moreover, because τ_V is weaker than the norm topology, it follows that $v_{k'}$ converges to v^δ with respect to τ_V and thus $F(u_{k'}) - v_{k'}$ converges to $F(\tilde{u}) - v^\delta$ with respect to τ_V. Because $\|\cdot\|_V$ and $\mathcal{R}$ are lower semi-continuous with respect to the τ_V and τ_U topologies, respectively, it follows that

$$
\begin{aligned}
\left\| F(\tilde{u}) - v^\delta \right\|^p &\leq \liminf_{k'} \left\| F(u_{k'}) - v_{k'} \right\|^p , \\
\mathcal{R}(\tilde{u}) &\leq \liminf_{k'} \mathcal{R}(u_{k'}) .
\end{aligned}
\tag{3.13}
$$

Using (3.13), (3.12), and the fact that $(v_{k'})$ converges to v^δ with respect to the norm topology, it follows that

$$
\begin{aligned}
\left\| F(\tilde{u}) - v^\delta \right\|^p + \alpha \mathcal{R}(\tilde{u}) &\leq \liminf_{k'} \left\| F(u_{k'}) - v_{k'} \right\|^p + \alpha \liminf_{k'} \mathcal{R}(u_{k'}) \\
&\leq \limsup_{k'} \left(\left\| F(u_{k'}) - v_{k'} \right\|^p + \alpha \mathcal{R}(u_{k'}) \right) \\
&\leq \lim_{k'} \left(\left\| F(u) - v_{k'} \right\|^p + \alpha \mathcal{R}(u) \right) \\
&= \left\| F(u) - v^\delta \right\|^p + \alpha \mathcal{R}(u) , \qquad u \in \mathcal{D} .
\end{aligned}
\tag{3.14}
$$

This implies that $\tilde{u}$ is a minimizer of $\mathcal{T}_{\alpha, v^\delta}$. Moreover, by taking $u = \tilde{u} \in \mathcal{D}$ on the right-hand side of (3.14), it follows that

$$
\left\| F(\tilde{u}) - v^\delta \right\|^p + \alpha \mathcal{R}(\tilde{u}) = \lim_{k'} \left(\left\| F(u_{k'}) - v_{k'} \right\|^p + \alpha \mathcal{R}(u_{k'}) \right) .
\tag{3.15}
$$

From (3.15) and (3.13), it follows that

$$
\begin{aligned}
\limsup_{k'} \alpha \mathcal{R}(u_{k'}) &\leq \\
&\leq \limsup_{k'} \left(\alpha \mathcal{R}(u_{k'}) + \left\| F(u_{k'}) - v_{k'} \right\|^p \right) - \liminf_{k'} \left\| F(u_{k'}) - v_{k'} \right\|^p \\
&\leq \left\| F(\tilde{u}) - v^\delta \right\|^p + \alpha \mathcal{R}(\tilde{u}) - \left\| F(\tilde{u}) - v^\delta \right\|^p = \alpha \mathcal{R}(\tilde{u}) ,
\end{aligned}
$$

which shows that $\left(\mathcal{R}(u_{k'}) \right)$ converges to $\mathcal{R}(\tilde{u})$. $\square$

In the Hilbert space setting with $\mathcal{R}(u) = \|u - u_0\|_U^2$, we deduce from Theorem 3.23 that a subsequence $(u_{k'})$ of (u_k) converges weakly to $\tilde{u}$ in U and that $\mathcal{R}(u_{k'}) \to \mathcal{R}(\tilde{u})$, which in this situation gives strong convergence of $(u_{k'})$ (see Lemma 8.48).

In the following we prove convergence, convergence rates, and stability estimates for variational regularization methods in Banach spaces.

In a Banach space setting, the concept of a minimal norm solution generalizes to $\mathcal{R}$-minimizing solutions:

Definition 3.24. *An element $u^\dagger \in \mathcal{D}$ is called an $\mathcal{R}$-minimizing solution of* (3.1) *if $F(u^\dagger) = v$ and*

$$\mathcal{R}(u^\dagger) = \min\{\mathcal{R}(u) : u \in \mathcal{D}(F), \ F(u) = v\} \ .$$

This solution concept generalizes the definition of a u_0-minimal norm solution in a Hilbert space setting.

Theorem 3.25. *Let Assumption 3.13 be satisfied. If there exists a solution of* (3.1) *in $\mathcal{D}$, then there exists an $\mathcal{R}$-minimizing solution of* (3.1).

Proof. The proof is along the lines of Lemma 3.2. $\square$

Theorem 3.26 (Convergence). *Let F, $\mathcal{R}$, $\mathcal{D}$, U, and V satisfy Assumption 3.13. Assume that* (3.1) *has a solution in $\mathcal{D}$ (which, according to Theorem 3.25, implies the existence of an $\mathcal{R}$-minimizing solution) and that $\alpha : (0, \infty) \to (0, \infty)$ satisfies*

$$\alpha(\delta) \to 0 \ and \ \frac{\delta^p}{\alpha(\delta)} \to 0 , \ as \ \delta \to 0 . \tag{3.16}$$

Moreover, assume that the sequence (δ_k) converges to 0, and that $v_k := v^{\delta_k}$ satisfies $\|v - v_k\| \leq \delta_k$.

Set $\alpha_k := \alpha(\delta_k)$. Then every sequence (u_k) of elements minimizing $\mathcal{T}_{\alpha_k, v_k}$ has a subsequence $(u_{k'})$ that converges with respect to τ_U. The limit $u^\dagger$ of every τ_U-convergent subsequence $(u_{k'})$ is an $\mathcal{R}$-minimizing solution of (3.1), *and $\mathcal{R}(u_k) \to \mathcal{R}(u^\dagger)$. If, in addition, the $\mathcal{R}$-minimizing solution $u^\dagger$ is unique, then $u_k \to u^\dagger$ with respect to τ_U.*

Proof. Let $u^\dagger$ denote an $\mathcal{R}$-minimizing solution of (3.1). From the definition of u_k it follows that

$$\|F(u_k) - v_k\|^p + \alpha_k \mathcal{R}(u_k) \leq \|F(u^\dagger) - v_k\|^p + \alpha_k \mathcal{R}(u^\dagger) \leq \delta_k^p + \alpha_k \mathcal{R}(u^\dagger) . \tag{3.17}$$

Because of (3.16), the right-hand side of (3.17) converges to 0, and hence $\|F(u_k) - v_k\| \to 0$. From the inequalities $\|F(u_k) - v\| \leq \|F(u_k) - v_k\| + \delta_k$ and (3.17), it follows that

$$\lim_k \|F(u_k) - v\| = 0 , \tag{3.18}$$

$$\limsup_k \mathcal{R}(u_k) \leq \mathcal{R}(u^\dagger) . \tag{3.19}$$

Using (3.18) and (3.19) and defining $\alpha^+ := \max\{\alpha_k : k \in \mathbb{N}\}$ gives

$$\limsup_k \left(\|F(u_k) - v\|^p + \alpha^+ \mathcal{R}(u_k)\right) \leq \alpha^+ \mathcal{R}(u^\dagger) =: M < \infty . \tag{3.20}$$

This shows that there exists $k_0 \in \mathbb{N}$ such that

$$u_k \in \mathcal{M}_{\alpha^+}(M+1), \quad k \geq k_0 .$$

Therefore, it follows from Item 6 in Assumption 3.13 that (u_k) has a subsequence that converges with respect to τ_U.

Let $(u_{k'})$ be a subsequence that converges to $\tilde{u} \in \mathcal{D}$ with respect to τ_U. Because F is continuous on $\mathcal{M}_{\alpha^+}(M+1)$ with respect to τ_U and τ_V, the sequence $\big(F(u_{k'})\big)$ converges to $F(\tilde{u})$ with respect to τ_V. Thus (3.18) implies that $F(\tilde{u}) = v$. From the lower semi-continuity of $\mathcal{R}$, (3.19), and the definition of $u^\dagger$, it follows that

$$\mathcal{R}(\tilde{u}) \leq \liminf_k \mathcal{R}(u_{k'}) \leq \limsup_k \mathcal{R}(u_{k'}) \leq \mathcal{R}(u^\dagger) \leq \mathcal{R}(\tilde{u}) .$$

This shows that $\tilde{u}$ is an $\mathcal{R}$-minimizing solution and that $\mathcal{R}(u_{k'}) \to \mathcal{R}(u^\dagger)$. From Lemma 8.2 it follows that, in fact, $\mathcal{R}(u_k) \to \mathcal{R}(u^\dagger)$.

Now assume that the $\mathcal{R}$-minimizing solution $u^\dagger$ is unique. Then every subsequence of (u_k) has itself a subsequence that converges to $u^\dagger$ with respect to τ_U. Thus it follows from Lemma 8.2 that $u_k \to u^\dagger$ with respect to τ_U. $\quad\square$

Remark 3.27. Let the assumptions of Theorem 3.26 hold and fix $\delta_0 > 0$. Let $\alpha_{\max} > 0$ be such that $\alpha = \alpha(\delta) \leq \alpha_{\max}$ for $\delta \leq \delta_0$, and let $\rho > \alpha_{\max}\mathcal{R}(u_\alpha)$. As in the proof of Theorem 3.26 (see (3.20)), it follows that $u_\alpha^\delta \in \mathcal{M}_{\alpha_{\max}}(\rho)$ for $\delta \leq \delta_0$. Similarly, as u_α is a minimizer of $\mathcal{T}_{\alpha,v}$, we also have that $u_\alpha \in \mathcal{M}_{\alpha_{\max}}(\rho)$. Therefore, under the assumptions of Theorem 3.26, we obtain

$$u^\dagger, u_\alpha^\delta, u_\alpha \in \mathcal{M}_{\alpha_{\max}}(\rho), \quad \delta \leq \delta_0 .$$

$$\diamond$$

In certain situations, see Proposition 3.32 below, we obtain even strong convergence of the sequence of minimizers of $\mathcal{T}_{\alpha_k, v_k}$. To that end we need some further notations.

Definition 3.28. *Let $\mathcal{R} : U \to \mathbb{R} \cup \{\infty\}$ be convex and proper. We define the directional Bregman distance of $\mathcal{R}$ at $u \in \mathcal{D}(\mathcal{R})$ by*

$$D_{\mathcal{R}}(\tilde{u}, u) := \mathcal{R}(\tilde{u}) - \mathcal{R}(u) - \mathcal{R}'(u; \tilde{u} - u), \qquad \tilde{u} \in U .$$

Here $\mathcal{R}'(u; \tilde{u} - u)$ denotes the one-sided directional derivative of $\mathcal{R}$ at u in direction $\tilde{u} - u$ (see Definition 10.31).

We emphasize that contrary to the Bregman distance, the directional Bregman distance is defined everywhere on $\mathcal{D}(\mathcal{R})$. Moreover, we have the inequality

$$D_{\mathcal{R}}(\tilde{u}, u) \leq D_\xi(\tilde{u}, u), \qquad \tilde{u} \in U , \; \xi \in \partial\mathcal{R}(u) .$$

Definition 3.29. *The functional $\mathcal{R}$ is totally convex at $u \in \mathcal{D}(\mathcal{R})$, if the modulus of convexity $\eta_u : \mathbb{R}_{>0} \to \bar{\mathbb{R}}_{>0}$ at u, defined by*

$$\eta_u(t) := \inf \{D_\mathcal{R}(\tilde{u}, u) : \tilde{u} \in \mathcal{D}(\mathcal{R}) , \ \|u - \tilde{u}\| = t\} , \qquad t \geq 0, \qquad (3.21)$$

is strictly positive for every $0 < t < \infty$ (see [72, 73]). Here, the infimum over the empty set is defined as ∞.

Note in particular that a functional that is totally convex everywhere is strictly convex.

Totally convex functionals have the nice property that convergence of a sequence in the directional Bregman distance already implies *strong* convergence. Before proving this result, we require some properties of the modulus of convexity.

Lemma 3.30. *Let $\mathcal{R} : U \to \mathbb{R} \cup \{\infty\}$ be convex and proper and $u \in \mathcal{D}(\mathcal{R})$. Then the modulus of convexity at u is an increasing non-negative function. If, in addition, $\mathcal{R}$ is totally convex at u, then the modulus of convexity is strictly increasing on the set $\{0 < t < \infty : \eta_u(t) < \infty\}$.*

The following proof is based on the ideas in [70].

Proof. For $h \in U$, the function $H_h : \mathbb{R}_{\geq 0} \to \mathbb{R} \cup \{\infty\}$ defined by $H_h(t) = D_\mathcal{R}(u + th, u)$ is convex and increasing and satisfies $H_h(0) = 0$. The convexity of H_h implies that

$$cH_h(t) = cH_h\left(\frac{1}{c}ct + \frac{c-1}{c}0\right) \leq H_h(ct) + (c-1)H_h(0) = H_h(ct) , \qquad c \geq 1 .$$

Because

$$\eta_u(t) = \inf\{H_h(t) : \|h\| = 1\} ,$$

it follows that η_u is increasing and non-negative, too, and satisfies

$$c\eta_u(t) \leq \eta_u(ct) , \qquad c \geq 1 .$$

Now assume that $\mathcal{R}$ is totally convex at u. Let $s > t > 0$. Because $s/t > 1$ and $\eta_u(t) > 0$, it follows that

$$\eta_u(s) = \eta_u\left(\frac{s}{t}t\right) \geq \frac{s}{t}\eta_u(t) = \eta_u(t) + \frac{s-t}{t}\eta_u(t) > \eta_u(t) ,$$

which proves the assertion.   □

Lemma 3.31. *Let $\mathcal{R} : U \to \mathbb{R} \cup \{\infty\}$ be convex and proper. Then the functional $\mathcal{R}$ is totally convex at $u \in \mathcal{D}(\mathcal{R})$, if and only if every sequence $(u_k) \subset \mathcal{D}(\mathcal{R})$ with $D_\mathcal{R}(u_k, u) \to 0$ satisfies $\|u_k - u\| \to 0$.*

Proof. Assume first that $\mathcal{R}$ is totally convex at u, and let η_u be its modulus of convexity (see (3.21)). Let $(u_k) \subset \mathcal{D}(\mathcal{R})$ satisfy $D_{\mathcal{R}}(u_k, u) \to 0$. Then the definition of η_u implies that

$$\lim_k \eta_u(\|u_k - u\|) \leq \lim_k D_{\mathcal{R}}(u_k, u) = 0 \, .$$

Because η_u is strictly increasing and non-negative, this implies that $\|u_k - u\| \to 0$.

In order to show the converse implication, assume to the contrary that $\eta_u(t) = 0$ for some $t > 0$. Then there exists a sequence (u_k) such that $D_{\mathcal{R}}(u_k, u) \to \eta_u(t) = 0$ and $\|u_k - u\| = t$ for all k, which is a contradiction to the assumption that every sequence $(\tilde{u}_k)$ with $D_{\mathcal{R}}(\tilde{u}_k, u) \to 0$ satisfies $\|\tilde{u}_k - u\| \to 0$. $\qquad\square$

Proposition 3.32 (Strong convergence). *Let the assumptions of Theorem 3.26 hold with τ_U being the weak topology on U. Assume that $\mathcal{R}$ is totally convex and that every $\mathcal{R}$-minimizing solution $u^\dagger$ of (3.1) satisfies $u^\dagger \in \mathcal{D}_B(\mathcal{R})$.*

Then for every sequence (u_k) of elements minimizing $\mathcal{T}_{\alpha_k, v_k}$, there exists a subsequence $(u_{k'})$ and an $\mathcal{R}$-minimizing solution $u^\dagger$ with $\|u_{k'} - u^\dagger\| \to 0$. If the $\mathcal{R}$-minimizing solution is unique, then $u_k \to u^\dagger$ with respect to the norm topology.

Proof. It follows from Theorem 3.26 that there exists a subsequence $(u_{k'})$ weakly converging to some $\mathcal{R}$-minimizing solution $u^\dagger$ such that $\mathcal{R}(u_{k'}) \to \mathcal{R}(u^\dagger)$.

Because $u^\dagger \in \mathcal{D}_B(\mathcal{R})$, it follows that there exists a subdifferential $\xi \in \partial\mathcal{R}(u^\dagger)$. From the weak convergence of $(u_{k'})$ and the convergence of $(\mathcal{R}(u_{k'}))$, it follows that $D_\xi(u_{k'}, u^\dagger) \to 0$. Consequently also $D_{\mathcal{R}}(u_{k'}, u^\dagger) \to 0$. Thus it follows from Lemma 3.31 that $\|u_{k'} - u^\dagger\| \to 0$.

If $u^\dagger$ is the unique $\mathcal{R}$-minimizing solution, then the convergence of (u_k) to $u^\dagger$ follows from Lemma 8.2. $\qquad\square$

Example 3.33. A frequently used regularization functional is the norm on the Banach space U, to some power q, more precisely, $\mathcal{R}(u) = \|u\|^q$ with $q > 1$. Assume now that the space U is reflexive and *strictly convex*, that is, $\|(u + \hat{u})/2\| < 1$, whenever u and $\hat{u}$ are different points on the unit sphere S_U (see [274, Prop. 5.1.2]). In this case, the total convexity of $\mathcal{R}$ can be shown to be equivalent to the *Radon–Riesz property*, which states that the assumptions $u_k \rightharpoonup u$ and $\|u_k\| \to \|u\|$ imply that $\|u_k - u\| \to 0$ (see [329, Thm. 3.2]).

As a consequence, Proposition 3.32 can be applied, showing that norm regularization on Banach spaces enjoying the Radon–Riesz property yields convergence results in the norm. In contrast, in general Banach spaces only convergence in the weak topology can be obtained (see Theorem 3.26).

The spaces $U = L^r(\Omega)$ or $U = l^r(\mathbb{N})$ with $1 < r < \infty$ are typical examples for Banach spaces satisfying these properties (see [274, Thms. 5.2.11, 5.2.18]). $\qquad\Diamond$

A Convergence Rates Result

This paragraph extends and modifies some convergence rates results presented in [215]. Throughout the whole section, we assume that the noisy data $v^\delta \in V$ satisfy

$$\left\| v^\delta - v \right\| \leq \delta \,. \tag{3.22}$$

For the derivation of convergence rates, we use the following assumptions:

Assumption 3.34

1. Let F, $\mathcal{R}$, $\mathcal{D}$, U, and V satisfy Assumption 3.13.
2. There exists an $\mathcal{R}$-minimizing solution $u^\dagger$ of (3.1), which is an element of the Bregman domain $\mathcal{D}_B(\mathcal{R})$.
3. There exist $\beta_1 \in [0,1)$, $\beta_2 \geq 0$, and $\xi^* \in \partial \mathcal{R}(u^\dagger)$ such that

$$\boxed{\left\langle \xi^*, u^\dagger - u \right\rangle_{U^*,U} \leq \beta_1 D_{\xi^*}(u, u^\dagger) + \beta_2 \left\| F(u) - F(u^\dagger) \right\|,} \tag{3.23}$$

for $u \in \mathcal{M}_{\alpha_{\max}}(\rho)$, where $\alpha_{\max}$, $\rho > 0$ satisfy the relation $\rho > \alpha_{\max} \mathcal{R}(u^\dagger)$.

In Item 2 of Assumption 3.34, the existence of an $\mathcal{R}$-minimizing solution is assumed, which under the included Assumption 3.13 already follows from the existence of a solution of (3.1) in $\mathcal{D}$ (see Theorem 3.25). Thus, the existence of an $\mathcal{R}$-minimizing solution can as well be replaced by the assumption that there exists a solution of (3.1) in $\mathcal{D}$.

For the following propositions, it is necessary to recall the definition of the dual adjoint operator $L^\#$ defined in Proposition 8.18.

Proposition 3.35. *Let F, $\mathcal{R}$, $\mathcal{D}$, U, and V satisfy Assumption 3.13. Assume that there exists an $\mathcal{R}$-minimizing solution $u^\dagger$ of (3.1), and that F is Gâteaux differentiable in $u^\dagger$.*

Moreover, assume that there exist $\gamma \geq 0$ and $\omega^* \in V^*$ with $\gamma \left\| \omega^* \right\| < 1$, such that

$$\xi^* := F'(u^\dagger)^\# \omega^* \in \partial \mathcal{R}(u^\dagger) \tag{3.24}$$

and there exists $\alpha_{\max} > 0$ satisfying $\rho > \alpha_{\max} \mathcal{R}(u^\dagger)$ such that

$$\left\| F(u) - F(u^\dagger) - F'(u^\dagger)(u - u^\dagger) \right\| \leq \gamma D_{\xi^*}(u, u^\dagger), \quad u \in \mathcal{M}_{\alpha_{\max}}(\rho) \,. \tag{3.25}$$

Then Assumption 3.34 holds.

Proof. We have

$$
\begin{aligned}
\left\langle \xi^*, u^\dagger - u \right\rangle_{U^*,U} &= \left\langle F'(u^\dagger)^\# \omega^*, u^\dagger - u \right\rangle_{U^*,U} \\
&= \left\langle \omega^*, F'(u^\dagger)(u^\dagger - u) \right\rangle_{V^*,V} \\
&\leq \left\| \omega^* \right\| \left\| F'(u^\dagger)(u^\dagger - u) \right\| \\
&\leq \left\| \omega^* \right\| \left\| F(u) - v \right\| + \left\| \omega^* \right\| \left\| F(u) - v - F'(u^\dagger)(u - u^\dagger) \right\| \\
&\leq \left\| \omega^* \right\| \left\| F(u) - v \right\| + \gamma \left\| \omega^* \right\| D_{\xi^*}(u, u^\dagger) \,.
\end{aligned}
$$

Setting $\beta_1 = \gamma \left\| \omega^* \right\|$ and $\beta_2 = \left\| \omega^* \right\|$, the assertion follows. $\qquad \square$

Remark 3.36. Let U and V be Hilbert spaces, and $\mathcal{R}(u) = \|u - u_0\|^2$. Then $\partial \mathcal{R}(u^\dagger) = \{\mathcal{J}_U 2(u^\dagger - u_0)\}$ and $D_{\xi^*}(u, u^\dagger) = \|u - u^\dagger\|^2$. Moreover, from Remark 8.30 it follows that $F^\# = \mathcal{J}_U F^*$. Thus (3.24) and (3.25) are equivalent to the assumptions

$$2(u^\dagger - u_0) = F'(u^\dagger)^* \omega$$

with $\gamma \|\omega\| < 1$, and

$$\left\| F(u) - F(u^\dagger) - F'(u^\dagger)(u - u^\dagger) \right\| \leq \gamma \left\| u^\dagger - u \right\|^2, \qquad u \in \mathcal{M}_{\alpha_{\max}}(\rho) .$$

Consequently, it follows from Proposition 3.35 that the condition (3.23) is a generalization of (3.4). $\diamond$

Remark 3.37. If in Proposition 3.35, $F = L \in L(U, V)$ is linear and bounded, then the choice $\gamma = 0$ in (3.25) is appropriate, and (3.24) is equivalent to

$$\partial \mathcal{R}(u^\dagger) \cap \operatorname{Ran}(L^\#) \neq \emptyset . \tag{3.26}$$

We stress that as $\gamma = 0$, the additional nearness condition $\gamma \|\omega^*\| < 1$ for some $\omega^* \in V^*$ is superfluous.

From Proposition 3.35, it follows that (3.26) implies (3.23). Below we show that also the converse direction is true, and thus (3.23) and (3.26) are equivalent. $\diamond$

Proposition 3.38. *Let F, $\mathcal{R}$, $\mathcal{D}$, U, and V satisfy Assumption 3.13. Assume that there exists an $\mathcal{R}$-minimizing solution $u^\dagger$ of (3.1) such that F and $\mathcal{R}$ are Gâteaux differentiable in $u^\dagger$. Then Assumption 3.34 implies the source condition*

$$\xi^* = \mathcal{R}'(u^\dagger) \in \operatorname{Ran}(F'(u^\dagger)^\#) . \tag{3.27}$$

Proof. Because $\mathcal{R}$ and F are Gâteaux differentiable at $u^\dagger$, it follows that

$$\lim_{t \to 0} \left(\frac{\mathcal{R}(u^\dagger - t\hat{u}) - \mathcal{R}(u^\dagger)}{t} + \langle \xi^*, \hat{u} \rangle \right) = 0 ,$$
$$\lim_{t \to 0} \left\| \frac{F(u^\dagger - t\hat{u}) - F(u^\dagger)}{t} + F'(u^\dagger)\hat{u} \right\| = 0 , \qquad \hat{u} \in U . \tag{3.28}$$

In particular, it follows that for every $\hat{u} \in U$, there exists $t_0 > 0$ such that $\alpha_{\max} \mathcal{R}(u^\dagger - t\hat{u}) + \left\| F(u^\dagger - t\hat{u}) - v^\delta \right\|^2 < \rho$ for all $0 \leq t < t_0$, which implies that $u^\dagger - t\hat{u} \in \mathcal{M}_{\alpha_{\max}}(\rho)$ for $0 \leq t < t_0$. Thus it follows from (3.23) that

$$\langle \xi^*, t\hat{u} \rangle \leq \beta_1 D_{\xi^*}(u^\dagger - t\hat{u}, u^\dagger) + \beta_2 \left\| F(u^\dagger - t\hat{u}) - F(u^\dagger) \right\|$$
$$= \beta_1 \left(\mathcal{R}(u^\dagger - t\hat{u}) - \mathcal{R}(u^\dagger) + \langle \xi^*, t\hat{u} \rangle \right) + \beta_2 \left\| F(u^\dagger - t\hat{u}) - F(u^\dagger) \right\| \tag{3.29}$$

for $0 \leq t < t_0$. Dividing (3.29) by t and letting $t \to 0^+$, we therefore obtain from (3.28) that

$$\langle \xi^*, \hat{u} \rangle \leq \beta_2 \left\| F'(u^\dagger)\hat{u} \right\| , \qquad \hat{u} \in U .$$

Thus it follows from Lemma 8.21 that $\xi^* \in \operatorname{Ran}(F'(u^\dagger)^\#)$. $\square$

The following proposition is a generalization of Proposition 3.35 that, in particular, also applies to non-Gâteaux differentiable functionals.

Proposition 3.39. *Let F, $\mathcal{R}$, $\mathcal{D}$, U, and V satisfy Items 1 and 2 in Assumption 3.34. Item 3 in Assumption 3.34 holds, if additionally to Items 1 and 2 the following conditions are satisfied:*

- *There exists a bounded embedding $i : V \to \tilde{V}$, where $\tilde{V}$ is a Banach space.*
- *$\mathcal{D}$ is locally starlike with respect to $u^\dagger$, that is, for every $u \in \mathcal{D}$ there exists $t_0 > 0$ such that*

$$u^\dagger + t\,(u - u^\dagger) \in \mathcal{D}\,, \qquad 0 \le t \le t_0\,.$$

- *F attains a one-sided directional derivative $F'(u^\dagger; u - u^\dagger)$ at $u^\dagger$ in direction $u - u^\dagger$, $u \in \mathcal{D}$, with respect to the norm topology on $\tilde{V}$, that is,*

$$\lim_{t \to 0^+} \left\| i \left(\frac{F(u^\dagger + t(u - u^\dagger)) - F(u^\dagger)}{t} - F'(u^\dagger; u - u^\dagger) \right) \right\|_{\tilde{V}} = 0\,, \quad u \in \mathcal{D}\,.$$

- *There exist $\gamma \ge 0$, $\tilde{\omega}^* \in \tilde{V}^*$, and $\xi^* \in \partial\mathcal{R}(u^\dagger)$, such that $\gamma\,\|\tilde{\omega}^*\|_{\tilde{V}^*} < 1$ and*

$$\left\| i\left(F(u) - F(u^\dagger) - F'(u^\dagger; u - u^\dagger) \right) \right\|_{\tilde{V}} \le \gamma D_{\xi^*}(u, u^\dagger)\,, \qquad (3.30)$$

$$\left\langle \xi^*, u - u^\dagger \right\rangle_{U^*, U} \le \left| \left\langle \tilde{\omega}^*, i\left(F'(u^\dagger; u - u^\dagger) \right) \right\rangle_{\tilde{V}^*, \tilde{V}} \right|\,, \qquad (3.31)$$

for $u \in \mathcal{M}_{\alpha_{\max}}(\rho)$.

Proof. Define $\beta_1 := \gamma\,\|\tilde{\omega}^*\|_{\tilde{V}^*} < 1$ and $\beta_2 := \left\| i^{\#}\tilde{\omega}^* \right\|_{V^*}$. From (3.30), the Cauchy–Schwarz inequality, and (3.31) it follows that

$$
\begin{aligned}
\langle \xi^*, u^\dagger - u \rangle_{U^*, U} &\le \left| \left\langle \tilde{\omega}^*, i\left(F'(u^\dagger; u - u^\dagger) \right) \right\rangle_{\tilde{V}^*, \tilde{V}} \right| \\
&\le \left\| i^{\#}\tilde{\omega}^* \right\|_{V^*} \left\| F(u) - F(u^\dagger) \right\|_V \\
&\quad + \left\| \tilde{\omega}^* \right\|_{\tilde{V}^*} \left\| i\left(F(u) - F(u^\dagger) - F'(u^\dagger; u - u^\dagger) \right) \right\|_{\tilde{V}} \\
&\le \beta_2 \left\| F(u) - F(u^\dagger) \right\|_V + \beta_1 D_{\xi^*}(u, u^\dagger)
\end{aligned}
$$

for $u \in \mathcal{M}_{\alpha_{\max}}(\rho)$. □

The relations between the different source conditions are summarized in Table 3.1.

Remark 3.40. Given a convex set D, let $F = L|_D$ be the restriction of a bounded linear operator L to D. As in Proposition 3.35 and Remark 3.37, it follows that (3.23) is satisfied if $\xi^* \in \mathrm{Ran}(L^{\#})$, where ξ^* is an element of the subdifferential of $\mathcal{R}$. ◇

Table 3.1. Relations between the different source conditions.

General $\mathcal{R}$	
F Gâteaux differentiable	$(3.23) \underset{\text{Pr. 3.38}}{\Longrightarrow} (3.27) = (3.24)$
	(3.24) and $(3.25) \underset{\text{Pr. 3.35}}{\Longrightarrow} (3.23)$
$F \in L(U, V)$	$(3.26) \underset{\text{Rem. 3.37}}{\Longleftrightarrow} (3.23)$

$\mathcal{R}(u) = \|u - u_0\|^2$	
F satisfies Assumption 3.7	$\left.\begin{array}{l}(3.3) \underset{\text{Ex. 3.18}}{\Longleftrightarrow} (3.25) \\ (3.4) \Longleftrightarrow (3.24)\end{array}\right\} \underset{\text{Pr. 3.35}}{\Longrightarrow} (3.23)$
$F = L \in L(U, V)$	$(3.4) \Longleftrightarrow (3.26) \Longleftrightarrow (3.23)$

Proposition 3.41. *Let F, $\mathcal{R}$, $\mathcal{D}$, U, and V satisfy Assumption 3.34. Moreover assume that $\alpha\beta_2 < 1$. Then $\mathcal{R}(u_\alpha^\delta) \leq \delta^p/\alpha + \mathcal{R}(u^\dagger)$.*

If $p = 1$, then

$$\left\| F(u_\alpha^\delta) - v^\delta \right\| \leq \frac{\delta(1 + \alpha\beta_2)}{1 - \alpha\beta_2}, \tag{3.32}$$

$$D_{\xi^*}(u_\alpha^\delta, u^\dagger) \leq \frac{\delta(1 + \alpha\beta_2)}{\alpha(1 - \beta_1)}. \tag{3.33}$$

If $p > 1$, then

$$\left\| F(u_\alpha^\delta) - v^\delta \right\| \leq \left[\frac{p}{p-1} \left(\delta^p + \alpha\delta\beta_2 + \frac{(\alpha\beta_2)^{p_*}}{p_*} \right) \right]^{1/p}, \tag{3.34}$$

$$D_{\xi^*}(u_\alpha^\delta, u^\dagger) \leq \frac{\delta^p + \alpha\delta\beta_2 + (\alpha\beta_2)^{p_*}/p_*}{\alpha(1 - \beta_1)}. \tag{3.35}$$

Proof. From the definition of u_α^δ and (3.22), it follows that

$$\left\| F(u_\alpha^\delta) - v^\delta \right\|^p + \alpha\mathcal{R}(u_\alpha^\delta) \leq \delta^p + \alpha\mathcal{R}(u^\dagger), \tag{3.36}$$

and therefore

$$\begin{aligned}\left\| F(u_\alpha^\delta) - v^\delta \right\|^p + \alpha D_{\xi^*}(u_\alpha^\delta, u^\dagger) \\ \leq \delta^p + \alpha\big(\mathcal{R}(u^\dagger) - \mathcal{R}(u_\alpha^\delta) + D_{\xi^*}(u_\alpha^\delta, u^\dagger)\big).\end{aligned} \tag{3.37}$$

Equation (3.36) implies $\mathcal{R}(u_\alpha^\delta) \leq \delta^p/\alpha + \mathcal{R}(u^\dagger)$.

Using the definition of the Bregman distance (3.8) and estimates (3.23) and (3.22), it follows that

$$\mathcal{R}(u^\dagger) - \mathcal{R}(u_\alpha^\delta) + D_{\xi^*}(u_\alpha^\delta, u^\dagger) = - \langle \xi^*, u_\alpha^\delta - u^\dagger \rangle_{U^*,U}$$
$$\leq \beta_1 D_{\xi^*}(u_\alpha^\delta, u^\dagger) + \beta_2 \left\| F(u_\alpha^\delta) - F(u^\dagger) \right\|$$
$$\leq \beta_1 D_{\xi^*}(u_\alpha^\delta, u^\dagger) + \beta_2 \left(\left\| F(u_\alpha^\delta) - v^\delta \right\| + \delta \right) .$$

Therefore, it follows from (3.37) that

$$\left\| F(u_\alpha^\delta) - v^\delta \right\|^p + \alpha D_{\xi^*}(u_\alpha^\delta, u^\dagger)$$
$$\leq \delta^p + \alpha \big(\beta_1 D_{\xi^*}(u_\alpha^\delta, u^\dagger) + \beta_2 \big(\left\| F(u_\alpha^\delta) - v^\delta \right\| + \delta \big) \big) . \quad (3.38)$$

1. **Case $p = 1$.** From (3.38), it follows that

$$(1 - \alpha\beta_2) \left\| F(u_\alpha^\delta) - v^\delta \right\| + \alpha(1 - \beta_1) D_{\xi^*}(u_\alpha^\delta, u^\dagger) \leq \delta(1 + \alpha\beta_2) . \quad (3.39)$$

Because $\beta_1 < 1$, it follows that the left-hand side in (3.39) is the sum of two non-negative numbers. This shows (3.32) and (3.33).

2. **Case $p > 1$.** From (3.38), it follows that

$$\left\| F(u_\alpha^\delta) - v^\delta \right\|^p - \alpha\beta_2 \left\| F(u_\alpha^\delta) - v^\delta \right\|$$
$$+ \alpha(1 - \beta_1) D_{\xi^*}(u_\alpha^\delta, u^\dagger) \leq \delta^p + \alpha\delta\beta_2 . \quad (3.40)$$

Young's inequality, $ab \leq a^p/p + b^{p_*}/p_*$ for $1/p + 1/p_* = 1$, with $a = \left\| F(u_\alpha^\delta) - v^\delta \right\|$ and $b = \alpha\beta_2$ gives

$$-\frac{1}{p} \left\| F(u_\alpha^\delta) - v^\delta \right\|^p \leq -\alpha\beta_2 \left\| F(u_\alpha^\delta) - v^\delta \right\| + (\alpha\beta_2)^{p_*}/p_* . \quad (3.41)$$

By adding $(\alpha\beta_2)^{p_*}/p_*$ to both sides of (3.40) and applying (3.41), it follows that

$$\left(1 - \frac{1}{p} \right) \left\| F(u_\alpha^\delta) - v^\delta \right\|^p + \alpha(1 - \beta_1) D_{\xi^*}(u_\alpha^\delta, u^\dagger)$$
$$\leq \delta^p + \alpha\delta\beta_2 + (\alpha\beta_2)^{p_*}/p^* . \quad (3.42)$$

Because $\beta_1 < 1$, the left-hand side of (3.42) is the sum of two non-negative terms, which shows (3.34) and (3.35).

$\square$

Theorem 3.42 (Convergence rates). *Let F, $\mathcal{R}$, $\mathcal{D}$, U, and V satisfy Assumption 3.34.*

1. *Case $p = 1$. Let $\alpha : (0, \infty) \to (0, \infty)$ satisfy $\alpha(\delta) \sim \delta^\varepsilon$ with $0 \leq \varepsilon < 1$. If $\varepsilon = 0$, assume additionally that $0 < \alpha(\delta)\beta_2 < 1$. Then*

$$\boxed{D_{\xi^*}(u_{\alpha(\delta)}^\delta, u^\dagger) = O(\delta^{1-\varepsilon}), \qquad \left\| F(u_{\alpha(\delta)}^\delta) - v^\delta \right\| = O(\delta) ,}$$

and there exists $c > 0$, such that $\mathcal{R}(u_{\alpha(\delta)}^\delta) \leq \mathcal{R}(u^\dagger) + \delta^{1-\varepsilon}/c$ for every δ with $\alpha(\delta) \leq \alpha_{max}$.

2. **Case** $p > 1$. *Let* $\alpha : (0, \infty) \to (0, \infty)$ *satisfy* $\alpha(\delta) \sim \delta^{p-1}$. *Then*

$$\boxed{D_{\xi^*}(u^\delta_{\alpha(\delta)}, u^\dagger) = O(\delta), \qquad \left\| F(u^\delta_{\alpha(\delta)}) - v^\delta \right\| = O(\delta),}$$

and there exists $c > 0$, *such that* $\mathcal{R}(u^\delta_{\alpha(\delta)}) \leq \mathcal{R}(u^\dagger) + \delta/c$ *for every* δ *with* $\alpha(\delta) \leq \alpha_{\max}$.

Proof. This is a direct consequence of Proposition 3.41.   □

Let U, V be Hilbert spaces and take $\mathcal{R}(u) = \|u - u_0\|^2_U$, where $\|\cdot\|_U$ denotes the norm on the Hilbert space U. Recall that in this case $D_{\xi^*}(u, u^\dagger) = \|u - u^\dagger\|^2_U$ (cf. Example 3.18). Therefore Theorem 3.42 is a generalization of Theorem 3.11.

In the sequel, we bring a series of comments highlighting the obtained results and embedding them in the literature.

Remark 3.43. Let $\alpha > 0$ be fixed and let Assumption 3.34 be satisfied.

- Let $p = 1$. If $\delta = 0$ and $\alpha\beta_2 < 1$, then (3.32) and (3.33) imply

$$\|F(u_\alpha) - v\| = 0 \quad \text{and} \quad D_{\xi^*}(u_\alpha, u^\dagger) = 0.$$

The last identity is the reason that regularization methods with $p = 1$ are in [63] called *exact penalization methods*. In the case of perturbed data, it follows from (3.32) and (3.33) that

$$\|F(u^\delta_\alpha) - v\| = O(\delta) \quad \text{and} \quad D_{\xi^*}(u^\delta_\alpha, u^\dagger) = O(\delta),$$

which is also a result stated in [63]. In particular, if $F : \mathcal{D}(F) \subset U \to V$ is an operator between a Hilbert space U and a Banach space V, then

$$\|F(u_\alpha) - v\| = 0 \qquad \text{and} \qquad \|u_\alpha - u^\dagger\| = 0$$

for $\delta = 0$ and $\alpha\beta_2 < 1$.

Consider for instance a linear operator $F = L : L^2(\Omega) \to L^1(\Omega)$ and L^1-L^2 regularization, which consists in minimization of the functional

$$\mathcal{T}_{\alpha,v^\delta}(u) = \int_\Omega |Lu - v^\delta| + \alpha \|u\|^2_2 .$$

For $1 \leq p < \infty$, let $\Im_p$ be the identification operator from $(L^p(\Omega))^*$ to $L^{p^*}(\Omega)$ (see Lemma 9.11) and define

$$L^* := \Im_2 L^\#(\Im_1)^{-1} : L^\infty(\Omega) \to L^2(\Omega).$$

In such a situation, $\partial\mathcal{R}(u^\dagger) = \{\xi^*\}$ with $\xi^* = 2\mathcal{J}_{L^2}(u^\dagger)$, where $\mathcal{J}_{L^2}$ is the duality mapping on $L^2(\Omega)$. Using the definition of $L^\#$ and (9.4), it follows that

$$\int_\Omega L^*\tilde\omega\, g = \left\langle L^\#(\Im_1)^{-1}\tilde\omega, g\right\rangle_{L^2(\Omega)^*, L^2(\Omega)}$$

$$= \left\langle (\Im_1)^{-1}\tilde\omega, Lg\right\rangle_{L^1(\Omega)^*, L^1(\Omega)} = \int_\Omega \tilde\omega\, Lg\,, \quad g \in L^2(\Omega)\,.$$

Assume now that $2u^\dagger = L^*\tilde\omega$, then

$$\left\langle \xi^*, u^\dagger - u\right\rangle_{L^2(\Omega)^*, L^2(\Omega)} = \int_\Omega L^*\tilde\omega\,(u^\dagger - u)$$

$$= \int_\Omega \tilde\omega\, L(u^\dagger - u) \le \|\tilde\omega\|_\infty \left\|L(u^\dagger - u)\right\|_1\,.$$

Therefore (3.23) is satisfied with $\beta_1 = 0$ and $\beta_2 = \|\tilde\omega\|_\infty$. If in addition $\alpha\|\tilde\omega\|_\infty < 1$, then $u_\alpha = u^\dagger$.

- Let $p > 1$. If $\delta = 0$ and $\alpha\beta_2 < 1$, then (3.34) and (3.35) imply

$$\boxed{\|F(u_\alpha) - v\| \le (\alpha\beta_2)^{1/(p-1)}\,, \quad D_{\xi^*}(u_\alpha, u^\dagger) \le \frac{\beta_2^{p_*}\alpha^{p_*-1}}{p_*(1-\beta_1)}\,.} \qquad (3.43)$$

$$\diamondsuit$$

Remark 3.44. Several convergence rates results of the form

$$\left\|F(u_\alpha^\delta) - v^\delta\right\| = O(\delta) \quad \text{and} \quad D_\xi(u_\alpha^\delta, u^\dagger) = O(\delta)$$

for Tikhonov regularization in a Banach space setting have been derived in the literature:

- In [105], a convergence rates result for regularization with $\mathcal{R}(u) = \|u\|_2^2 + |Du|$ has been proven. However, the convergence rates have not been expressed in terms of Bregman distances, but in the L^2 norm.
- In [63, Sect. 3.3], it has been assumed that U is a Banach space, V a Hilbert space, that F is Fréchet differentiable, and that there exist $\gamma > 0$, $\omega \in V$, and $\xi^* \in \partial\mathcal{R}(u^\dagger)$, which satisfy

$$F'(u^\dagger)^\#\omega^* = \xi^* \quad \text{with } \omega^* = \mathcal{J}_V\omega\,, \qquad (3.44)$$

where $\mathcal{J}_V$ is the duality mapping from V into V^*, and

$$\left\langle F(u) - F(u^\dagger) - F'(u^\dagger)(u - u^\dagger), \omega\right\rangle_V \le \gamma\left\|F(u) - F(u^\dagger)\right\|\|\omega\|\,. \qquad (3.45)$$

This is a special case of Assumption 3.34: Setting $\beta_2 := (1 + \gamma)\|\omega\|$ and $\beta_1 = 0$, it follows from (3.45) and (3.44) that

$$-\left\langle \xi^*, u - u^\dagger\right\rangle_{U^*, U}$$

$$\le -\left\langle F'(u^\dagger)^\#\omega^*, u - u^\dagger\right\rangle_{U^*, U} = -\left\langle \omega, F'(u^\dagger)(u - u^\dagger)\right\rangle_{V^*, V}$$

$$\le -\left\langle \omega, F'(u^\dagger)(u - u^\dagger) + F(u^\dagger) - F(u) + F(u) - F(u^\dagger)\right\rangle_{V^*, V}$$

$$\le \beta_2\left\|F(u) - F(u^\dagger)\right\|\,.$$

Thus (3.23) holds. Note that in this situation, no smallness condition is associated to $\gamma \left\| \omega \right\|_V$, as (3.45) is already scaling invariant.

- In [332], we have assumed that U and V are both Banach spaces, F is Fréchet differentiable, there exists $\omega^* \in V^*$ satisfying

$$F'(u^\dagger)^\# \omega^* = \xi^* \in \partial\mathcal{R}(u^\dagger) \quad \text{and} \quad \gamma \left\| \omega^* \right\|_{V^*} < 1 \,,$$

and

$$\left\| F(u) - F(u^\dagger) - F'(u^\dagger)(u - u^\dagger) \right\| \leq \gamma D_{\xi^*}(u, u^\dagger) \,.$$

Under these assumptions, we were able to prove that the assertions of Theorem 3.42 are valid. Theorem 3.42, however, is applicable to the more general situation of Proposition 3.39, where we only assume that F attains a one-sided directional derivative satisfying (3.30) and (3.31).

$\diamond$

In the following, we present a stability estimate in Banach spaces. The result is a generalization of the work published in [332] and of Theorem 3.12.

Proposition 3.45. *Let F, $\mathcal{R}$, U, V, and $\mathcal{D}$ satisfy Assumption 3.34. Moreover, we assume that $\mathcal{M}_{\alpha_{\max}}(\rho) \subset \mathcal{D}_B(\mathcal{R})$ and that there exist $\beta_1, \beta_2 > 0$ with $2^{p-1}\beta_1 < 1$ such that for every $u_2 \in \mathcal{M}_{\alpha_{\max}}(\rho)$, there exists $\xi_2^* \in \partial\mathcal{R}(u_2)$ satisfying*

$$\boxed{\left| \langle \xi_2^*, u_1 - u_2 \rangle_{U^*,U} \right| \leq \beta_1 D_{\xi_2^*}(u_1, u_2) + \beta_2 \left\| F(u_1) - F(u_2) \right\|} \tag{3.46}$$

for all $u_1 \in \mathcal{M}_{\alpha_{\max}}(\rho)$.

Then, for $p = 1$ we have

$$
\begin{aligned}
\left\| F(u_\alpha^\delta) - F(u_\alpha) \right\| &\leq \frac{2\delta}{1 - \alpha\beta_2} \,, \\
D_{\xi_\alpha^*}(u_\alpha^\delta, u_\alpha) &\leq \frac{2}{1 - \beta_1} \frac{\delta}{\alpha} \,.
\end{aligned}
\tag{3.47}
$$

Moreover, for $p > 1$ there exists $C > 0$ such that

$$
\begin{aligned}
\left\| F(u_\alpha^\delta) - F(u_\alpha) \right\| &\leq C\left(\alpha^{1/(p-1)} + \delta \right) \,, \\
D_{\xi_\alpha^*}(u_\alpha^\delta, u_\alpha) &\leq \frac{C}{\alpha}\left(\alpha^{p/(p-1)} + \delta^p \right) \,.
\end{aligned}
\tag{3.48}
$$

Proof. We have shown in Remark 3.27 that for sufficiently small δ, the functions u_α^δ, u_α, and $u^\dagger$ are elements of $\mathcal{M}_{\alpha_{\max}}(\rho)$. Then the assumption $\mathcal{M}_{\alpha_{\max}}(\rho) \subset \mathcal{D}_B(\mathcal{R})$ ensures that at each of the three functions, the subdifferential of $\mathcal{R}$ is non-empty. Therefore (3.46) is valid for u_α^δ, u_α, and $u^\dagger$.

From the definition of u_α^δ, it follows that

$$\left\| F(u_\alpha^\delta) - v^\delta \right\|^p + \alpha\mathcal{R}(u_\alpha^\delta) \leq \left\| F(u_\alpha) - v^\delta \right\|^p + \alpha\mathcal{R}(u_\alpha) \,.$$

From the definition of u_α^δ, it follows that

$$
\frac{1}{2^{p-1}} \left\| F(u_\alpha^\delta) - F(u_\alpha) \right\|^p + \alpha D_{\xi_\alpha^*}(u_\alpha^\delta, u_\alpha)
$$

$$
\leq \left\| F(u_\alpha) - v^\delta \right\|^p + \left\| F(u_\alpha^\delta) - v^\delta \right\|^p + \alpha D_{\xi_\alpha^*}(u_\alpha^\delta, u_\alpha)
$$

$$
= \left\| F(u_\alpha) - v^\delta \right\|^p + \left\| F(u_\alpha^\delta) - v^\delta \right\|^p +
$$

$$
+ \alpha \left(\mathcal{R}(u_\alpha^\delta) - \mathcal{R}(u_\alpha) - \langle \xi_\alpha^*, u_\alpha^\delta - u_\alpha \rangle_{U^*, U} \right) \tag{3.49}
$$

$$
\leq 2 \left\| F(u_\alpha) - v^\delta \right\|^p - \alpha \langle \xi^*, u_\alpha^\delta - u_\alpha \rangle_{U^*, U}
$$

$$
\leq 2^p \left\| F(u_\alpha) - v \right\|^p + 2^p \delta^p +
$$

$$
+ \alpha \beta_1 D_{\xi_\alpha^*}(u_\alpha^\delta, u_\alpha) + \alpha \beta_2 \left\| F(u_\alpha^\delta) - F(u_\alpha) \right\| .
$$

1. **Case $p = 1$.** From (3.49) and (3.32), which states that $\| F(u_\alpha) - v \| = 0$, it follows that

$$
(1 - \alpha \beta_2) \left\| F(u_\alpha^\delta) - F(u_\alpha) \right\| + (1 - \beta_1)\alpha \, D_{\xi_\alpha^*}(u_\alpha^\delta, u_\alpha) \leq 2\delta .
$$

This shows (3.47).

2. **Case $p > 1$.** From (3.49) and (3.43), which states that $\| F(u_\alpha) - v \| \leq \sqrt[p]{\beta_2} \alpha^{1/(p-1)}$, it follows that

$$
\left\| F(u_\alpha^\delta) - F(u_\alpha) \right\|^p + \alpha \, 2^{p-1} D_{\xi_\alpha^*}(u_\alpha^\delta, u_\alpha)
$$

$$
\leq 2^{2p-1} (\beta_2 \alpha)^{p/(p-1)} + 2^{2p-1} \delta^p +
$$

$$
+ 2^{p-1} \alpha \beta_1 D_{\xi_\alpha^*}(u_\alpha^\delta, u_\alpha) + 2^{p-1} \alpha \beta_2 \left\| F(u_\alpha) - F(u_\alpha^\delta) \right\| .
$$

Again we can apply Young's inequality and obtain

$$
\left(1 - \frac{1}{p} \right) \left\| F(u_\alpha^\delta) - F(u_\alpha) \right\|^p + 2^{p-1} \alpha (1 - 2^{p-1} \beta_1) D_{\xi_\alpha^*}(u_\alpha^\delta, u_\alpha)
$$

$$
\leq 2^{2p-1} (\alpha \beta_2)^{p/p-1} + 2^{p-1} \delta^p + \frac{2^p (p-1)}{p} (\alpha \beta_2)^{p/p-1} .
$$

This shows (3.48). $\qquad\qquad\qquad\qquad\qquad\qquad\qquad\qquad\qquad\qquad\qquad\qquad$ $\square$

Theorem 3.46 (Stability estimates). *Let the assumptions of Proposition 3.45 be satisfied.*

Then, for $p = 1$ and a parameter choice $\alpha(\delta) \sim \delta^\varepsilon$ with $0 < \varepsilon < 1$, we have

$$
\boxed{D_{\xi_{\alpha(\delta)}^*}(u_{\alpha(\delta)}^\delta, u_{\alpha(\delta)}) = O(\delta^{1-\varepsilon}), \quad \text{for some } \xi_{\alpha(\delta)}^* \in \partial \mathcal{R}(u_{\alpha(\delta)}) .}
$$

For $p > 1$ and a parameter choice $\alpha(\delta) \sim \delta^{p-1}$, we have

$$
\boxed{D_{\xi_{\alpha(\delta)}^*}(u_{\alpha(\delta)}^\delta, u_{\alpha(\delta)}) = O(\delta), \quad \text{for some } \xi_{\alpha(\delta)}^* \in \partial \mathcal{R}(u_{\alpha(\delta)}) .}
$$

Proof. This is a direct consequence of Proposition 3.45. $\qquad\qquad\qquad\qquad$ $\square$

3.3 Regularization with Sparsity Constraints

Let (ϕ_i) be an orthonormal basis of the Hilbert space U. The goal of *sparsity regularization* is to find an approximative solution u_α^δ of (3.1) such that only finitely many coefficients $\langle u_\alpha^\delta, \phi_i \rangle$ of the series expansion of u_α^δ with respect to (ϕ_i) are different from zero (see [77,126,136]). For this purpose, we investigate the following regularization method:

$$u_\alpha^\delta = \arg\min \mathcal{T}_{\alpha,v^\delta}^{\mathrm{sp}}(u) := \arg\min \left(\left\| F(u) - v^\delta \right\|_V^p + \alpha \mathcal{R}^{\mathrm{sp}}(u) \right),$$

where

$$\mathcal{R}^{\mathrm{sp}}(u) := \sum_i w_i \left| \langle u, \phi_i \rangle \right|^q .$$

In the following, we apply the general results of the previous section concerning existence, stability, convergence, and convergence rates to sparsity regularization.

We make the following assumptions:

Assumption 3.47

1. *U is a Hilbert space, V is a reflexive Banach space, and τ_U and τ_V are the weak topologies on U and V, respectively.*
2. *(ϕ_i) is an orthonormal basis of U.*
3. *The exponents p and q satisfy $p \geq 1$ and $q \in [1,2]$.*
4. *The weights (w_i) satisfy $w_{\min} \leq w_i < \infty$ for some constant $w_{\min} > 0$.*
5. *The operator $F : \mathcal{D}(F) \subset U \to V$ is weakly continuous and its domain $\mathcal{D}(F)$ is weakly sequentially closed.*
6. *The set $\mathcal{D} := \mathcal{D}(F) \cap \mathcal{D}(\mathcal{R}^{\mathrm{sp}})$ is not empty.*

We stress that we do not assume that U is separable. In fact, the assumption also applies to every non-separable Hilbert space U, because according to Theorem 8.36, such a space has an (uncountable) orthonormal basis. In this case, the uncountable sum in the definition of $\mathcal{R}^{\mathrm{sp}}(u)$ is defined as the supremum of all finite partial sums.

Theorem 3.48 (Well-posedness). *Let F, U, V, (ϕ_i), (w_i), p, and q satisfy Assumption 3.47. Then, minimizing $\mathcal{T}_{\alpha,v^\delta}^{\mathrm{sp}}$ is well-defined (in the sense of Theorem 3.22), stable (in the sense of Theorem 3.23), and convergent (in the sense of Theorem 3.26).*

Proof. It suffices to verify Assumption 3.13. Noting that $\|\cdot\|_V$ is sequentially lower semi-continuous (cf. Lemma 10.6), it remains to verify that $\mathcal{R}^{\mathrm{sp}}$ is weakly sequentially lower semi-continuous and that the level sets $\mathcal{M}_\alpha(M)$ are sequentially pre-compact.

In order to show that $\mathcal{R}^{\mathrm{sp}}$ is weakly sequentially lower semi-continuous, assume that (u_k) weakly converges to u. The weak continuity of $u \mapsto |\langle u, \phi_i \rangle|^q$ implies that for all i

$$\lim_k w_i |\langle u_k, \phi_i \rangle|^q = w_i |\langle u, \phi_i \rangle|^q \, .$$

Together with Fatou's Lemma 9.8, it follows that

$$\liminf_k \mathcal{R}^{\mathrm{sp}}(u_k) = \liminf_k \sum_i w_i |\langle u_k, \phi_i \rangle|^q$$

$$\geq \sum_i \liminf_k w_i |\langle u_k, \phi_i \rangle|^q = \sum_i w_i |\langle u, \phi_i \rangle|^q = \mathcal{R}^{\mathrm{sp}}(u) \, ,$$

which shows that $\mathcal{R}^{\mathrm{sp}}$ is sequentially weakly lower semi-continuous.

Let $\alpha, M > 0$. In order to show that $\mathcal{M}_\alpha(M)$ is sequentially pre-compact, we use the fact that

$$\|u\| = \left(\sum_i |\langle u, \phi_i \rangle|^2 \right)^{1/2} \leq \left(\sum_i |\langle u, \phi_i \rangle|^q \right)^{1/q} \leq w_{\min}^{-1/q} \mathcal{R}^{\mathrm{sp}}(u) \, .$$

Therefore, every sequence in $\mathcal{M}_\alpha(M)$ is bounded in U and thus has a weakly convergent subsequence. □

Theorem 3.48 ensures weak convergence of the regularized solutions as $\delta \to 0$. The following result shows that in the context of sparsity regularization, we can obtain strong convergence.

Theorem 3.49 (Strong convergence). *Let F, U, V, (ϕ_i), (w_i), p, and q satisfy Assumption 3.47. Assume that (3.1) has a solution in $\mathcal{D}$ and that $\alpha : (0, \infty) \to (0, \infty)$ satisfies*

$$\alpha(\delta) \to 0 \text{ and } \frac{\delta^p}{\alpha(\delta)} \to 0, \text{ as } \delta \to 0 \, .$$

Moreover, assume that the sequence (δ_k) converges to 0, that $v_k := v^{\delta_k}$ satisfies $\|v - v_k\| \leq \delta_k$, and that (u_k) is a sequence of elements minimizing $\mathcal{T}_{\alpha(\delta_k), v_k}$.

Then there exist an $\mathcal{R}^{\mathrm{sp}}$-minimizing solution $u^\dagger$ and a subsequence $(u_{k'})$ of (u_k) such that $\|u_{k'} - u^\dagger\| \to 0$. If, in addition, the $\mathcal{R}^{\mathrm{sp}}$-minimizing solution $u^\dagger$ is unique, then $\|u_k \to u^\dagger\| \to 0$.

Proof. Theorem 3.48 implies that there there exist an $\mathcal{R}^{\mathrm{sp}}$-minimizing solution $u^\dagger$ and a subsequence of (u_k), which we again denote by (u_k), such that $u_k \rightharpoonup u^\dagger$ and $\mathcal{R}^{\mathrm{sp}}(u_k) \to \mathcal{R}^{\mathrm{sp}}(u^\dagger)$. Below we verify that $\|u_k\| \to \|u^\dagger\|$, which according to Lemma 8.48 implies that $\|u_k - u^\dagger\| \to 0$.

Because (u_k) weakly converges to $u^\dagger$, it follows that $\langle u_k, \phi_i \rangle \to \langle u, \phi_i \rangle$ for all i, and that there exists $C_1 > 0$ such that $\|u_k\| \leq C_1$ for all k. Because $\|u_k\|^2 = \sum_i |\langle u_k, \phi_i \rangle|^2$, this implies that also $|\langle u_k, \phi_i \rangle| \leq C_1$ for all k and i.

Because $q \leq 2$, the function

$$(x, y) \mapsto \frac{x^2 - y^2}{x^q - y^q}, \qquad x, y \geq 0,$$

is continuous, and therefore it is bounded on every bounded subset of $\mathbb{R}_{\geq 0} \times \mathbb{R}_{\geq 0}$. Consequently

$$\left| |\langle u_k, \phi_i \rangle|^2 - |\langle u^\dagger, \phi_i \rangle|^2 \right| \leq C_2 \left| |\langle u_k, \phi_i \rangle|^q - |\langle u^\dagger, \phi_i \rangle|^q \right|$$

for some constant $C_2 > 0$ and all i. Thus,

$$\left| \|u_k\|^2 - \|u^\dagger\|^2 \right| \leq \sum_i \left| |\langle u_k, \phi_i \rangle|^2 - |\langle u^\dagger, \phi_i \rangle|^2 \right|$$

$$\leq C_2 \sum_i \left| |\langle u_k, \phi_i \rangle|^q - |\langle u^\dagger, \phi_i \rangle|^q \right| . \quad (3.50)$$

Now define

$$c_{k,i} := \min \left\{ |\langle u_k, \phi_i \rangle|, |\langle u^\dagger, \phi_i \rangle| \right\} .$$

From the weak convergence of u_k to $u^\dagger$, it follows that $c_{k,i} \rightarrow |\langle u^\dagger, \phi_i \rangle|$. Thus the Dominated Convergence Theorem 9.9 implies that $\sum_i c_{k,i}^q \rightarrow \sum_i |\langle u^\dagger, \phi_i \rangle|^q$. Consequently,

$$\lim_k \sum_i \left| |\langle u_k, \phi_i \rangle|^q - |\langle u^\dagger, \phi_i \rangle|^q \right| = \lim_k \sum_i \left(|\langle u_k, \phi_i \rangle|^q + |\langle u^\dagger, \phi_i \rangle|^q - 2c_{k,i}^q \right) = 0 .$$

$$(3.51)$$

Equations (3.50) and (3.51) imply that $\|u_k\| \rightarrow \|u^\dagger\|$, which concludes the proof. $\qquad \square$

The subdifferential of $\mathcal{R}^{\mathrm{sp}}$ at $u^\dagger$ is given by

$$\partial \mathcal{R}^{\mathrm{sp}}(u^\dagger) = \left\{ \xi^* \in U^* : \langle \xi^*, \phi_i \rangle \in w_i q \, \mathrm{sgn}(\langle u^\dagger, \phi_i \rangle) \, |\langle u^\dagger, \phi_i \rangle|^{q-1} \right\} , \quad (3.52)$$

where sgn is the set-valued function

$$\mathrm{sgn}(x) := \begin{cases} \{-1\}, & \text{if } x < 0, \\ [-1, 1], & \text{if } x = 0, \\ \{+1\}, & \text{if } x > 0, \end{cases} \quad (3.53)$$

and $\langle \xi^*, \phi_i \rangle$ is written for the evaluation of ξ^* at ϕ_i. We emphasize that $q \, \mathrm{sgn}(x) \, |x|^{q-1} \subset \mathbb{R}$ is the subdifferential at $x \in \mathbb{R}$ of the functional $\hat{x} \mapsto |\hat{x}|^q$.

The Bregman distance of $\mathcal{R}^{\mathrm{sp}}$ at $u^\dagger \in \mathcal{D}(\mathcal{R}^{\mathrm{sp}})$ and $\xi^* \in \partial \mathcal{R}^{\mathrm{sp}}(u^\dagger)$ is

$$D_{\xi^*}(u, u^\dagger) = \sum_i w_i \, d_{\langle \xi^*, \phi_i \rangle / w_i}(\langle u, \phi_i \rangle, \langle u^\dagger, \phi_i \rangle), \qquad u \in U,$$

with

$$d_\eta(y, x) := |y|^q - |x|^q - \eta(y - x), \quad x, y \in \mathbb{R}, \eta \in q \operatorname{sgn}(x) |x|^{q-1}. \quad (3.54)$$

Note that $d_\eta(y, x)$ is the Bregman distance of $\hat{x} \mapsto |\hat{x}|^q$ at x and η. Moreover, from (3.52), it follows that $\langle \xi^*, \phi_i \rangle w_i^{-1}$ is an element of the subdifferential of $\hat{x} \mapsto |\hat{x}|^q$, whenever $\xi^* \in \partial \mathcal{R}^{\mathrm{sp}}(u^\dagger)$.

Remark 3.50. From Lemma 3.16, it follows that the Bregman domain $\mathcal{D}_B(\mathcal{R}^{\mathrm{sp}})$ is dense in $\mathcal{D}(\mathcal{R}^{\mathrm{sp}})$. However, $\mathcal{D}(\mathcal{R}^{\mathrm{sp}})$ is strictly larger than $\mathcal{D}_B(\mathcal{R}^{\mathrm{sp}})$, unless $\dim(U) < \infty$, or $q = 2$ and the weights w_i are bounded.

Indeed, assume that $\dim(U) = \infty$ and $1 \leq q < 2$. Let (c_i) be such that $\sum_i |c_i|^q < \infty$ and $\sum_i |c_i|^{2q-2} = \infty$. Such a sequence exists, because by assumption $2q - 2 < q$. Let now $u := \sum_i w_i^{-1/q} c_i \phi_i$. Because the weights w_i are bounded below and $q < 2$, it follows that $u \in U$, and by definition we have $\mathcal{R}^{\mathrm{sp}}(u) = \sum_i |c_i|^q < \infty$. Thus $u \in \mathcal{D}(\mathcal{R}^{\mathrm{sp}})$.

Now assume that $\xi^* \in \partial \mathcal{R}^{\mathrm{sp}}(u) \subset U$. Using (3.52), it follows that

$$\infty > \|\xi^*\|^2 = \sum_i w_i^2 q^2 |\langle u, \phi_i \rangle|^{2q-2} = q^2 \sum_i w_i^{2/q} c_i^{2q-2} \geq q^2 w_{\min}^{2/q} \sum_i c_i^{2q-2},$$

which contradicts the assumption that $\sum_i c_i^{2q-2} = \infty$. Consequently, it follows that $\partial \mathcal{R}^{\mathrm{sp}}(u) = \emptyset$.

Similarly, in case $q = 2$ and the weights w_i are unbounded, there exist c_i such that $\sum_i c_i^2 < \infty$ and $\sum_i w_i c_i^2 = \infty$. Again the choice $u = \sum_i w_i^{-1} c_i^2 \phi_i$ yields an element of U that lies in $\mathcal{D}(\mathcal{R}^{\mathrm{sp}})$ but not in $\mathcal{D}_B(\mathcal{R}^{\mathrm{sp}})$. ◇

Remark 3.51. In the following, we summarize some facts to be used in later results:

In the special case $q = 1$, we have

$$\mathcal{D}_B(\mathcal{R}^{\mathrm{sp}}) = \{ u \in U : \{ i : \langle u, \phi_i \rangle \neq 0 \} \text{ is finite} \},$$

$$d_\eta(y, x) = \begin{cases} |y| - \eta y, & \text{if } x = 0, \\ 2|y|, & \text{if } x \neq 0 \text{ and } \operatorname{sgn} y \neq \operatorname{sgn} x, \\ 0, & \text{if } x \neq 0 \text{ and } \operatorname{sgn} y = \operatorname{sgn} x. \end{cases}$$

For every $\xi^* \in \partial \mathcal{R}(u^\dagger)$, we have $\|\xi^*\|^2 = \sum_i |\langle \xi^*, \phi_i \rangle|^2 < \infty$. Consequently,

$$I_{\xi^*} := \{ i : |\langle \xi^*, \phi_i \rangle| \geq w_{\min} \} \quad (3.55)$$

is a finite set. Moreover, the maximum

$$m_{\xi^*} := \max \{ |\langle \xi^*, \phi_i \rangle| : i \notin I_{\xi^*} \}$$

is attained and satisfies $m_{\xi^*} < w_{\min}$. Note that $\langle u^\dagger, \phi_i \rangle = 0$ for all $i \notin I_{\xi^*}$. ◇

Below, convergence rates will be obtained under the following assumptions:

Assumption 3.52

1. F, U, V, (ϕ_i), (w_i), p, and q satisfy Assumption 3.47.
2. There exists an $\mathcal{R}^{\mathrm{sp}}$-minimizing solution $u^\dagger \in \mathcal{D}_B(\mathcal{R}^{\mathrm{sp}})$.
3. There exist $\beta_1 \in [0, 1)$, $\beta_2 \geq 0$, and $\xi^* \in \partial\mathcal{R}^{\mathrm{sp}}(u^\dagger)$, such that

$$\boxed{\langle \xi^*, u^\dagger - u \rangle \leq \beta_1 D_{\xi^*}(u, u^\dagger) + \beta_2 \left\| F(u) - F(u^\dagger) \right\|, \qquad u \in \mathcal{M}_{\alpha_{\max}}(\rho) .}$$
(3.56)

Here $\alpha_{\max}$, $\rho > 0$ are assumed to satisfy the relation $\rho > \alpha_{\max}\mathcal{R}(u^\dagger)$.

For $q = 1$, let the following additional assumptions be satisfied:

4. The operator F is Gâteaux differentiable in $u^\dagger$.
5. There exist constants γ_1, $\gamma_2 \geq 0$ such that for all $u \in \mathcal{M}_{\alpha_{\max}}(\rho)$, we have

$$\boxed{\left\| F(u) - F(u^\dagger) - F'(u^\dagger)(u - u^\dagger) \right\| \leq \gamma_1 D_{\xi^*}(u, u^\dagger) + \gamma_2 \| F(u) - F(u^\dagger) \| .}$$
(3.57)

6. The restriction of $F'(u^\dagger)$ to $U_{\xi^*} := \left\{ \sum_{i \in I_{\xi^*}} x_i \phi_i : x_i \in \mathbb{R} \right\}$ is injective. Here I_{ξ^*} is the finite set defined in (3.55).

The following auxiliary lemma is used to prove the convergence rates results for sparsity constraints.

Lemma 3.53. *Assume that $q \in (1, 2]$. Then, for every x, $y \in \mathbb{R}$, we have*

$$c_q |x - y|^2 \leq d_\eta(y, x) ,$$

where $\eta = q\,\mathrm{sgn}(x) |x|^{q-1}$ and $c_q := q(q-1)\max\{|x|, |y|\}^{q-2}/2$.

Proof. Define the function $\Phi : \mathbb{R} \to \mathbb{R}$ by $\Phi(t) := |t|^q$. For $t \neq 0$, we have $\Phi'(t) = q\,\mathrm{sgn}(t) |t|^{q-1}$ and $\Phi''(t) = q(q-1) |t|^{q-2}$. Because $q > 1$, the derivatives Φ' and Φ'' are locally integrable. Therefore, the fundamental theorem of integral calculus (see [210, Thm. 18.17]) implies

$$|y|^q = \Phi(y) = \Phi(x) + \int_x^y \Phi'(t)\, \mathrm{d}t$$

$$= \Phi(x) + \int_x^y \left(\Phi'(x) + \int_x^t \Phi''(s)\, \mathrm{d}s \right) \mathrm{d}t$$

$$= \Phi(x) + (y - x)\Phi'(x) + \int_x^y \Phi''(s)(y - s)\, \mathrm{d}s$$

$$= |x|^q + q\,\mathrm{sgn}(x) |x|^{q-1} (y - x) + q(q-1) \int_x^y |s|^{q-2} (y - s)\, \mathrm{d}s .$$

Because $q \leq 2$, it follows that

$$\int_x^y |s|^{q-2} (y - s) \, ds \geq \max\{|x|, |y|\}^{q-2} \int_x^y (y - s) \, ds$$
$$= \max\{|x|, |y|\}^{q-2}(y - x)^2/2 \, .$$

Consequently,

$$d_\eta(y, x) = q(q-1) \int_x^y |s|^{p-2} (y - s) \, ds$$
$$\geq q(q-1) \max\{|x|, |y|\}^{q-2}(y - x)^2/2 = c_q \, (y - x)^2 \, ,$$

which shows the assertion.   □

Theorem 3.42 gives rise to convergence rates with respect to the Bregman distance. Below we also verify convergence rates with respect to the Hilbert space norm.

Theorem 3.54 (Convergence rates). *Let Assumption 3.52 hold. Assume that $\alpha(\delta) \sim \delta^{p-1}$ if $p > 1$, and $\alpha(\delta) = \alpha_0$ with $0 < \alpha_0\beta_2 < 1$ if $p = 1$.*
Then

$$D_{\xi^*}(u_{\alpha(\delta)}^\delta, u^\dagger) = O(\delta), \qquad and \qquad \|F(u_{\alpha(\delta)}^\delta) - v^\delta\| = O(\delta) \, . \qquad (3.58)$$

Moreover, there exists $c > 0$, such that $\mathcal{R}(u_{\alpha(\delta)}^\delta) \leq \mathcal{R}(u^\dagger) + \delta/c$ for every δ with $\alpha(\delta) \leq \alpha_{\max}$, and

$$\begin{aligned}
\|u_{\alpha(\delta)}^\delta - u^\dagger\| &= O(\sqrt{\delta}), &\quad if \ q > 1, \\
\|u_{\alpha(\delta)}^\delta - u^\dagger\| &= O(\delta), &\quad if \ q = 1 \, .
\end{aligned} \qquad (3.59)$$

In particular, if $p = 1$ and α_0 is sufficiently small, then the method is an exact penalization method (cf. Remark 3.43).

Proof. The rates in (3.58) are an immediate consequence of Theorem 3.42.

To prove (3.59), we first consider the case $q > 1$. Lemma 3.53 and (3.58) imply that

$$\begin{aligned}
\left\|u_{\alpha(\delta)}^\delta - u^\dagger\right\|^2 &= \sum_i |\langle u_{\alpha(\delta)}^\delta - u^\dagger, \phi_i \rangle|^2 \\
&\leq c_q^{-1} \sum_i d_{\langle \xi^*, \phi_i \rangle/w_i}\left(\langle u_{\alpha(\delta)}^\delta, \phi_i \rangle, \langle u^\dagger, \phi_i \rangle \right) \\
&\leq w_{\min}^{-1} c_q^{-1} \sum_i w_i \, d_{\langle \xi^*, \phi_i \rangle/w_i}\left(\langle u_{\alpha(\delta)}^\delta, \phi_i \rangle, \langle u^\dagger, \phi_i \rangle \right) \\
&= w_{\min}^{-1} c_q^{-1} D_{\xi^*}\left(u_{\alpha(\delta)}^\delta, u^\dagger \right) = O(\delta) \, .
\end{aligned}$$

The above estimate required the fact that the coefficients $\langle u_{\alpha(\delta)}^\delta, \phi_i \rangle$ and $\langle u^\dagger, \phi_i \rangle$ are uniformly bounded, and consequently the constant c_q of Lemma 3.53 can be chosen independently of α and i.

Next we verify (3.59) for $q = 1$. By the triangle inequality,

$$\left\| u_{\alpha(\delta)}^\delta - u^\dagger \right\| \leq \left\| P_{\xi^*} \left(u_{\alpha(\delta)}^\delta - u^\dagger \right) \right\| + \left\| (I - P_{\xi^*}) \, u_{\alpha(\delta)}^\delta \right\|, \tag{3.60}$$

where

$$P_{\xi^*} : U \to U_{\xi^*}, \qquad u \mapsto \sum_{i \in I_{\xi^*}} \langle u, \phi_i \rangle \, \phi_i,$$

$$I - P_{\xi^*} : U \to U_{\xi^*}^\perp, \qquad u \mapsto \sum_{i \notin I_{\xi^*}} \langle u, \phi_i \rangle \, \phi_i,$$

denote the projections on U_{ξ^*} and $U_{\xi^*}^\perp$, respectively. From Remark 3.51, it follows that, for $i \notin I_{\xi^*}$, we have $|\langle \xi^*, \phi_i \rangle| \leq m_{\xi^*} < w_{\min} \leq w_i$ and $\langle u^\dagger, \phi_i \rangle = 0$. Therefore,

$$
\begin{aligned}
D_{\xi^*}(u_{\alpha(\delta)}^\delta, u^\dagger) &\geq \sum_{i \notin I_{\xi^*}} w_i \, d_{\langle \xi^*, \phi_i \rangle / w_i} \left(\langle u_{\alpha(\delta)}^\delta, \phi_i \rangle, \langle u^\dagger, \phi_i \rangle \right) \\
&= \sum_{i \notin I_{\xi^*}} w_i |\langle u_{\alpha(\delta)}^\delta, \phi_i \rangle| - \langle \xi^*, \phi_i \rangle \langle u_{\alpha(\delta)}^\delta, \phi_i \rangle \\
&\geq (w_{\min} - m_{\xi^*}) \sum_{i \notin I_{\xi^*}} |\langle u_{\alpha(\delta)}^\delta, \phi_i \rangle| \\
&\geq (w_{\min} - m_{\xi^*}) \left(\sum_{i \notin I_{\xi^*}} |\langle u_{\alpha(\delta)}^\delta, \phi_i \rangle|^2 \right)^{1/2}.
\end{aligned}
$$

with $w_{\min} - m_{\xi^*} > 0$. This implies that

$$\left\| (I - P_{\xi^*}) \, u_{\alpha(\delta)}^\delta \right\| = \left(\sum_{i \notin I_{\xi^*}} |\langle u_{\alpha(\delta)}^\delta, \phi_i \rangle|^2 \right)^{1/2} \leq \frac{D_{\xi^*}(u_{\alpha(\delta)}^\delta, u^\dagger)}{w_{\min} - m_{\xi^*}}. \tag{3.61}$$

The restriction of $F'(u^\dagger)$ to U_{ξ^*} is an isomorphism between the finite dimensional Hilbert spaces U_{ξ^*} and $F'(u^\dagger)U_{\xi^*}$ and thus has a bounded inverse. If we denote the norm of its inverse by $C := \left\| (F'(u^\dagger)|_{U_{\xi^*}})^{-1} \right\|$, then

$$
\begin{aligned}
\left\| P_{\xi^*}(u_{\alpha(\delta)}^\delta - u^\dagger) \right\| &\leq C \left\| F'(u^\dagger)(P_{\xi^*} u_{\alpha(\delta)}^\delta - u^\dagger) \right\| \\
&\leq C \left\| F'(u^\dagger)(u_{\alpha(\delta)}^\delta - u^\dagger) + F'(u^\dagger)(I - P_{\xi^*}) u_{\alpha(\delta)}^\delta \right\| \\
&\leq C \left(\left\| F(u_{\alpha(\delta)}^\delta) - F(u^\dagger) \right\| + \left\| F'(u^\dagger) \right\| \left\| (I - P_{\xi^*}) u_{\alpha(\delta)}^\delta \right\| \right. \\
&\qquad \left. + \left\| F(u_{\alpha(\delta)}^\delta) - F(u^\dagger) - F'(u^\dagger)(u_{\alpha(\delta)}^\delta - u^\dagger) \right\| \right).
\end{aligned}
$$

Together with (3.57) and (3.61), the above inequality implies that

$$\left\| P_{\xi^*}\left(u^{\delta}_{\alpha(\delta)} - u^{\dagger}\right)\right\| \leq C(1 + \gamma_2)\left\| F(u^{\delta}_{\alpha(\delta)}) - F(u^{\dagger})\right\|$$
$$+ C\left(\gamma_1 + \frac{\left\| F'(u^{\dagger})\right\|}{w_{\min} - m_{\xi^*}}\right) D_{\xi^*}(u^{\delta}_{\alpha(\delta)}, u^{\dagger}). \quad (3.62)$$

Combining (3.60), (3.61), (3.62), and (3.58) concludes the proof.   □

Remark 3.55. If F is Gâteaux differentiable, we can apply Proposition 3.35 and find that (3.56) holds, if there exist $\omega^* \in V^*$ and $\gamma \geq 0$ with $\gamma \|\omega^*\| < 1$, such that

$$\left\langle F'(u^{\dagger})^{\#}\omega^*, \phi_i\right\rangle \in w_i \, q \, \mathrm{sgn}(\langle u^{\dagger}, \phi_i\rangle)\left|\langle u^{\dagger}, \phi_i\rangle\right|^{q-1}, \quad (3.63)$$

and

$$\left\| F(u) - F(u^{\dagger}) - F'(u^{\dagger})(u - u^{\dagger})\right\| \leq \gamma \sum_i w_i \, d_{\langle\xi^*, \phi_i\rangle/w_i}\left(\langle u, \phi_i\rangle, \langle u^{\dagger}, \phi_i\rangle\right),$$

for $u \in \mathcal{M}_{\alpha_{\max}}(\rho)$ with $\xi^* := F'(u^{\dagger})^{\#}\omega^*$.

   Equation (3.63) is a condition postulated in [262] to obtain convergence rates for *linear problems*.   ◇

Example 3.56 (Soft thresholding). Let $p = 2$, $q = 1$, and let $F = \mathrm{Id}$ be the identity operator. We consider minimizing

$$\mathcal{T}^{\mathrm{sp}}_{\alpha, v^{\delta}}(u) = \sum_i \left|\langle u - v^{\delta}, \phi_i\rangle\right|^2 + \alpha \sum_i w_i \left|\langle u, \phi_i\rangle\right|$$

over the Hilbert space U. Assumption 3.47 is clearly satisfied. With the parameter choice $\alpha(\delta) \sim \delta$, Theorem 3.54 implies the convergence rate

$$\left\| u^{\delta}_{\alpha(\delta)} - u^{\dagger}\right\|_2 \leq \left\| \mathrm{Id}\, u^{\delta}_{\alpha(\delta)} - v^{\delta}\right\|_2 + \left\| v^{\delta} - \mathrm{Id}\, u^{\dagger}\right\|_2 = O(\delta).$$

The unique minimizer of $\mathcal{T}^{\mathrm{sp}}_{\alpha, v^{\delta}}$ is given by

$$u^{\delta}_{\alpha} = \sum_i S_{\alpha w_i}\left(\langle v^{\delta}, \phi_i\rangle\right)\phi_i,$$

where the non-linear *soft thresholding* function $S_{\lambda} : \mathbb{R} \to \mathbb{R}$, $\lambda \geq 0$, is defined as

$$S_{\lambda}(x) = \begin{cases} x + \lambda/2, & \text{if } x \leq -\lambda/2, \\ 0, & \text{if } |x| < \lambda/2, \\ x - \lambda/2, & \text{if } x \geq \lambda/2. \end{cases} \quad (3.64)$$

In many applications, soft thresholding is used with (ϕ_i) being a wavelet basis (see [89, 135, 137]). For detailed information on wavelets and wavelet bases, see, e.g., [110, 125, 265].   ◇

L^1 Regularization

Another sparse regularization method is L^1 regularization consisting in minimizing the functional

$$\mathcal{T}^{\mathrm{SP}}_{\alpha,v^\delta}(u) := \left\| F(u) - v^\delta \right\|_V^p + \alpha \mathcal{R}^{\mathrm{SP}}(u),$$

where

$$\mathcal{R}^{\mathrm{SP}} : U \to \mathbb{R} \cup \{\infty\}, \qquad \mathcal{R}^{\mathrm{SP}}(u) := \int_\Omega w\, |Qu|.$$

Here $Q : U \to L^2(\Omega)$ is a linear isomorphism and $w : \Omega \to \mathbb{R}$ is a positive measurable function. The functional $\mathcal{T}^{\mathrm{SP}}_{\alpha,v^\delta}$ is useful for sparse reconstructions, as Qu^δ_α (with $u^\delta_\alpha = \arg\min \mathcal{T}^{\mathrm{SP}}_{\alpha,v^\delta}$) has significant domains where it is zero.

In the following, we apply the general results of Section 3.2, concerning existence (see Theorem 3.22), stability (see Theorem 3.23), convergence (see Theorem 3.26), and convergence rates (see Theorem 3.42).

We make the following assumptions:

Assumption 3.57

1. U and V are reflexive Banach spaces, and τ_U and τ_V denote the weak topologies on U and V, respectively.
2. The set $\Omega \subset \mathbb{R}^n$, $n \in \mathbb{N}$, is open.
3. $Q : U \to L^2(\Omega)$ is linear, bounded, and has a bounded inverse $Q^{-1} : L^2(\Omega) \to U$.
4. The function $w : \Omega \to \mathbb{R}$ is measurable and $w_{\inf} := \mathrm{ess\,inf}_\Omega\, w > 0$.
5. The exponent p is larger or equal to 1.
6. The operator $F : \mathcal{D}(F) \subset U \to V$ is weakly continuous and its domain $\mathcal{D}(F) \subset U$ is weakly sequentially closed.
7. The level sets $\mathcal{M}_\alpha(M)$, α, $M > 0$, are weakly sequentially pre-compact.
8. The set $\mathcal{D} := \mathcal{D}(F) \cap \mathcal{D}(\mathcal{R}^{\mathrm{SP}})$ is not empty.

Theorem 3.58. *Let F, U, V, and p satisfy Assumption 3.57. Then minimizing $\mathcal{T}^{\mathrm{SP}}_{\alpha,v^\delta}$ over $\mathcal{D}(F)$ is well-defined (in the sense of Theorem 3.22), stable (in the sense of Theorem 3.23), and convergent (in the sense of Theorem 3.26).*

Proof. In order to show the theorem, we have to verify Assumption 3.13.

We recall that $\|\cdot\|_V$ is sequentially lower semi-continuous with respect to τ_V (see Lemma 10.6).

Because $\mathcal{R}^{\mathrm{SP}}$ is convex, for proving its weak lower semi-continuity it is sufficient to show that it is lower semi-continuous (see Lemma 10.6). Let therefore (u_k) converge to u with respect to the norm topology on U. Because Q is linear and bounded, it follows that (Qu_k) strongly converges in $L^2(\Omega)$ to Qu. Therefore, after possibly passing to a subsequence, we may assume without loss of generality that (Qu_k) converges to Qu pointwise almost everywhere. Then Fatou's Lemma 9.8 implies that

$$\liminf_k \mathcal{R}^{\mathrm{SP}}(u_k) = \liminf_k \int_\Omega w\,|Qu_k|$$

$$\geq \int_\Omega \liminf_k w\,|Qu_k| = \int_\Omega w\,|Qu| = \mathcal{R}^{\mathrm{SP}}(u)\,.$$

Thus $\mathcal{R}^{\mathrm{SP}}$ is weakly sequentially lower semi-continuous on $\mathcal{D}(F) \subset U$. $\square$

Remark 3.59. The subdifferential of $\mathcal{R}^{\mathrm{SP}}$ at $u^\dagger$ is given by

$$\partial\mathcal{R}^{\mathrm{SP}}(u^\dagger) = \left\{ \xi^* \in U^* : \left(Q^\# \mathcal{J}_{L^2(\Omega)}\right)^{-1} \xi^* \in w\,\mathrm{sgn}(Qu^\dagger) \right\},$$

where sgn is the set-valued function defined in (3.53), $\mathcal{J}_{L^2(\Omega)}$ the isometric isomorphism of Theorem 8.25, and $Q^\#$ the dual adjoint of Q. Therefore, the Bregman domain of $\mathcal{R}^{\mathrm{SP}}$ is given by

$$\mathcal{D}_B(\mathcal{R}^{\mathrm{SP}}) = \left\{ u \in U : \int_{\{Qu \neq 0\}} w^2 < \infty \right\}.$$

In the case that w is essentially bounded, $\mathcal{D}_B(\mathcal{R}^{\mathrm{SP}})$ consists of all $u \in U$, where $\mathcal{L}^n\big(\{Qu \neq 0\}\big) < \infty$. $\Diamond$

Remark 3.60 (Bregman distance of $\mathcal{R}^{\mathrm{SP}}$). The Bregman distance of $\mathcal{R}^{\mathrm{SP}}$ at $u^\dagger \in \mathcal{D}(\mathcal{R}^{\mathrm{SP}})$ and $\xi^* \in U^*$ is

$$D_{\xi^*}(u, u^\dagger) = \int_\Omega w\,d_{\xi/w}(Qu, Qu^\dagger)\,,$$

where (compare with (3.54))

$$\xi := \left(Q^\# \mathcal{J}_{L^2(\Omega)}\right)^{-1} \xi^* \in w\,\mathrm{sgn}(Qu^\dagger)\,,$$

and

$$d_\eta\big(Qu, Qu^\dagger\big)(\mathbf{x}) := |Qu(\mathbf{x})| - |Qu^\dagger(\mathbf{x})| - \eta(u^\dagger(\mathbf{x}))\,Q\big(u(\mathbf{x}) - u^\dagger(\mathbf{x})\big)\,.$$

$\Diamond$

Now, in addition to Assumption 3.57, let us assume that there exists an $\mathcal{R}^{\mathrm{SP}}$-minimizing solution $u^\dagger$. Then Proposition 3.41 guarantees convergence rates and is applicable if in addition the condition (3.23) is satisfied, which reads as follows: There exist $\xi \in w\,\mathrm{sgn}(Qu^\dagger)$, $\beta_1 \in [0,1)$, and $\beta_2 \geq 0$, such that

$$\boxed{\begin{aligned} \int_\Omega \xi\,Q(u^\dagger - u) &\leq \beta_1 \int_\Omega w\,d_{\xi/w}(Qu, Qu^\dagger) \\ &\quad + \beta_2\,\big\|F(u) - F(u^\dagger)\big\|_V\,, \quad u \in \mathcal{M}_{\alpha_{\max}}(\rho)\,, \end{aligned}} \tag{3.65}$$

where $\alpha_{\max}$, $\rho > 0$ satisfy the relation $\rho > \alpha_{\max} \mathcal{R}(u^\dagger)$.

The following example is the continuous version of Example 3.61.

Example 3.61 (Continuous soft thresholding). Let $p = 2$, $U = V$, $F = \mathrm{Id}$ being the identity operator, and assume that $Q^{-1} = Q^*$. We consider minimizing

$$\mathcal{T}^{\mathrm{SP}}_{\alpha,v^\delta}(u) = \left\| u - v^\delta \right\|^2 + \alpha \int_\Omega w \, |Qu| \tag{3.66}$$

over U. Assumption 3.57 is clearly satisfied and guarantees well-posedness of minimizing $\mathcal{T}^{\mathrm{SP}}_{\alpha,v^\delta}$. Moreover, if $u^\dagger$ satisfies (3.65), then the choice $\alpha(\delta) \sim \delta$ implies the convergence rate

$$\left\| u^\delta_{\alpha(\delta)} - u^\dagger \right\| \leq \left\| \mathrm{Id}\, u^\delta_{\alpha(\delta)} - v^\delta \right\| + \delta = O(\delta)\,.$$

The assumption $Q^{-1} = Q^*$ implies that $\|u\| = \|Qu\|$, $u \in U$, and therefore the functional in (3.66) can be rewritten as

$$\mathcal{T}^{\mathrm{SP}}_{\alpha,v^\delta}(u) = \int_\Omega \left(Qu - Qv^\delta \right)^2 + \alpha w \, |Qu|\,.$$

Now one notes that minimizing $\mathcal{T}^{\mathrm{SP}}_{\alpha,v^\delta}$ decomposes into pointwise minimization of the integrand. Therefore, the unique minimizer is given by *continuous soft thresholding*

$$u^\delta_\alpha = Q^* \left(S_{\alpha w} \left(Q v^\delta \right) \right),$$

where

$$S_{\alpha w} \left(Q v^\delta \right)(\mathbf{x}) := S_{\alpha w(\mathbf{x})} \left(Q v^\delta(\mathbf{x}) \right)$$

and S_λ, $\lambda \geq 0$, is the soft thresholding function defined in (3.64). $\Diamond$

3.4 Linear Inverse Problems with Convex Constraints

In this section, we apply the theoretical results of Sections 3.1 and 3.2 to three imaging examples presented in Chapter 1. The problems we are considering can be formulated in the form (3.1), where $F := L|_{\mathcal{D}(F)}$ is the restriction of a linear operator $L : U \to V$ to the set $\mathcal{D}(F) \subset U$.

Here we make the following assumptions:

Assumption 3.62

1. U and V are Hilbert spaces.
2. $L : U \to V$ is a bounded linear operator.
3. $F := L|_{\mathcal{D}(F)}$, where $\emptyset \neq \mathcal{D}(F)$ is closed and convex.

We analyze variational regularization methods consisting in minimization of the functional

$$\mathcal{T}_{\alpha,v^\delta}(u) = \left\| F(u) - v^\delta \right\|^2 + \alpha \mathcal{R}(u) , \qquad (3.67)$$

and study the effect of different regularization terms $\mathcal{R}$. Note that the minimizers of $\mathcal{T}_{\alpha,v^\delta}$ in general depend non-linearly on v^δ, unless $\mathcal{D}(F) \subset U$ is a linear subspace and $\mathcal{R}(u)$ is a quadratic functional on U.

Let $\Omega \subset \mathbb{R}^n$ be bocL. In the remainder of this section, we denote

$$L_\Omega^p := \left\{ u \in L^p(\mathbb{R}^n) : u = 0 \text{ on } \mathbb{R}^n \setminus \Omega \right\}, \quad p \geq 1 ,$$
$$W_\Omega^{s,2} := \left\{ u \in L_\Omega^2 : u|_\Omega \in W_0^{s,2}(\Omega) \right\}, \qquad s \geq 0 .$$

The space $W_\Omega^{s,2}$ with $\langle \cdot, \cdot \rangle_{s,2}$ is a Hilbert space, see Theorem 9.41. We note that $L_\Omega^2 = W_\Omega^{0,2}$. The same spaces can be obtained by extending functions $u \in W_0^{s,2}(\Omega)$ to $\mathbb{R}^n$ setting $u(\mathbf{x}) = 0$ for $\mathbf{x} \notin \Omega$.

Quadratic Regularization

In this subsection, we consider *quadratic regularization*, where $\Omega \subset \mathbb{R}^n$, $n \in \mathbb{N}$, is bocL, and

$$U = W_\Omega^{l,2} , \qquad \mathcal{R}(u) = |u|_{l,2}^2 = \left\| \nabla^l u \right\|_2^2 , \qquad \text{for some } l \in \mathbb{N}_0 .$$

The following proposition provides existence, stability, and convergence of quadratic regularization.

Proposition 3.63 (Well-posedness). *Let Assumption 3.62 hold. Then minimization of $\mathcal{T}_{\alpha,v^\delta}$ over $\mathcal{D}(F)$ is* well-defined *(in the sense of Theorem 3.3)*, stable *(in the sense of Theorem 3.4), and* convergent *(in the sense of Theorem 3.5).*

Proof. We verify Assumption 3.1. Then the results of Section 3.1 concerning existence, stability, and convergence of minimizing $\mathcal{T}_{\alpha,v^\delta}$ can be applied. Because the operator $L : U \to V$ is bounded, it is also weakly continuous, see Lemma 8.49. The set $\mathcal{D}(F)$ is closed and convex and thus also weakly closed (Lemma 8.50). Weak closedness of $\mathcal{D}(F)$ and weak continuity of L imply that $F = L|_{\mathcal{D}(F)}$ is sequentially weakly closed. Thus Assumption 3.1 is satisfied. $\qquad \square$

Proposition 3.64 (Convergence rates). *Let Assumption 3.62 hold. In addition, we assume that there exists a minimal norm solution $u^\dagger \in \mathcal{D}(F)$ of (3.1) (with respect to $|\cdot|_{l,2}$) satisfying*

$$u^\dagger \in \operatorname{Ran}(L^*) . \qquad (3.68)$$

Then, for $\alpha \sim \delta$, we have

$$\left| u_\alpha^\delta - u^\dagger \right|_{l,2} = O(\sqrt{\delta}) \quad and \quad \left\| F(u_\alpha^\delta) - v^\delta \right\| = O(\delta) .$$

Proof. Proposition 3.63 states that minimizing $\mathcal{T}_{\alpha,v^\delta}$ over U is well-posed. Below we verify Items 2 and 3 in Assumption 3.34. According to Remark 3.14, Item 1 holds if and only if Assumption 3.1 holds, which has already been shown in the proof of Proposition 3.63. Then Theorem 3.42 applies, showing the assertion.

- The functional $\mathcal{R}$ is the squared norm on U, and thus the Bregman domain $\mathcal{D}_B(\mathcal{R})$ of $\mathcal{R}$ is equal to U (see Lemma 3.16). Therefore we have $u^\dagger \in \mathcal{D}_B(\mathcal{R})$, showing Item 2 in Assumption 3.34.
- The subdifferential of $\mathcal{R}$ at $u^\dagger$ consists of the single element $\xi^* = 2\mathcal{J}_U u^\dagger$, see Example 3.18. Equation (3.68) states that there exists $\omega \in V$, such that $2u^\dagger = L^*\omega$ and consequently

$$\langle \xi^*, u^\dagger - u \rangle_{U^*,U} = \langle L^*\omega, u^\dagger - u \rangle_U \leq \|\omega\|_V \|L(u - u^\dagger)\|_V , \quad u \in U .$$

This implies that Item 3 in Assumption 3.34 holds with $\beta_1 = 0$ and $\beta_2 = \|\omega\|_V$.

$\square$

Remark 3.65. The functional $\mathcal{R}(u) = |u|^2_{l,2}$ is Gâteaux differentiable on U. Proposition 3.38 therefore implies that if $\mathcal{D}(F) = U$, then (3.68) is equivalent to (3.23). $\diamond$

The choice $U = W^{l,2}_\Omega$, with $l \geq 1$, implies zero values of the minimizer on $\partial\Omega$, which is inappropriate in some applications. Instead, if we additionally assume that the operator L does not annihilate polynomials up to degree $l-1$, then Propositions 3.63 and 3.64 still hold true for $U = W^{l,2}(\Omega)$. This is a consequence of the following proposition.

Proposition 3.66. *Let $\mathcal{R} = |\cdot|^2_{l,2}$ denote the squared semi-norm on $U = W^{l,2}(\Omega)$ with $l \geq 1$. If the operator L satisfies $Lq \neq 0$ for all polynomials $q : \Omega \to \mathbb{R}$ of degree at most $l-1$, then the level sets $\mathcal{M}_\alpha(M) = \mathrm{level}_M(\mathcal{T}_{\alpha,v})$ are sequentially pre-compact with respect to the weak topology on U.*

Proof. Denote by $\mathcal{Q}_{l-1}$ the space of polynomials $q : \Omega \to \mathbb{R}$ of degree at most $l-1$. Because $\mathcal{Q}_{l-1}$ is a finite dimensional vector space and $L|_{\mathcal{Q}_{l-1}}$ is linear and injective, it follows that there exists $C_1 > 0$ such that

$$\|Lq\|_V \geq C_1 \|q\|_{l,2} , \quad q \in \mathcal{Q}_{l-1} .$$

Let now α, $M > 0$, and assume that (u_k) is a sequence in $\mathcal{M}_\alpha(M)$, which especially implies that $(|u_k|_{l,2})$ is bounded. There exist polynomials $q_k \in \mathcal{Q}_{l-1}$ such that

$$\int_\Omega \partial^\gamma q_k = \int_\Omega \partial^\gamma u_k , \quad |\gamma| \leq l-1, \ k \in \mathbb{N} . \tag{3.69}$$

In particular, $\tilde{u}_k := u_k - q_k \in W^{l,2}_\diamond(\Omega)$ and $|\tilde{u}_k|_{l,2} = |u_k|_{l,2}$. Therefore $(\tilde{u}_k)$ is a bounded sequence in $W^{l,2}_\diamond(\Omega)$. Consequently, it follows from Theorem 9.42 that

$$\|\tilde{u}_k\|_{l,2} \leq C \, |\tilde{u}_k|_{l,2} = C \, |u_k|_{l,2} \leq C_2 \,, \qquad k \in \mathbb{N} \,, \tag{3.70}$$

for a certain constant $C_2 > 0$. Moreover, it follows from (3.69) and (3.70) that

$$
\begin{aligned}
\mathcal{T}_{\alpha,v}(u_k) &= \|(L\tilde{u}_k - v) + Lq_k\|_V^2 + \alpha \mathcal{R}(\tilde{u}_k) \\
&\geq \left(\|Lq_k\|_V - \|L\tilde{u}_k - v\|_V\right)^2 \\
&\geq \|Lq_k\|_V \left(\|Lq_k\|_V - 2\|L\tilde{u}_k - v\|_V\right) \\
&\geq C_1 \|q_k\|_{l,2}\left(C_1 \|q_k\|_{l,2} - 2(C_2 \|L\| + \|v\|_V)\right) .
\end{aligned}
$$

Because $\left(\mathcal{T}_{\alpha,v}(u_k)\right)$ is bounded, it follows that $(\|q_k\|_{l,2})$ must be bounded by some constant C_3. Thus one concludes that

$$\|u_k\|_{l,2} \leq \|\tilde{u}_k\|_{l,2} + \|q_k\|_{l,2} \leq C_2 + C_3 \,.$$

From Corollary 8.52, it follows that (u_k) has a weakly convergent subsequence in $U = W^{l,2}(\Omega)$. $\qquad\square$

Total Variation Regularization

Let $\Omega \subset \mathbb{R}^2$ be bocL and $U = L_\Omega^2$. For regularization we use the BV^l semi-norm, $l \in \mathbb{N}$, that is, $\mathcal{R}(u) = \mathcal{R}_l(u) = \left|D^l u\right|(\mathbb{R}^2)$.

Proposition 3.67 (Well-posedness). *Let Assumption 3.62 hold. Then minimization of $\mathcal{T}_{\alpha,v^\delta}$ over U is* well-defined *(in the sense of Theorem 3.22),* stable *(in the sense of Theorem 3.23), and* convergent *(in the sense of Theorem 3.26).*

Proof. In order to apply the general results of Section 3.2 guaranteeing existence, stability, and convergence, we first have to define the necessary spaces and topologies and then have to verify Assumption 3.13.

- Let τ_U and τ_V be the weak topologies on U and V, respectively. These topologies are weaker than the norm topologies on U and V, as required in Item 1 in Assumption 3.13.
- Every norm is continuous and convex, and therefore it follows from Lemma 10.6 that $\|\cdot\|_V$ is sequentially weakly lower semi-continuous.
- As in the proof of Proposition 3.63, one shows that the operator $L|_{\mathcal{D}(F)}$ is weakly continuous and that $\mathcal{D}(F)$ is weakly closed.
- According to Proposition 10.8, the functional $\mathcal{R}_l$ is convex and lower semi-continuous on U.
- Let α, $M > 0$, and let (u_k) be a sequence in $\mathcal{M}_\alpha(M)$. Then $\left(\mathcal{R}_l(u_k)\right)$ is bounded and from Theorems 9.86 and 9.87 it follows that (u_k) is bounded with respect to $\|\cdot\|_2$. Therefore (u_k) has a subsequence that weakly converges in U (see Corollary 8.52), showing that the sets $\mathcal{M}_\alpha(M)$ are weakly sequentially pre-compact.

Therefore, Assumption 3.13 is satisfied and the assertions follow.   □

Theorem 3.26 requires the existence of a solution of (3.1) in $\mathcal{D} = \mathcal{D}(F) \cap \mathcal{D}(\mathcal{R}_l)$. Thus, for the application of the convergence result of Proposition 3.67, the existence of a solution of (3.1) with finite l-th order total variation is necessary. In the following, for the sake of simplicity of notation, we employ Convention 10.17 and consider the subdifferential $\partial \mathcal{R}_l(u)$ as a subset of L^2_Ω and not as a subset of $(L^2_\Omega)^*$.

Proposition 3.68 (Convergence rates). *Let Assumption 3.62 hold. Assume that there exist an $\mathcal{R}_l$-minimizing solution $u^\dagger \in \mathcal{D}(F) \cap \mathcal{D}_B(\mathcal{R}_l)$ of (3.1) and an element*

$$\xi \in \text{Ran}(L^*) \cap \partial \mathcal{R}_l(u^\dagger) . \tag{3.71}$$

Then, with the parameter choice $\alpha \sim \delta$, we have

$$D_\xi(u_\alpha^\delta, u^\dagger) = O(\delta) \quad \text{and} \quad \|F(u_\alpha^\delta) - v^\delta\| = O(\delta) .$$

Proof. In order to apply the convergence rates result of Theorem 3.42, we have to show that Assumption 3.34 is satisfied. We first note that Item 1 has been verified in the proof of Proposition 3.67, and Item 2 is already assumed. Because the operator F is the restriction of a bounded linear operator to a convex set, Item 3 in Assumption 3.34 follows from (3.71), see Remark 3.40.   □

Remark 3.69. If the operator L satisfies $Lq \neq 0$ for polynomials q up to degree $l - 1$, then we can choose the BV^l semi-norm as regularizing functional on $L^2(\Omega)$, and the assertions of Propositions 3.67 and 3.68 remain valid. This is a consequence of the following proposition, which is based on [1, Lemma 4.1] and [376, Prop. 3.1].   ◇

Proposition 3.70. *Let $U = L^2(\Omega)$ and $\mathcal{R}(u) = \mathcal{R}_l(u) = |D^l u| (\Omega)$ be the BV^l semi-norm. If the operator L satisfies $Lq \neq 0$ for all polynomials $q : \Omega \to \mathbb{R}$ of degree at most $l - 1$, then the level sets $\mathcal{M}_\alpha(M) = \text{level}_M(\mathcal{T}_{\alpha,v})$ are sequentially pre-compact with respect to the weak topology on $L^2(\Omega)$.*

Proof. The proof is essentially the same as for Proposition 3.66. An estimate analogous to (3.70), with the Sobolev semi-norm replaced by the BV^l semi-norm, follows from Theorem 9.86.   □

In many applications, $\text{Ran}(L^*)$ consists of smooth functions. In order to show that the convergence rates result of Proposition 3.68 is applicable, we therefore have to show that also $\partial \mathcal{R}_1(u^\dagger)$ can contain smooth elements.

Lemma 3.71. *Let $u \in C_0^1(\mathbb{R}^2)$ and set $E[u] := \{\mathbf{x} : \nabla u(\mathbf{x}) \neq 0\}$. Assume that there exists an element $\psi \in C_0^1(\mathbb{R}^2; \mathbb{R}^2)$ with $|\psi| \leq 1$ and*

$$\psi(\mathbf{x}) = -\frac{\nabla u(\mathbf{x})}{|\nabla u(\mathbf{x})|}, \qquad \mathbf{x} \in E[u] . \tag{3.72}$$

Then $\nabla \cdot (\psi) \in \partial \mathcal{R}_1(u) \subset L^2(\mathbb{R}^2)$. In particular $u \in \mathcal{D}_B(\mathcal{R}_1)$.

Proof. Because $u \in C_0^1(\mathbb{R}^2)$, there exists $r > 0$ such that $\operatorname{supp} u \subset B_r(0)$. Let $\mathbf{n}$ denote the outward unit normal to $B_r(0)$. Assume that $\boldsymbol{\psi} \in C_0^1(\mathbb{R}^2; \mathbb{R}^2)$ satisfies (3.72) and $|\boldsymbol{\psi}| \leq 1$. From (9.13), (3.72), and the assumption $\boldsymbol{\psi} \in C_0^1(\mathbb{R}^2; \mathbb{R}^2)$, it follows that

$$\int_{\mathbb{R}^2} u \, \nabla \cdot (\boldsymbol{\psi}) = - \int_{B_r(0)} \boldsymbol{\psi} \cdot \nabla u + \int_{\partial B_r(0)} u \, \mathbf{n} \cdot \boldsymbol{\psi} \, d\mathcal{H}^{n-1}$$

$$= \int_{E[u]} \frac{\nabla u}{|\nabla u|} \cdot \nabla u = \int_{E[u]} |\nabla u| = \mathcal{R}_1(u) \, .$$

Moreover, because $|\boldsymbol{\psi}| \leq 1$ and $\boldsymbol{\psi} \in C_0^1(\mathbb{R}^2; \mathbb{R}^2)$, we obtain for $w \in L^2(\mathbb{R}^2)$,

$$\int_{\mathbb{R}^2} (w - u) \, \nabla \cdot (\boldsymbol{\psi}) = \int_{\mathbb{R}^2} w \, \nabla \cdot (\boldsymbol{\psi}) - \mathcal{R}_1(u)$$

$$\leq \sup \left\{ \int_{\mathbb{R}^2} w \nabla \cdot (\boldsymbol{\phi}) : \boldsymbol{\phi} \in C_0^1(\mathbb{R}^2; \mathbb{R}^2), |\boldsymbol{\phi}| \leq 1 \right\} - \mathcal{R}_1(u) \qquad (3.73)$$

$$= \mathcal{R}_1(w) - \mathcal{R}_1(u) \, .$$

Consequently, $\nabla \cdot (\boldsymbol{\psi}) \in \partial \mathcal{R}_1(u) \subset L^2(\mathbb{R}^2)$ and, in particular, $u \in \mathcal{D}_B(\mathcal{R}_1)$. $\quad\square$

Remark 3.72. Let $u \in C_0^2(\mathbb{R}^2)$ and $\mathbf{x} \in E[u]$. From the implicit function theorem [228, Thm. 10.1], it follows that the level set $\operatorname{level}_{u(\mathbf{x})}(u)$ is locally C^2 and that $-\nabla \cdot (\boldsymbol{\psi}) (\mathbf{x})$ is the curvature of the level line $\partial \operatorname{level}_{u(\mathbf{x})}(u)$ at $\mathbf{x}$, see Lemma 9.30. $\qquad\qquad\qquad\qquad\qquad\qquad\qquad\qquad\qquad\qquad\qquad\qquad\quad\Diamond$

The following example shows that there exist functions u, for which we can find $\boldsymbol{\psi} \in C_0^\infty(\mathbb{R}^2; \mathbb{R}^2)$ satisfying the assumptions of Lemma 3.71.

Example 3.73. Consider the mollifier $\rho \in C_0^\infty(\mathbb{R}^2)$ defined in (9.19). Let a, μ be positive numbers, and let $\mathbf{x}_0 \in \mathbb{R}^2$. Then $u := \chi_{B_{a+\mu}(\mathbf{x}_0)} * \rho_\mu$ and $\operatorname{supp}(u) = \overline{B_{a+2\mu}(\mathbf{x}_0)}$. Here ρ_μ is as in Definition 9.51.

If we write $u(\mathbf{x}) = f(|\mathbf{x} - \mathbf{x}_0|)$, then f is equal to 1 on $[0, a]$, is strictly decreasing on $(a, a + 2\mu)$, and vanishes for $r \geq a + 2\mu$. From the chain rule it follows that

$$\nabla u(\mathbf{x}) = \frac{\mathbf{x} - \mathbf{x}_0}{|\mathbf{x} - \mathbf{x}_0|} f'(|\mathbf{x} - \mathbf{x}_0|), \qquad \mathbf{x} \neq \mathbf{x}_0 \, .$$

In particular,

$$\frac{\nabla u(\mathbf{x})}{|\nabla u(\mathbf{x})|} = \frac{\mathbf{x} - \mathbf{x}_0}{|\mathbf{x} - \mathbf{x}_0|}, \qquad \mathbf{x} \in E[u] \, ,$$

where $E[u] = \{\mathbf{x} : |\mathbf{x} - \mathbf{x}_0| \in (a, a + 2\mu)\}$ is as in Lemma 3.71. Let $g \in C_0^\infty(\mathbb{R}_{>0})$ be such that $|g| \leq 1$ and $g(r) = 1$ for $r \in (a, a + 2\mu)$ (such a function can for instance be constructed by convolution of a characteristic function with a mollifier). Then the vector field $\boldsymbol{\psi}$, defined by

$$\psi(\mathbf{x}) := \begin{cases} -\dfrac{\mathbf{x} - \mathbf{x}_0}{|\mathbf{x} - \mathbf{x}_0|} \, g(|\mathbf{x} - \mathbf{x}_0|), & \text{if } \mathbf{x} \in \mathbb{R}^2 \setminus \{\mathbf{x}_0\}, \\ 0, & \text{if } \mathbf{x} = \mathbf{x}_0, \end{cases}$$

satisfies $|\psi| \leq 1$ and (3.72). Consequently, Lemma 3.71 implies that

$$\xi := \nabla \cdot (\psi) \in \partial \mathcal{R}_1(u)$$

and, in particular, $u \in \mathcal{D}_B(\mathcal{R}_1)$.   ◇

In the results above, we have constructed $u \in C_0^1(\mathbb{R}^2)$ for which $\partial \mathcal{R}_1(u)$ contains smooth elements. The following example provides a discontinuous function u, for which $C_0^\infty(\mathbb{R}^2) \cap \partial \mathcal{R}_1(u) \neq \emptyset$.

Example 3.74. Let u denote the characteristic function of an open and bounded set $D \subset \mathbb{R}^2$ with C^∞ boundary ∂D. The outward unit normal $\mathbf{n}$ can be extended to a compactly supported C^∞ vector field ψ with $|\psi| \leq 1$. Then $\nabla \cdot (\psi) \in C_0^\infty(\mathbb{R}^2)$, and from the Gauss–Green Theorem 9.31 it follows that

$$\int_{\mathbb{R}^2} u \, \nabla \cdot (\psi) = \int_D \nabla \cdot (\psi) = \int_{\partial D} \psi \cdot \mathbf{n} \, d\mathcal{H}^{n-1} = \int_{\partial D} d\mathcal{H}^{n-1} = \mathcal{R}_1(u).$$

As for (3.73) one shows that $\int_{\mathbb{R}^2} (w - u) \, \nabla \cdot (\psi) \leq \mathcal{R}_1(w) - \mathcal{R}_1(u)$ for $w \in L^2(\mathbb{R}^2)$. Therefore

$$\xi := \nabla \cdot (\psi) \in \partial \mathcal{R}_1(u) \cap C_0^\infty(\mathbb{R}^2; \mathbb{R}^2)$$

and, in particular, $u \in \mathcal{D}_B(\mathcal{R}_1)$.   ◇

In the following, we analyze regularization methods for solving three linear inverse problems with convex constraints introduced in Chapter 1.

Reconstruction from Chopped and Nodded Images

The first concrete case example we consider is Problem 1.1, which consists in reconstructing an image from chopped and nodded data. This problem has been considered before in [50–52].

We assume that $\Omega \subset \mathbb{R}^2$ is bocL. For $\mathbf{h} \in \mathbb{R}^2$, let

$$D_{\mathbf{h}} : L^2(\mathbb{R}^2) \to L^2(\mathbb{R}^2),$$
$$u \mapsto (D_{\mathbf{h}} u)(\mathbf{x}) := 2u(\mathbf{x}) - u(\mathbf{x} + \mathbf{h}) - u(\mathbf{x} - \mathbf{h}), \qquad \mathbf{x} \in \mathbb{R}^2,$$

denote the second-order finite difference operator in direction $\mathbf{h}$. If $\Omega \subset \mathbb{R}^2$ denotes the section of the sky under observation, then the observed data are given by $(D_{\mathbf{h}} u)|_\Omega$.

We recall the data presented in Section 1.2: Figure 1.5 shows an intensity function u and simulated chopped and nodded data v, which in addition are distorted by Gaussian noise.

We consider solving the operator equation $Lu = v$, where

$$L : U \to L^2(\Omega), \qquad u \mapsto (D_{\mathbf{h}}\, u)\,|_\Omega\,,$$

and analyze two regularization methods for its stable solution:

- $W^{1,2}$ regularization: We take $U = W_\Omega^{1,2}$, $\mathcal{R}(u) = |u|_{1,2}^2$, and $\mathcal{D}(F) :=$ $\{u \in U : u \geq 0\}$.
- BV regularization: We take $U = L_\Omega^2$ and $\mathcal{R} = \mathcal{R}_1$, the total variation semi-norm of functions on $\mathbb{R}^n$, and $\mathcal{D}(F) := \{u \in U : u \geq 0\}$.

The choice of $\mathcal{D}(F)$ takes into account that an image u represents intensities recorded by CCD sensors (see [40, 223, 359]) and therefore is a non-negative function.

The chopping and nodding operator $D_{\mathbf{h}}$ is linear and bounded, and $\mathcal{D}(F)$ is convex and closed in U. Therefore Assumption 3.62 is satisfied, and hence Propositions 3.63 and 3.67 can be applied:

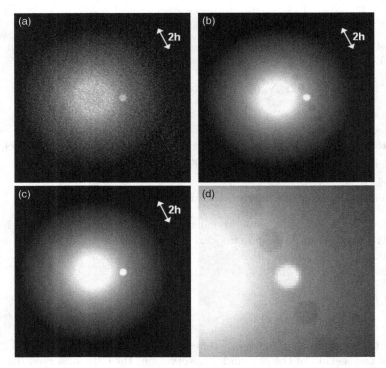

Fig. 3.2. Reconstructed data. (**a**) Reconstruction without regularization; (**b**) $W^{1,2}$ regularization; (**c**) BV regularization; (**d**) magnification of the ghosts, i.e., negative counterparts of the spot of high intensity, which show up in the $W^{1,2}$ reconstruction. The white arrows in the images indicate the double chopping throw $2\mathbf{h}$.

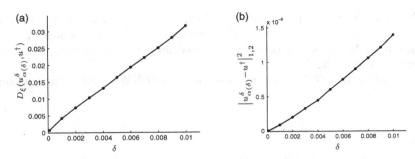

Fig. 3.3. Convergence study for the reconstruction from chopped and nodded data. (a) Bregman distance for BV regularization; (b) residual for $W^{1,2}$ reconstruction. The numerical results support the convergence rates stated in Propositions 3.64 and 3.68, respectively.

Proposition 3.75 (Well-posedness). *Minimizing T_{α,v^δ} is well-defined, stable, and convergent for $W^{1,2}$ and BV regularization.*

Note that for the convergence result, the existence of a solution $u^\dagger$ with finite energy $\mathcal{R}(u)$ is required.

Figure 3.2 shows different reconstructions with the data represented in Fig. 1.5. The numerical solution without regularization is the top left image in Fig. 3.2. The noise in the data is significantly amplified in the reconstruction, showing the ill-conditioning of the discretized problem. The numerical result of $W^{1,2}$ regularization is shown in Fig. 3.2, top right. In the reconstruction, *ghosts* (as described in [51]) appear near the spot of high intensity, which can be better recognized in the magnification of the reconstructed image, Fig. 3.2, bottom right. BV regularization provides a numerical solution without ghosts, see Fig. 3.2, bottom left.

A convergence study is shown in Fig. 3.3. We have added noise of different amount δ to the numerically simulated data and have chosen the regularization parameter $\alpha(\delta) = c\delta$. Then, the error between $u^\dagger$ and the reconstruction $u^\delta_{\alpha(\delta)}$ is plotted as a function of δ. For BV regularization, the error is measured in terms of the Bregman distance between $u^\dagger$ and $u^\delta_{\alpha(\delta)}$ (according to Definition 3.15), see Fig. 3.3, left, and for $W^{1,2}$ regularization it is measured with respect to $|\cdot|^2_{1,2}$, see Fig. 3.3, right. The experimental results indicate the convergence rates stated in Propositions 3.64 and 3.68.

Inpainting

As described in Chapter 1, the task of inpainting is to fill in information into a data set such that it nicely aligns with the neighborhood.

We denote by $\emptyset \neq \Omega_I$ a compactly supported subset of Ω. We refer to Ω_I as the *inpainting domain*, which is assumed to be bocL. Image data v^δ are given on $\Omega \backslash \Omega_I$ and have to be extended onto Ω_I, where image data are missing or not available.

In mathematical terms, the problem of inpainting is stated as the equation

$$Lu = v\,,$$

where

$$L : U \subset L^2(\Omega) \to L^2(\Omega \setminus \Omega_I)\,, \qquad L(u) = u|_{\Omega \backslash \Omega_I}\,.$$

We make different model assumptions on functional properties of u in the inpainting domain, which are reflected by the assumption $u \in W^{l,2}(\Omega)$ or $u \in BV^l(\Omega)$, $l \in \mathbb{N}$. The model assumptions constitute certain *a priori* knowledge on the data in the inpainting domain. The smoother the function in the inpainting domain should look like, the higher the order of the Sobolev or BV space that should be chosen.

For inpainting, we minimize (3.67) in the following situations:

- $W^{l,2}$ inpainting: $U = W^{l,2}(\Omega)$ and $\mathcal{R}(u) = |u|_{l,2}^2$, $l \in \mathbb{N}$.
- BV^l inpainting: $U = L^2(\Omega)$ and $\mathcal{R}(u) = \mathcal{R}_l(u) = |D^l u|\,(\Omega)$, $l \in \mathbb{N}$, the BV^l semi-norm.

The regularized solution u_α^δ provides data in the inpainting domain, and outside it approximates the data v^δ. Use of the BV semi-norm regularization for inpainting has been studied in [97].

Theorem 3.76 (Well-posedness). *Minimizing $\mathcal{T}_{\alpha,v^\delta}$ is well-defined, stable, and convergent for $W^{l,2}$ and BV^l regularization.*

Proof. Let U and $V = L^2(\Omega \setminus \Omega_I)$ be equipped with their weak topologies. In the proof of Proposition 3.67, it has already been shown that $\|\cdot\|_V$ is weakly sequentially lower semi-continuous. The weak continuity of F and the weak closedness of $\mathcal{D}(F)$ have been shown in the proof of Proposition 3.63.

For $W^{l,2}$ inpainting, the functional $\mathcal{R}$ is convex and lower semi-continuous, according to Proposition 10.7. Lemma 10.6 then implies the weak lower semi-continuity of $\mathcal{R}$. Because $Lq = q|_{\Omega_I} \neq 0$ for all polynomials $q \neq 0$, the weak sequential pre-compactness of the level sets $\mathcal{M}_\alpha(M) = \text{level}_M(\mathcal{T}_{\alpha,v})$ follows from Proposition 3.66.

For BV^l inpainting, the lower semi-continuity of $\mathcal{R}$ follows from Proposition 10.8 and Lemma 10.6, and the weak sequential pre-compactness of the level sets follows from Proposition 3.70.

Therefore Assumptions 3.13 are verified, and the results of Theorems 3.22 (existence), 3.23 (stability), and 3.26 (convergence) hold.   □

Remark 3.77. The $\mathcal{R}$-minimizing solution $u^\dagger$ in Theorem 3.76 has minimal $\mathcal{R}$ energy under all functions u in U that satisfy

$$u = v \quad \text{a.e. on } \Omega \setminus \Omega_I \, .$$

For $W^{1,2}$ inpainting, the $\mathcal{R}$-minimizing solution satisfies

$$u^\dagger = \arg\min \left\{ \int_\Omega |\nabla u|^2 : u = v \text{ a.e. on } \Omega \setminus \Omega_I \right\} \, .$$

It is well-known that in this case $u^\dagger$ is the solution of Laplace's equation on Ω_I with Dirichlet boundary conditions $u^\dagger = v$ on $\partial \Omega_I$. Therefore, $u^\dagger$ is also called *harmonic inpainting*. Analogously, one sees that the $\mathcal{R}$-minimizing solution of $W^{2,2}$ inpainting can be characterized as solution of the biharmonic equation with corresponding boundary conditions.

For BV inpainting, it follows that the $\mathcal{R}$-minimizing solution $u^\dagger$ is given by

$$u^\dagger = \arg\min \{ |Du| \, (\Omega) : u = v \text{ a.e. on } \Omega \setminus \Omega_I \} \, . \tag{3.74}$$

From (3.74), it follows that $u^\dagger$ needs not necessarily coincide with v on the boundary of Ω_I. $\diamond$

Example 3.78. Results for $W^{l,2}$ and BV^l inpainting with $l = 1, 2$ can be seen in Fig. 3.4. Because only the BV semi-norm allows for discontinuities on sets with positive $\mathcal{H}^1$ measure, only the BV inpainting preserves the edges from the original image and creates a new edge in the inpainting domain. $\diamond$

Thermoacoustic CT and the Circular Radon Transform

Now we study variational regularization methods for solving Problem 1.5, an inverse problem of thermoacoustic CT.

The problem we consider is to solve the operator equation for the *circular Radon transform*

$$R_{\text{circ}} \, u = v \tag{3.75}$$

in a stable way, where

$$R_{\text{circ}} : L^2(\mathbb{R}^2) \to V := L^2\big(S^1 \times (0,2)\big) \, ,$$
$$u \mapsto (R_{\text{circ}} \, u)(\mathbf{z}, t) := t \int_{S^1} u(\mathbf{z} + t\boldsymbol{\omega}) \, \mathrm{d}\mathcal{H}^1(\boldsymbol{\omega}) \, . \tag{3.76}$$

Lemma 3.79. *The circular Radon transform, as defined in (3.76), is well-defined, bounded, and satisfies* $\|R_{\text{circ}}\| \leq 2\pi$.

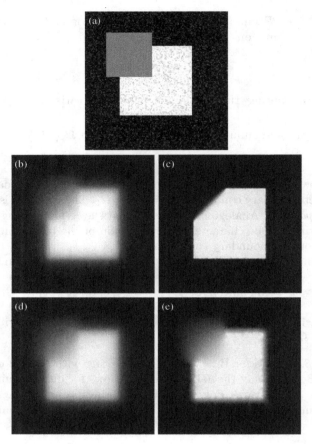

Fig. 3.4. Results of different inpainting functionals. (**a**) Noisy image to be inpainted. The gray area highlights the inpainting domain. (**b**) $W^{1,2}$ inpainting. (**c**) BV inpainting. (**d**) $W^{2,2}$ inpainting. (**e**) BV^2 inpainting.

Proof. Let $u \in L^2(\mathbb{R}^2)$. From the Cauchy–Schwarz inequality, it follows that

$$\|\mathrm{R}_{\mathrm{circ}}\, u\|^2 = \int_{S^1} \int_0^2 t^2 \left(\int_{S^1} \chi_\Omega(\mathbf{z} + t\boldsymbol{\omega}) u(\mathbf{z} + t\boldsymbol{\omega})\, \mathrm{d}\mathcal{H}^1(\boldsymbol{\omega}) \right)^2 \mathrm{d}t\, \mathrm{d}\mathcal{H}^1(\mathbf{z})$$

$$\leq \pi \int_{S^1} \int_0^2 t^2 \left(\int_{S^1} u^2(\mathbf{z} + t\boldsymbol{\omega})\, \mathrm{d}\mathcal{H}^1(\boldsymbol{\omega}) \right) \mathrm{d}t\, \mathrm{d}\mathcal{H}^1(\mathbf{z})\, .$$

In the domain of definition, the estimate $t^2 \leq 2t$ holds. This together with Fubini's Theorem 9.15 gives

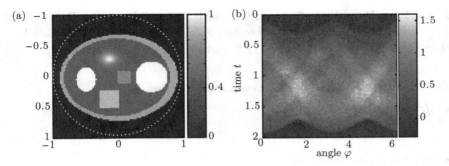

Fig. 3.5. Example of circular Radon transform data. (**a**) Phantom. (**b**) Noisy data of $(R_{circ} u)((\cos\varphi, \sin\varphi), t)$ are obtained by adding Gaussian noise with variance 5% of the maximum of $R_{circ} u$.

$$\|R_{circ} u\|^2 \leq 2\pi \int_{S^1} \left(\int_0^2 t \int_{S^1} u(\mathbf{z} + t\boldsymbol{\omega})^2 \, d\mathcal{H}^1(\boldsymbol{\omega}) \, dt \right) d\mathcal{H}^1(\mathbf{z})$$

$$= 2\pi \int_{S^1} \|u\|^2 \, d\mathcal{H}^1(\mathbf{z}) = (2\pi)^2 \|u\|^2 .$$

This shows the assertion. □

Figure 3.5 shows a density function u and the according circular Radon transform $R_{circ} u$ with Gaussian noise added. The latter are the data from which the density has to be recovered.

In order to obtain convergence rates, we will in particular make use of the Sobolev space estimate for the circular Radon transform from [315] (see also [4, Prop. 21]).

In the following, let $\Omega := B_1(0)$ and $\Omega_\varepsilon := B_{1-\varepsilon}(0)$.

Proposition 3.80 (Sobolev space estimate). *Let $\varepsilon \in (0,1)$. Then there exists a constant $C_\varepsilon > 0$, such that*

$$C_\varepsilon^{-1} \|R_{circ} u\|_2 \leq \|i^*(u)\|_{1/2,2} \leq C_\varepsilon \|R_{circ} u\|_2 , \quad u \in L^2_{\Omega_\varepsilon} , \tag{3.77}$$

where i^* is the adjoint of the embedding $i : W_\Omega^{1/2,2} \to L^2_\Omega$.

Note that the $W^{-1/2,2}$ norm of a function $u \in L^2_{\Omega_\varepsilon}$, considered as a functional on $W_\Omega^{1/2,2}$, equals $\|i^*(u)\|_{1/2,2}$.

The constant C_ε in (3.77) depends on ε, and no estimate of the form (3.77) is known that holds uniformly for all $u \in L^2_\Omega$.

Proposition 3.81. *For every $\varepsilon \in (0,1)$, we have*

$$\mathrm{Ran}(R^*_{circ}) \cap L^2_{\Omega_\varepsilon} = W_{\Omega_\varepsilon}^{1/2,2} .$$

Proof. From Proposition 3.80 and Corollary 8.32, it follows that $\mathrm{Ran}(\mathrm{R}^*_{\mathrm{circ}}) \cap L^2_{\Omega_\varepsilon} = \mathrm{Ran}((i^*)^*) \cap L^2_{\Omega_\varepsilon}$. From Lemma 8.28, it follows that $(i^*)^* = i$. This shows that $\mathrm{Ran}(\mathrm{R}^*_{\mathrm{circ}}) = \mathrm{Ran}(i) \cap L^2_{\Omega_\varepsilon}$, which proves the assertion. □

We consider three types of variational regularization methods:

- L^2 regularization: Let

$$U = L^2_\Omega, \quad \mathcal{R}(u) = \|u\|^2_2, \text{ and } L = \mathrm{R}_{\mathrm{circ}}.$$

- $W^{1,2}$ regularization: Let

$$U = W^{1,2}_\Omega, \quad \mathcal{R}(u) = |u|^2_{1,2}, \text{ and } L = \mathrm{R}_{\mathrm{circ}} \circ j,$$

  where j is the embedding $j : W^{1,2}_\Omega \to L^2_\Omega$.

- BV regularization: Let

$$U = L^2_\Omega, \quad \mathcal{R}(u) = \mathcal{R}_1(u), \text{ and } L = \mathrm{R}_{\mathrm{circ}}.$$

Proposition 3.82 (Well-posedness). *Minimizing* $\mathcal{T}_{\alpha,v^\delta}$ *is well-defined, stable, and convergent for* L^2, $W^{1,2}$, *and* BV *regularization.*

Proof. The circular Radon transform L is linear and bounded. Therefore Assumption 3.62 is satisfied, and hence Propositions 3.63 and 3.67 can be applied and guarantee well-posedness. □

According to Proposition 3.80, the solution $u^\dagger$ of (3.75), provided it exists and has compact support in Ω, is unique. The convergence result for BV regularization requires that the unique solution $u^\dagger$ of (3.75) is an element of $\mathcal{D}(\mathcal{R}_1)$.

Proposition 3.83 (Convergence rates). *Let* $\varepsilon \in (0,1)$ *and* $u^\dagger$ *be the solution of* (3.75). *Then we have the following convergence rates result:*

1. L^2 *regularization: If* $u^\dagger \in W^{1,2}_{\Omega_\varepsilon}$, *then*

$$\left\| u^\delta_{\alpha(\delta)} - u^\dagger \right\|^2_2 = O(\delta) \qquad \text{for } \alpha(\delta) \sim \delta.$$

2. $W^{1,2}$ *regularization: If* $u^\dagger \in j^*\big(W^{1/2,2}_{\Omega_\varepsilon}\big)$, *then*

$$\left| u^\delta_{\alpha(\delta)} - u^\dagger \right|^2_{1,2} = O(\delta) \qquad \text{for } \alpha(\delta) \sim \delta. \tag{3.78}$$

  Note that $w = j^*(v)$ *solves the Dirichlet problem* $-\Delta w = v$ *on* Ω, *and* $w = 0$ *on* $\mathbb{R}^2 \setminus \Omega$.

3. BV *regularization: If* $\xi \in \partial\mathcal{R}_1(u^\dagger) \cap W^{1/2,2}_{\Omega_\varepsilon}$, *then*

$$D_\xi(u^\delta_{\alpha(\delta)}, u^\dagger) = O(\delta) \qquad \text{for } \alpha(\delta) \sim \delta.$$

  Here D_ξ *is the Bregman distance of* $\mathcal{R}_1$ *at* u *and* ξ.

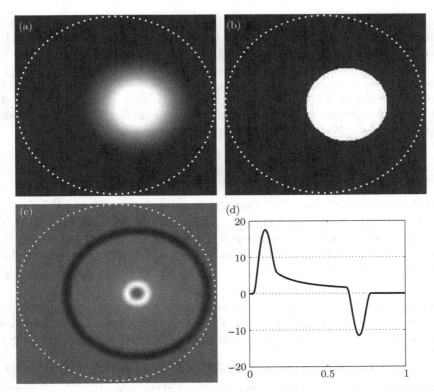

Fig. 3.6. (a) Density functions for Example 3.84. (b) Density functions for Example 3.85. (c) Element $\xi \in \partial \mathcal{R}_1(u^\dagger)$ that is considered for the convergence rate studies shown in Fig. 3.9. (d) Radial profile of ξ with respect to $(0.2, 0)$.

Proof. From Proposition 3.81, it follows that $W_{\Omega_\varepsilon}^{1/2,2} \subset \mathrm{Ran}(\mathrm{R}_{\mathrm{circ}}^*)$. Therefore Propositions 3.64 and 3.68 imply the rates stated in (3.78). $\qquad\square$

In the following numerical experiments, we compare the results of minimizing $\mathcal{T}_{\alpha,v^\delta}$ using L^2, $W^{1,2}$, and BV regularization. In all examples, data v^δ have been generated by adding Gaussian noise to the simulated data $\mathrm{R}_{\mathrm{circ}}\, u$.

In the first two examples (phantoms shown in Fig. 3.6), the convergence rates conditions of Proposition 3.83 are checked analytically. Moreover, numerical experiments are performed to support the theoretical results. There we use the parameter choice

$$\alpha(\delta) = \begin{cases} 4\,\delta, & \text{for } L^2 \text{ regularization}, \\ \delta/4, & \text{for } W^{1,2} \text{ regularization}, \\ \delta/200, & \text{for } BV \text{ regularization}. \end{cases} \qquad (3.79)$$

The last test example concerns reconstructing the phantom shown in Fig. 3.5.

Example 3.84 (Reconstruction of a C^∞ function). We use $u^\dagger = u$, which is the density function of Example 3.73 with the parameters $\mathbf{x}_0 = (0.2, 0)$, $a = 0.1$, and $\mu = 0.3$.

As shown in Example 3.73, there exists an element $\xi \in C_\Omega^\infty(\mathbb{R}^2) \cap \partial\mathcal{R}_1(u^\dagger)$. The functions $u^\dagger$ and ξ are depicted in Fig. 3.6. Because $u^\dagger$ is an element of each of the spaces L_Ω^2 and $W_\Omega^{1,2}$ (in other words, there exists a solution of the operator equation in U), well-posedness of minimizing $\mathcal{T}_{\alpha,v^\delta}$ follows from Proposition 3.82. Moreover, the inclusion

$$\xi \in j^*(W_\Omega^{1/2,2}) \subset W_\Omega^{1/2,2}$$

and Proposition 3.83 imply the convergence rate $\left|u_{\alpha(\delta)}^\delta - u^\dagger\right|_{l,2}^2 = O(\delta)$ for L^2 and $W^{1,2}$ regularization, and $D_\xi(u_{\alpha(\delta)}^\delta, u^\dagger) = O(\delta)$ for BV regularization.

Numerical results of minimizing $\mathcal{T}_{\alpha,v^\delta}$ with $\delta = 0.15$ are depicted in Fig. 3.7. The value $\delta = 0.15$ corresponds to approximately 10% noise in the data, that is, $\delta \approx \|\mathrm{R}_{\mathrm{circ}}\, u^\dagger\|_2/10$.   ◇

Example 3.85 (Reconstruction of a characteristic function). Let $u^\dagger := \chi_D$ be the density function of Example 3.74, with D being the open disk with radius 0.4 centered at $(0.2, 0)$. As shown in Example 3.74, there exists $\xi \in \partial\mathcal{R}_1(u^\dagger) \cap C_\Omega^\infty(\mathbb{R}^2)$.

Then, minimizing $\mathcal{T}_{\alpha,v^\delta}$ is well-defined and stable for L^2, $W^{1,2}$, and BV regularization. The function $u^\dagger$ is not contained in the space $W_\Omega^{1/2,2}$ and therefore neither the convergence result for $W^{1,2}$ nor the convergence rates result for L^2 regularization are applicable. The relation

$$\xi \in C_\Omega^\infty(\mathbb{R}^2) \subset W_\Omega^{1/2,2}$$

and Proposition 3.83 imply the convergence rate $D_\xi(u_{\alpha(\delta)}^\delta, u^\dagger) = O(\delta)$ for BV regularization. Numerical results of minimizing $\mathcal{T}_{\alpha,v^\delta}$ with $\delta = 0.15$, corresponding to 10% noise, are depicted in Fig. 3.8.   ◇

Figure 3.9 depicts the the differences between the reconstructions and the exact solution in dependence of δ, for the phantoms of Examples 3.84 and 3.85. The regularization parameter is chosen according to (3.79).

Example 3.86. The last test example concerns the reconstruction of a density function consisting of a superposition of characteristic functions and one smooth function. The phantom is depicted in Fig. 3.5, and the obtained reconstructions from noisy data with $\delta = 0.22$ using different regularization methods are depicted in Fig. 3.10. The value $\delta = 0.22$ corresponds to approximately 8% noise in the data.   ◇

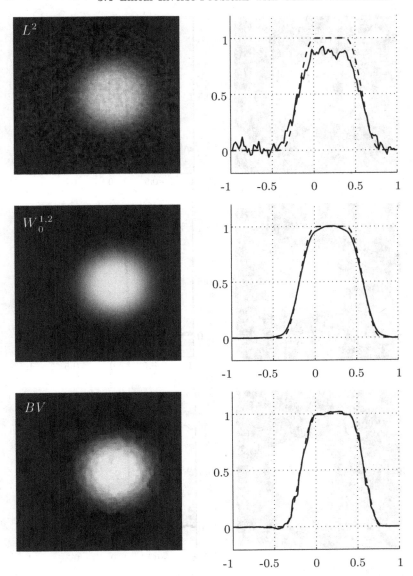

Fig. 3.7. Reconstruction of a C^∞ function from distorted data with 10% noise. *Left:* Reconstructed densities. *Right:* Profiles of density function and reconstructions along the horizontal center line.

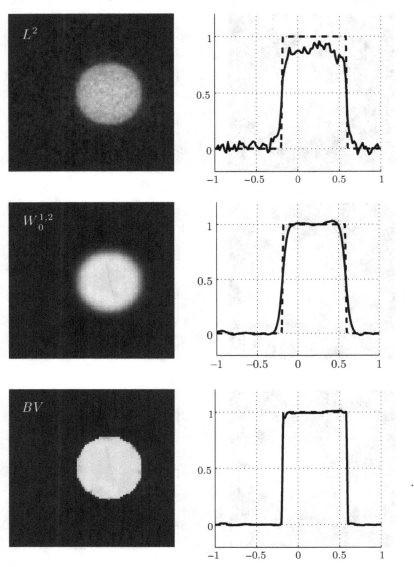

Fig. 3.8. Reconstruction of a characteristic function of a disk from distorted data with 10% noise. *Left:* Reconstructed densities. *Right:* Profiles of density function and reconstructions along the horizontal center line.

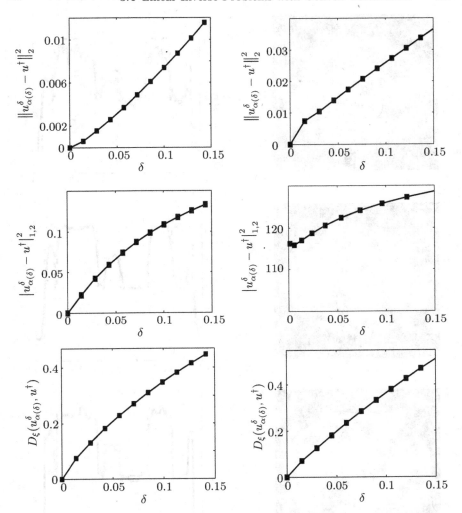

Fig. 3.9. Convergence study for the C^∞ function of Example 3.84 (*left*) and the characteristic function of Example 3.85 (*right*). *Top*: L^2 regularization. Note that for the characteristic function we have convergence, but no convergence rate. *Middle*: $W^{1,2}$ regularization. In the case of the characteristic function, no convergence can be shown. *Bottom*: BV regularization.

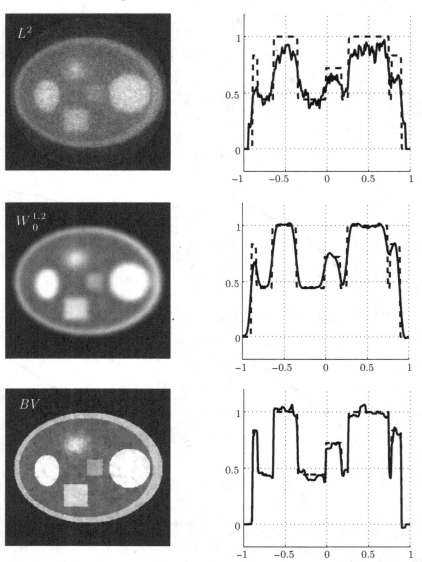

Fig. 3.10. Reconstruction from noisy data of the phantom depicted in Fig. 3.5. *Left*: Reconstructions for L^2, $W^{1,2}$, and BV regularization. *Right*: Profiles of phantom and reconstruction along the horizontal center line.

3.5 Schlieren Tomography

In the following, we consider Problem 1.8, consisting in reconstructing a function from squared linear projections. This is an example of a non-linear inverse problem.

The following notations will hold throughout this section: $\Omega := B_1(0)$ and $\Sigma := S^1 \times (-1, 1)$. For $\mathbf{n} \in S^1$, denote by $\mathbf{n}^\perp$ a unit vector satisfying $\mathbf{n} \cdot \mathbf{n}^\perp = 0$.

The *schlieren transform* S is a composition of the (linear) Radon transform (considered as an operator from L_Ω^4 to $L^4(\Sigma)$)

$$(R_{\text{line}} u)(\mathbf{n}, r) := \int_{\mathbb{R}} u(r\mathbf{n} + s\mathbf{n}^\perp) \, ds, \quad \mathbf{n} \in \Sigma,$$

and the quadratic operator

$$Q : L^4(\Sigma) \to L^2(\Sigma), \qquad Q v = v^2,$$

mapping a function $v \in L^4(\Sigma)$ to its pointwise square v^2, that is,

$$S : L_\Omega^4 \to L^2(\Sigma), \qquad S u = (Q \circ R_{\text{line}}) u = (R_{\text{line}} u)^2. \tag{3.80}$$

Lemma 3.87. *The schlieren transform as defined in (3.80) is well-defined and continuous with respect to the norm topologies on L_Ω^4 and $L^2(\Sigma)$.*

Proof. It is sufficient to show that R_{line} and Q are well-defined and continuous with respect to the norm topologies. Then $S = Q \circ R_{\text{line}}$ is well-defined and continuous, too.

The fact that Q is well-defined follows from the identity $\|Q v\|_2^2 = \int_\Sigma v^4 = \|v\|_4^4$. Moreover, the Cauchy–Schwarz inequality implies that

$$\|Q(v + h) - Q v\|_2^2 = \left(\int_\Sigma (2vh + h^2)^2 \right)^2$$
$$= \left(\int_\Sigma h^2 (2v + h)^2 \right)^2 \leq \|h\|_4^4 \int_\Sigma (2v + h)^4, \quad v, h \in L^4(\Sigma).$$

For $\|h\|_4 \to 0$, the right-hand side in the above inequality goes to zero, showing that Q is continuous at $v \in L^4(\Sigma)$.

It remains to verify that R_{line} is well-defined and continuous. To that end, let $u \in L_\Omega^4$. From the Cauchy–Schwarz inequality and Fubini's Theorem 9.15, it follows that

$$\|R_{\text{line}} u\|_4^4 = \int_{S^1} \int_{-1}^1 \left(\int_{\mathbb{R}} \chi_\Omega(r\mathbf{n} + s\mathbf{n}^\perp) u(r\mathbf{n} + s\mathbf{n}^\perp) \, ds \right)^4 dr \, d\mathcal{H}^1(\mathbf{n})$$
$$\leq 4 \int_{S^1} \int_{-1}^1 \left(\int_{\mathbb{R}} \chi_\Omega(r\mathbf{n} + s\mathbf{n}^\perp) u^2(r\mathbf{n} + s\mathbf{n}^\perp) \, ds \right)^2 dr \, d\mathcal{H}^1(\mathbf{n})$$
$$\leq 8 \int_{S^1} \left(\int_{\mathbb{R}} \int_{\mathbb{R}} u^4(r\mathbf{n} + s\mathbf{n}^\perp) \, ds \, dr \right) d\mathcal{H}^1(\mathbf{n}) = 16\pi \|u\|_4^4.$$

This shows that R_{line} is well-defined and continuous with respect to the norm topologies on L_Ω^4 and $L^4(\Sigma)$. $\qquad\qquad\qquad\qquad\qquad\qquad\qquad\qquad\square$

In the following, we analyze and evaluate variational regularization methods for the regularized inversion of the schlieren transform, consisting in minimization of $\mathcal{T}_{\alpha,v^\delta}$ (as defined in (3.7)), where $\mathcal{R}$ is either the squared Sobolev semi-norm $|\cdot|_{1,2}^2$ or the BV semi-norm $\mathcal{R}_1$.

- For $W^{1,2}$ regularization, we minimize $\mathcal{T}_{\alpha,v^\delta}$ with

$$F = \mathrm{S} \circ i : W_\Omega^{1,2} \to L^2(\Sigma)\,,$$

  $\mathcal{R}(u) = |u|_{1,2}^2$ and $i : W_\Omega^{1,2} \to L_\Omega^4$. According to Theorem 9.39, i is bounded.
- For BV regularization, we minimize $\mathcal{T}_{\alpha,v^\delta}$ with

$$F = \mathrm{S}\,|_{\mathcal{D}(F)} : \mathcal{D}(F) \subset L_\Omega^4 \to L^2(\Sigma)$$

  and $\mathcal{R} = \mathcal{R}_1$ over $\mathcal{D}(F) := \left\{u \in L_\Omega^4 : \|u\|_\infty < C\right\}$. Here $C > 0$ is a fixed constant.

Proposition 3.88 (Quadratic regularization). *Minimizing $\mathcal{T}_{\alpha,v^\delta}$ with $F = \mathrm{S} \circ i$ and $\mathcal{R}(u) = |u|_{1,2}^2$ is well-defined (in the sense of Theorem 3.3), stable (in the sense of Theorem 3.4), and convergent (in the sense of Theorem 3.5).*

Proof. It suffices to show that F is weakly closed. Then Assumption 3.1 is satisfied and allows application of the results of Section 3.1 concerning well-posedness of minimizing $\mathcal{T}_{\alpha,v^\delta}$.

The Sobolev space estimate for the linear Radon transform (see, e.g., [288, Chap. II, Thm. 5.1]) implies that

$$R_{\text{line}} : W_\Omega^{1,2} \to W_0^{1,2}(\Sigma)\,,$$

where $W_0^{1,2}(\Sigma) = W_0^{1,2}\big(S^1 \times (-1,1)\big)$ is the periodic Sobolev space of first order, is compact and therefore weakly-strongly continuous. The embedding of $W_0^{1,2}(\Sigma)$ into $L^4(\Sigma)$ is bounded (cf. Theorem 9.38). This and the continuity of Q imply that $F = \mathrm{Q} \circ R_{\text{line}}$ is weakly-strongly continuous and, in particular, weakly closed. $\qquad\qquad\qquad\qquad\qquad\qquad\qquad\qquad\qquad\qquad\square$

Proposition 3.89 (BV regularization). *Minimization of $\mathcal{T}_{\alpha,v^\delta}$ over $\mathcal{D}(F)$ with $F := \mathrm{S}\,|_{\mathcal{D}(F)}$ and $\mathcal{R} = \mathcal{R}_1$ is well-defined (in the sense of Theorem 3.22), stable (in the sense of Theorem 3.23), and convergent (in the sense of Theorem 3.25).*

Proof. In order to apply the general results of Section 3.2 guaranteeing well-posedness of minimizing $\mathcal{T}_{\alpha,v^\delta}$, we verify Assumption 3.13 with τ_U and τ_V being the strong topologies on $U = L_\Omega^4$ and $V = L^2(\Sigma)$, respectively.

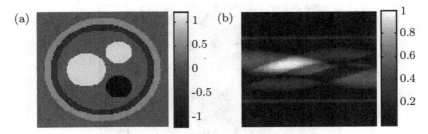

Fig. 3.11. Example of schlieren data. (a) Pressure function; (b) simulated schlieren data with 15% Gaussian noise added.

- Every norm is continuous; in particular $\|\cdot\|_V$ is sequentially lower semi-continuous. Proposition 10.8 states that the functional $\mathcal{R}_1$ is convex and lower semi-continuous.
- According to Lemma 3.87, the operator S (and therefore $F = \mathrm{S}\,|_{\mathcal{D}(F)}$) is continuous with respect to the topologies τ_U and τ_V. Moreover, the domain $\mathcal{D}(F)$ is closed with respect to τ_U.
- It remains to show that the level sets $\mathcal{M}_\alpha(M)$ with α, $M > 0$ are sequentially pre-compact. To that end, let (u_k) be a sequence in $\mathcal{M}_\alpha(M)$. In particular, we then have that $\sup_k \{\mathcal{R}_1(u_k)\} \leq M/\alpha$ and $u_k \in \mathcal{D}(F)$. Therefore,

$$\sup_k \{\|u_k\|_1 + \mathcal{R}_1(u_k)\} < \infty,$$

and from Lemmas 9.69 and 9.68 it follows that (u_k) has a subsequence $(u_{k'})$ that converges to some $u \in \mathcal{D}(\mathcal{R}_1)$ with respect to the L^1 norm. Consequently

$$\|u_{k'} - u\|_4^4 = \int_\Omega |u_{k'} - u|^3 \, |u_{k'} - u| \leq 8C^3 \, \|u_{k'} - u\|_1 \to 0,$$

which concludes the proof. □

Note that the convergence result of Theorem 3.26 requires the existence of a solution of (3.1) in $\mathcal{D}(\mathcal{R}_1)$, which means a solution of (3.1) with finite total variation.

Example 3.90. As a test example, we consider the reconstruction from the density function depicted in Fig. 3.11. The function u and its Radon transform $\mathrm{R}_{\text{line}}\, u$ contain negative and positive values. We added 15% Gaussian noise to the data, that is, $\|\mathrm{S}\, u - v^\delta\|_2 / \|\mathrm{S}\, u\|_2 = 0.15$.

The results of numerically minimizing $\mathcal{T}_{\alpha, v^\delta}$ for $W^{1,2}$ and BV regularization methods are depicted in Fig. 3.12.   ◇

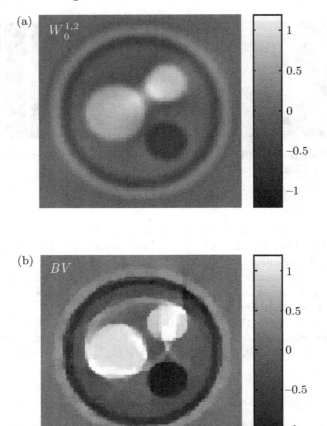

Fig. 3.12. Reconstruction of the density function depicted in Fig. 3.11. (a) $W^{1,2}$ regularization; (b) BV regularization.

3.6 Further Literature on Regularization Methods for Inverse Problems

Several authors have considered Tikhonov type regularization methods for the solution of ill-posed variational inequalities, which consist in finding $u \in U$ solving

$$\langle F(u) - v, \tilde{u} - u \rangle_{U^*, U} \geq 0, \qquad \tilde{u} \in U .$$

The basic assumption taken in this theory is that $F : U \to U^*$ is a *monotone* operator on a reflexive Banach space U.

Regularization techniques for solving variational inequalities consist in calculating u_α^δ solving

$$\langle F(u) - v^\delta + \alpha \mathcal{J}(u), \tilde{u} - u \rangle_{U^*,U} \geq 0 , \qquad \tilde{u} \in U ,$$

where $\mathcal{J}$ denotes the normalized duality mapping on U (see Definition 10.23). We refer to the recent monograph [5] and to the original references [260, 261, 285].

Very relevant for appropriate filtering are stopping criteria. Generally speaking, there are two classes of strategies for the choice of the regularization parameter, which are *a priori* and *a posteriori* strategies (see [152] for a survey). In this book, we have concentrated on *a priori* stopping criteria. The most famous *a posteriori* criterion is Morozov's discrepancy principle [277], which is understood quite well analytically. Especially for denoising, several parameter choice strategies, partially heuristically motivated, have been proposed. Especially in the computer vision area, stopping time selection criteria for diffusion filtering have been considered instead of parameter choice strategies (see, for example, [282]). In our recent work [173, 174] on stopping criteria for denoising applications, we have been concerned with exploiting the synergy with mathematical models for Bingham fluids (see [53] for an early reference on Bingham models). Thereby we have made use of analytical results in [280, 281], which allow for predicting the yield of flows. Conceptually similar results have been derived in the image processing context for total variation flow denoising, for instance in the papers [18–22, 43, 363], including a number of analytically calculated solutions.

In the context of non-linear inverse problems and flows, probably the first analysis of optimal stopping times has been given in [370].

An additional convergence rates result for Tikhonov regularization in Banach spaces has been proved in [330].

The term "inpainting" has first been used in [47]. There a purely numerical scheme was implemented, which was later shown to be related to the Navier–Stokes equations [46]. Inpainting based on different variational formulations has been investigated in a series of papers [35, 94, 96, 155, 272, 273]. Recently, there has been some research in inpainting based on sparse representation of images [91, 145, 170].

4

Convex Regularization Methods for Denoising

Variational regularization techniques are a common tool for solving *denoising* problems. We consider minimizing a scale-dependent family of functionals

$$\rho(u, u^\delta) + \alpha \mathcal{R}(u) := \int_\Omega \phi(u, u^\delta) + \alpha \int_\Omega \psi(\mathbf{x}, u, \nabla u, \ldots, \nabla^l u) \qquad (4.1)$$

with $\alpha > 0$.

Although denoising can be considered as an inverse problem and variational regularization methods for inverse problems have already been studied in Chapter 3, it is appropriate to reconsider these variational techniques from a point of view of *convex analysis*, as additional results can be derived.

Zero-Order Regularization

We call models of the form (4.1) *zero-order regularization* if ψ only depends on u, and, in general, *l-th order regularization* if l is the highest order of differentiation of u the integrand ψ depends on.

A prominent example of a zero-order regularization model is *maximum entropy regularization*, which consists in minimization of the functional

$$\mathcal{T}^{\mathrm{ME}}_{\alpha, u^\delta}(u) := \frac{1}{p} \int_{\mathbb{R}} \left| u - u^\delta \right|^p + \alpha \mathcal{R}(u)$$

over a set of non-negative functions u on $\mathbb{R}$, where

$$\mathcal{R}(u) = \begin{cases} \int_{\mathbb{R}} u \log u, & \text{if } u \geq 0 \text{ a.e., and } u \log u \in L^1(\mathbb{R}), \\ \infty, & \text{otherwise}. \end{cases}$$

We refer to [142, 154] for two references that deal with an analysis of maximum entropy regularization.

Least Squares Regularization

Regularization functionals with a fit-to-data function

$$\phi\big(\cdot, u^{\delta}(\mathbf{x})\big) := \frac{1}{2}\big(\cdot - u^{\delta}(\mathbf{x})\big)^2$$

are called *least squares* regularization methods.

Anisotropic and Isotropic Regularization

In image analysis, the gradient of an image u is a particularly important feature, as high gradients indicate edges and corners of the objects shown in the image. In the area of image processing, mainly first-order regularization models are used with the goal to penalize high gradients and thus to enforce *smooth* images.

We call a first-order regularization model *isotropic* if

$$\psi\left(\mathbf{x}, u, \nabla u\right) = \widehat{\psi}(\mathbf{x}, u, |\nabla u|) \,. \tag{4.2}$$

The terminology *isotropic* regularization method refers to the fact that the regularization term is invariant with respect to orientations of the gradient. We call first-order regularization functionals *anisotropic* if they cannot be written in the form (4.2).

Quadratic Regularization

We refer to quadratic regularization models when ψ is quadratic, that is, ψ has the form $\psi(\mathbf{x}, u, \nabla u, \dots, \nabla^l u) = \psi(\mathbf{x}, \mathbf{s}) = \mathbf{p}^T \mathbf{s} + \mathbf{s}^T Q \mathbf{s}$ with $\mathbf{p} = \mathbf{p}(\mathbf{x})$ and $Q = Q(\mathbf{x})$ positive semi-definite.

Some examples have been summarized in Table 4.1. Because variational regularization has been studied in a variety of settings such as continuous or discrete, in many cases it is almost impossible to refer to the original references. Therefore, we mention but a few that have been important to us. When references appear in the tables below, they might refer to a discrete, continuous, or semi-discrete regularization setting, thus they appear unbalanced. Of course, the primary setting of this book concerns continuous formulations. Prominent examples of convex, first-order, non-quadratic regularization functionals for denoising are summarized in Table 4.2.

Example 4.1. One important issue in image denoising is the preservation of edges, i.e., regions where the norm of the gradient of the image u becomes large. The idea is to weight ψ in dependence of ∇u: whenever $|\nabla u|$ becomes large, the regularization term should become small. Because also noise induces high gradients, it is not possible to extract edge information directly from noisy data. Instead, one pre-smoothes the data and uses the result as a guess for the true position of the edges.

Table 4.1. Isotropic versus anisotropic regularization methods. Here we use the abbreviation $\mathbf{t} := \nabla u$.

Quadratic Regularization	ψ	Note
Isotropic	$|\mathbf{t}|^2$	[328, 351, spline context]
Weighted isotropic	$\beta(\mathbf{x})|\mathbf{t}|^2$	cf. Example 4.1
Anisotropic	$\mathbf{t}^T A(\mathbf{x})\mathbf{t}$	[349]

Table 4.2. First-order regularization models. Here we use the abbreviations $\mathbf{t} := \nabla u$ and $t := |\nabla u|$, respectively.

Isotropic	$\hat{\psi}$	Note
Huber	$t \mapsto \begin{cases} t^2, & |t| \leq 1 \\ 2|t| - 1, & |t| \geq 1 \end{cases}$	[219, 250]
Rudin–Osher–Fatemi (ROF)	t	[339]
Bregman distance	$t + s(\mathbf{x})u$	[61, 62]
Weighted ROF	$\beta(\mathbf{x})t$	[106, 364]
Weighted quadratic	$\beta(\mathbf{x})t^2$	cf. Example 4.1
Bouman–Sauer	$t^\beta, \ 1 < \beta < 2$	[56]
Hyper surfaces	$\sqrt{\beta + t^2}$	[1, 54, 103, 286]
Anisotropic	ψ	
Esedoglu–Osher	$|\mathbf{t}|_p$	[308]
Anisotropic non-quadratic	$\sqrt{\mathbf{t}^T A(\mathbf{x})\mathbf{t}}$	

We consider two first-order regularization models for image denoising, which use $\nabla(\rho * u^\delta)$ for weighted regularization, where ρ is a mollifier (see Definition 9.51).

Let $\Omega \subset \mathbb{R}^2$. We define

$$g(r) := \frac{1}{1 + r^2/\lambda^2}, \qquad r \in \mathbb{R}, \tag{4.3}$$

where $\lambda > 0$.

1. The regularization model with

$$\psi(\mathbf{x}, \nabla u) = \psi(\mathbf{x}, \mathbf{t}) := g(|\nabla(\rho * u^\delta)|)|\mathbf{t}|^2, \tag{4.4}$$

is an isotropic regularization model (cf. [386], where ψ as in (4.4) is used for vector-valued data). The weight $g(|\nabla(\rho * u^\delta)|)$ becomes small near regions where $|\nabla(\rho * u^\delta)|$ is large, and is approximately 1 in regions where $\nabla(\rho * u^\delta)$ is almost 0.

2. Let $\mathbf{v} = (v_1, v_2)^T$ be defined as

$$\mathbf{v} := \begin{cases} \dfrac{\nabla(\rho * u^\delta)}{|\nabla(\rho * u^\delta)|}, & \text{if } |\nabla(\rho * u^\delta)| > 0, \\[2ex] \mathbf{e}_1, & \text{else .} \end{cases}$$

We set

$$A := \begin{pmatrix} v_1 & -v_2 \\ v_2 & v_1 \end{pmatrix} \begin{pmatrix} g(|\nabla(\rho * u^\delta)|) & 0 \\ 0 & 1 \end{pmatrix} \begin{pmatrix} v_1 & v_2 \\ -v_2 & v_1 \end{pmatrix} . \qquad (4.5)$$

Note that A is positive definite. The regularization model with

$$\psi(\mathbf{x}, \mathbf{t}) := \mathbf{t}^T A(\mathbf{x})\mathbf{t}$$

is anisotropic. In addition to the dependence of the weight on the size of the gradient of $\nabla(\rho * u^\delta)$, also the components of ∇u orthogonal and normal to $\nabla(\rho * u^\delta)$ are treated differently. $\qquad \diamond$

From the numerical examples below, it is evident that the solutions of quadratic higher-order regularization methods are rather over-smoothed, and edges and corners are blurred. Compare for instance the quadratically filtered and the BV filtered image in Fig. 4.1. In order to avoid this undesirable effect, non-quadratic regularization methods are useful.

In the following, we treat non-quadratic variational methods for denoising. We present a detailed analysis of variational methods consisting in minimizing

$$\boxed{\begin{aligned} &\mathcal{T}_{\alpha,u^\delta}^{p,l} : L^p(\Omega) \to \mathbb{R} \cup \{\infty\}, \\ &u \mapsto \frac{1}{p} \int_\Omega |u - u^\delta|^p + \alpha \, |D^l u| \, (\Omega) =: \mathcal{S}_p(u) + \alpha \mathcal{R}_l(u) . \end{aligned}} \qquad (4.6)$$

Here $\alpha > 0$, and $\mathcal{R}_l(u) = |D^l u| \, (\Omega)$ denotes the l-th order total variation of u (cf. (9.24)). Important tools in the analysis of these variational regularization methods are dual norms, in particular the G-norm and the $*$-number introduced below.

The function $\mathcal{T}_{\alpha,u^\delta}^{2,1}$ is called the ROF-functional: We assume for the sake of simplicity that $\int_\Omega u^\delta = 0$. The original model in [339] consists in minimization of $\mathcal{R}_1$ subject to the constraints that

$$\int_\Omega u = \int_\Omega u^\delta = 0 \quad \text{and} \quad \int_\Omega (u - u^\delta)^2 = \delta^2 ,$$

where $\Omega \subset \mathbb{R}^2$ is bocL. Under the assumption that $\|u^\delta\| > \delta$, it follows (see [90]) that the relaxed model where $\mathcal{R}_1$ is minimized with respect to

$$\int_\Omega u = \int_\Omega u^\delta = 0 \quad \text{and} \quad \int_\Omega (u - u^\delta)^2 \le \delta^2 \qquad (4.7)$$

is equivalent. It is also remarkable that the constraint optimization problems are equivalent to minimization of $\mathcal{T}^{2,1}_{\alpha,u^\delta}$ (see [22, 90]). Actually, in both references the equivalence problem has been treated in a more general setting for deconvolution and deblurring problems. A deblurring approach based on total variation has been considered in [338].

Another important class of regularization methods for denoising is *metrical regularization*, where minimizers of a scale-dependent family of functionals depending on a metric ρ are used for the approximation of u^δ. The most prominent examples of such regularization methods use the L^1-metric $\rho(u, u^\delta) = \int_\Omega |u - u^\delta|$ (see [6], where L^1-BV regularization was used for the first time in the discrete setting), or the L^2-metric $\rho(u, u^\delta) = \sqrt{\int_\Omega (u - u^\delta)^2}$ (see, for example, [350]).

Numerical Examples

In this section, we study and numerically compare isotropic and anisotropic first-order regularization models for denoising images, where ψ is one of the following functions (cf. Tables 4.1 and 4.2):

isotropic quadratic: $\psi(\mathbf{t}) = |\mathbf{t}|^2$,

weighted isotr. quadr.: $\psi(\mathbf{x}, \mathbf{t}) = g(\mathbf{x}) |\mathbf{t}|^2$,   where g is defined in (4.3),

ROF-functional: $\psi(\mathbf{t}) = |\mathbf{t}|$,

anisotropic quadratic: $\psi(\mathbf{x}, \mathbf{t}) = \mathbf{t}^T A(\mathbf{x})\mathbf{t}$,   where A is defined as in (4.5).

For the numerical experiments, in order to solve the variational optimization problem $\frac{1}{2} \left\| u - u^\delta \right\|^2 + \alpha \mathcal{R}(u) \to \min$, the inclusion equation

$$0 \in u - u^\delta + \alpha \partial \mathcal{R}(u) \tag{4.8}$$

is considered, where $\partial \mathcal{R}(u)$ is the subdifferential of $\mathcal{R}(u) := \int_\Omega \psi(\mathbf{x}, \nabla u)$. Because the functionals $\mathcal{R}(u)$ are convex, it follows that solving (4.8) is equivalent to solving the according minimization problems (see Lemma 10.15).

The subdifferential of $\mathcal{R}$ takes the form of a non-linear differential operator satisfying homogeneous Neumann boundary conditions on $\partial \Omega$ (cf. Example 10.41).

Note that (4.8) for $\psi(\mathbf{x}, \mathbf{t}) = g(\mathbf{x}) |\mathbf{t}|^2$ can be interpreted as one time-discrete step of the Perona–Malik diffusion [84, 320] and for $\psi(\mathbf{x}, \mathbf{t}) = \mathbf{t}^T A\mathbf{t}$ as a time-discrete step of the anisotropic diffusion proposed in [385].

For comparison, we use the ultrasound test data shown in Fig. 1.1. The results with different regularization methods are shown in Fig. 4.1. The speckle noise, characteristic for ultrasound images, is removed by each of the models. It can be observed that isotropic quadratic regularization blurs edges, which are better preserved by all other models. Anisotropic quadratic diffusion prefers filtering orthogonal to the gradients, so that edges appear smoother.

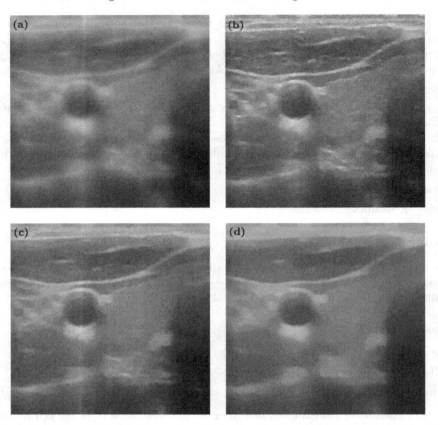

Fig. 4.1. The effect of different regularization methods: (**a**) Quadratic isotropic regularization with $\psi(\mathbf{t}) = |\mathbf{t}|^2$; (**b**) quadratic isotropic regularization with $\psi(\mathbf{x}, \mathbf{t}) = g(\mathbf{x})\,|\mathbf{t}|^2$; (**c**) quadratic anisotropic regularization; (**d**) minimization of the ROF-functional.

4.1 The *-Number

Starting point for the following is [275], where the minimizer of the ROF-functional $\mathcal{T}_{\alpha,u^\delta}^{2,1}$ with $\Omega = \mathbb{R}^2$ is characterized using the dual norm of $W^{1,1}(\mathbb{R}^2)$, which is called the G-norm. In [24], a characterization of minimizers of $\mathcal{T}_{\alpha,u^\delta}^{2,1}$ defined on $\Omega \subset \mathbb{R}^2$ being bocL is derived; in [98], a characterization is used that applies both to bounded and unbounded domains. In [301], we derived a characterization of minimizers of ROF-like functionals with penalization by the total variation of second-order derivatives. In [310], we characterized minimizers of regularization functionals with anisotropic total variation penalization term.

Convention 4.2 *In the remainder of this chapter, we use the following convention. We assume that $1 \leq p \leq \infty$ and $l \in \mathbb{N}$, and either Ω is bocL or $\Omega = \mathbb{R}^n$.*

- *If Ω is bocL, we consider the Sobolev spaces $\mathcal{W}^{l,p} := W_{\diamond}^{l,p}(\Omega)$ and the space of functions with derivatives of finite total variation $\mathcal{BV}^l := BV_{\diamond}^l(\Omega)$.*
- *For $\Omega = \mathbb{R}^n$, we consider the Sobolev space $\mathcal{W}^{l,p} := \widehat{W}^{l,p}(\mathbb{R}^n)$ as defined in (9.14) and the space of functions of finite total variation $\mathcal{BV}^l := \widehat{BV}^l(\mathbb{R}^n)$.*

Both Sobolev spaces are associated with the norm $\left\| \nabla^l u \right\|_p$; both spaces of functions of bounded total variation are associated with the norm $\mathcal{R}_l(u)$. We refer to Theorems 9.42 and 9.86, and Lemmas 9.43 and 9.87 from which the norm property follows.

G-Norm

Y. Meyer [275] defined the G-space

$$G := \left\{ v : v = \nabla \cdot (\mathbf{v}), \ \mathbf{v} \in L^\infty(\mathbb{R}^2; \mathbb{R}^2) \right\}$$

with the norm

$$\|v\|_G := \inf \left\{ \|\mathbf{v}\|_\infty : v = \nabla \cdot (\mathbf{v}) \right\}.$$

This definition was adopted in [24] to the case where the domain $\Omega \subset \mathbb{R}^2$ is bocL. The basic definition is the same, but boundary conditions have to be taken into account. There the following definition is used:

$$G := \left\{ v = \nabla \cdot (\mathbf{v}) \in L^2(\Omega) : \mathbf{v} \in L^\infty(\Omega; \mathbb{R}^2), \ \mathbf{v} \cdot \mathbf{n} = 0 \text{ on } \partial\Omega \right\}, \quad (4.9)$$

and again

$$\|v\|_G := \inf \left\{ \|\mathbf{v}\|_\infty : v = \nabla \cdot (\mathbf{v}) \right\}.$$

In both definitions, the divergence $\nabla \cdot (\mathbf{v})$ has to be understood in a weak sense, and in (4.9) the *normal trace* is understood distributionally. More precisely, $v = \nabla \cdot (\mathbf{v})$ with $\mathbf{v} \cdot \mathbf{n} = 0$ on $\partial\Omega$, if

$$\int_\Omega \mathbf{v} \cdot \nabla\phi = - \int_\Omega v\phi, \qquad \phi \in C_0^\infty(\mathbb{R}^n). \quad (4.10)$$

Now note that it follows from Theorem 9.47 that for every $L \in (\mathcal{W}^{1,1})^*$ there exists $\mathbf{v} \in L^\infty(\Omega; \mathbb{R}^2)$ such that

$$Lu = \int_\Omega \mathbf{v} \cdot \nabla u, \qquad u \in \mathcal{W}^{1,1}. \quad (4.11)$$

Moreover,

$$\|L\|_{(\mathcal{W}^{1,1})^*} = \min \left\{ \|\mathbf{v}\|_\infty : \mathbf{v} \text{ satisfies } (4.11) \right\}. \quad (4.12)$$

Comparing the definition of the G-norm and (4.10) with equations (4.11) and (4.12), one sees that one can regard the G-norm as the dual of the norm on $\mathcal{W}^{1,1}$.

We have used this approach in [310], where we have defined the G-norm on $(\mathcal{W}^{1,1})^*$ with $\Omega = \mathbb{R}^n$, setting for given $1 \leq s \leq \infty$

$$\|L\|_{G^s} := \inf \left\{ \||\mathbf{v}|_s\|_\infty : Lu = \int_{\mathbb{R}^n} \mathbf{v} \cdot \nabla u \right\} .$$

In the above definition, instead of the Euclidean norm, the s-norm of the vector valued function $\mathbf{v}$ is used. This definition can be used to characterize minimizers of regularization functionals with an anisotropic total variation regularization penalization term.

The next definition provides a generalization of the G-norm to both higher dimensions and higher-order derivatives.

Definition 4.3. *Let $l \in \mathbb{N}$ and $1 \leq p < \infty$. The G-norm of $L \in (\mathcal{W}^{l,p})^*$ is defined as*

$$\|L\|_G := \min \left\{ \|\mathbf{v}\|_{p_*} : Lu = \int_\Omega \mathbf{v} \cdot \nabla^l u, \ u \in \mathcal{W}^{l,p} \right\} .$$

Here the minimum is taken over all $\mathbf{v} \in L^{p_*}(\Omega; \mathbb{R}^{\mathcal{N}(l)})$, where $\mathcal{N}(l)$ denotes the number of multi-indices of length l (see (8.4)).

Remark 4.4. From Theorems 9.46 and 9.47, it follows that the G-norm coincides with the dual norm on $(\mathcal{W}^{l,p})^*$. In particular,

$$\|L\|_G = \sup \left\{ \langle L, u \rangle_{(\mathcal{W}^{l,p})^*, \mathcal{W}^{l,p}} : u \in \mathcal{W}^{l,p}, \ \left\|\nabla^l u\right\|_p \leq 1 \right\} .$$

$\diamond$

Remark 4.4 implies that the G-norm is useful for the analysis of regularization functionals with regularization term $\left\|\nabla^l u\right\|_p$. In the following, we generalize the concept to work with arbitrary norm-like regularization functionals.

Definition of the $*$-Number

Let X be a linear space. Recall that a functional $\mathcal{R} : X \to \mathbb{R} \cup \{\infty\}$ is *positively homogeneous*, if

$$\mathcal{R}(tu) = |t|\, \mathcal{R}(u), \qquad u \in X, \ t \in \mathbb{R} .$$

Here, the product $0 \cdot \infty$ is defined as 0.

Definition 4.5. *Let $(X, \mathcal{R})$ be a pair consisting of a locally convex space X and a positively homogeneous and convex functional $\mathcal{R} : X \to \mathbb{R} \cup \{\infty\}$. We define the ∗-number of $u^* \in X^*$ with respect to $(X, \mathcal{R})$ by*

$$\|u^*\|_* := \|u^*\|_{*, X^*, \mathcal{R}} := \sup \left\{ \langle u^*, u \rangle_{X^*, X} : u \in X, \ \mathcal{R}(u) \leq 1 \right\} .$$

If $X = L^p(\Omega)$ for some $\Omega \subset \mathbb{R}^n$ and $1 \leq p < \infty$, we define the ∗-number of $u^* \in L^{p^*}(\Omega)$ by

$$\|u^*\|_* := \|u^*\|_{*, L^{p^*}, \mathcal{R}} := \sup \left\{ \int_\Omega u^* u : u \in L^p(\Omega), \ \mathcal{R}(u) \leq 1 \right\} .$$

The two definitions for the ∗-number for $X = L^p(\Omega)$ are consistent if we identify $(L^p(\Omega))^*$ with $L^{p^*}(\Omega)$ (see Lemma 9.11).

Lemma 4.6. *Let $(X, \mathcal{R})$ be as in Definition 4.5, and let*

$$\mathcal{P} := \{p \in X : \mathcal{R}(p) = 0\} .$$

Because $\mathcal{R}$ is positively homogeneous and convex, it follows that $\mathcal{P}$ is a linear subspace of X. Denote by

$$\mathcal{P}^\perp := \left\{ u^* \in X^* : \langle u^*, p \rangle_{X^*, X} = 0 , p \in \mathcal{P} \right\} .$$

Then $\|u^*\|_* = \infty$ for all $u^* \notin \mathcal{P}^\perp$.

Proof. Let $u^* \notin \mathcal{P}^\perp$. Then there exists $p \in P$ such that $\langle u^*, p \rangle_{X^*, X} \neq 0$. Because $p \in P$, it follows that $\mathcal{R}(p) = 0$. Consequently,

$$\|u^*\|_* = \sup \left\{ \langle u^*, u \rangle_{X^*, X} : \mathcal{R}(u) \leq 1 \right\} \leq \sup_{t \in \mathbb{R}} \langle u^*, tp \rangle_{X^*, X} = \infty ,$$

which proves the assertion. □

The following results show that the ∗-number is a generalization of the G-norm.

Theorem 4.7. *Let U be a subspace of the normed linear space X. Assume that U is a Banach space with norm $\|\cdot\|_U$, and that the inclusion $i : U \to X$ is continuous with respect to the norms $\|\cdot\|_U$ and $\|\cdot\|_X$. Let*

$$\mathcal{R}(u) = \begin{cases} \|u\|_U, & \text{if } u \in U, \\ \infty, & \text{if } u \in X \setminus U . \end{cases}$$

Then

$$\|u^*\|_* = \left\| i^\#(u^*) \right\|_{U^*}, \qquad u^* \in X^*,$$

where $i^\# : U^* \to X^*$ denotes the dual-adjoint of the inclusion i (see Proposition 8.18).

Proof. Recall that the dual-adjoint $i^{\#} : X^* \to U^*$ of the inclusion mapping is defined implicitly by

$$\langle u^*, i(v) \rangle_{X^*,X} = \langle i^{\#}(u^*), v \rangle_{U^*,U}, \qquad u^* \in X^*, \; v \in U.$$

Thus, for $u^* \in X^*$,

$$
\begin{aligned}
\|u^*\|_* &= \sup \left\{ \langle u^*, u \rangle_{X^*,X} : u \in X, \; \mathcal{R}(u) \leq 1 \right\} \\
&= \sup \left\{ \langle u^*, i(v) \rangle_{X^*,X} : v \in U, \; \|v\|_U \leq 1 \right\} \\
&= \sup \left\{ \langle i^{\#}(u^*), v \rangle_{U^*,U} : v \in U, \; \|v\|_U \leq 1 \right\} \\
&= \left\| i^{\#}(u^*) \right\|_{U^*}.
\end{aligned}
$$

$\square$

Corollary 4.8. *Assume that either $n = 1$ and $1 \leq p < \infty$, or $n > 1$ and $1 \leq p \leq n/(n-1)$. Let $X = L^p(\Omega)$, and $\mathcal{R}(u) = \|\nabla u\|_p$ if $u \in \mathcal{W}^{1,p}$ and $\mathcal{R}(u) = \infty$ else. Then $\|u^*\|_* = \left\| i^{\#}(u^*) \right\|_G$, where $i^{\#} : \left(L^p(\Omega) \right)^* \to (\mathcal{W}^{1,p})^*$ denotes the dual-adjoint of the embedding $i : \mathcal{W}^{1,p} \to X$.*

Proof. This is a consequence of Theorem 4.7 combined with the Sobolev Embedding Theorem 9.38. $\square$

Corollary 4.9. *Assume that either $n = 1$ and $1 \leq p < \infty$, or $n > 1$ and $1 \leq p \leq n/(n-1)$. Let $X = L^p(\Omega)$, and $\mathcal{R}(u) = \mathcal{R}_1(u)$, the total variation semi-norm on $L^p(\Omega)$. Then $\|u^*\|_* = \left\| i^{\#}(u^*) \right\|_G$, where $i^{\#} : \left(L^p(\Omega) \right)^* \to (\mathcal{W}^{1,1})^*$ denotes the dual-adjoint of the inclusion $i : \mathcal{W}^{1,1} \to X$.*

Proof. From Corollary 4.8, it follows that

$$\left\| i^{\#}(u^*) \right\|_G = \sup \left\{ \int_{\Omega} u^* u : u \in X \cap \mathcal{W}^{1,1}, \; \|\nabla u\|_1 \leq 1 \right\}.$$

Consequently, we have to show that

$$
\begin{aligned}
\|u^*\|_* &= \sup \left\{ \int_{\Omega} u^* u : u \in X, \; \mathcal{R}_1(u) \leq 1 \right\} \\
&= \sup \left\{ \int_{\Omega} u^* u : u \in X \cap \mathcal{W}^{1,1}, \; \|\nabla u\|_1 \leq 1 \right\}.
\end{aligned}
$$

This equality, however, is a direct consequence of the density result Theorem 9.71. $\square$

4.2 Characterization of Minimizers

In the following, we characterize the minimizers of the family of functionals

$$\mathcal{T}_\alpha(u) := \mathcal{S}(u) + \alpha \mathcal{R}(u), \qquad \alpha > 0,$$

where both $\mathcal{S}$ and $\mathcal{R}$ are proper and convex. For this purpose, we make the following assumptions:

Assumption 4.10

1. X *is a Banach space.*
2. $\mathcal{R}, \mathcal{S} : X \to \mathbb{R} \cup \{\infty\}$ *are convex, proper, and bounded from below.*
3. *The set* $\mathcal{D} := \mathcal{D}(\mathcal{S}) \cap \mathcal{D}(\mathcal{R})$ *is non-empty.*

For the next results, note that the one-sided directional derivatives $\mathcal{S}'(u; h)$, $\mathcal{R}'(u; h)$ exist for every u, $h \in X$ (see Definition 10.31).

Theorem 4.11. *Let $\mathcal{R}$ and $\mathcal{S}$ satisfy Assumption 4.10. Then $u = u_\alpha$ minimizes $\mathcal{T}_\alpha$ if and only if $u \in \mathcal{D}$ satisfies*

$$-\mathcal{S}'(u; h) \le \alpha \mathcal{R}'(u; h), \quad h \in X. \qquad (4.13)$$

Proof. For $u \in X \setminus \mathcal{D}$, by assumption either $\mathcal{R}(u) = \infty$ or $\mathcal{S}(u) = \infty$, showing that a minimizer u_α must be an element of $\mathcal{D}$. Moreover, from the minimality of u_α and the definition of the directional derivatives of $\mathcal{R}$ and $\mathcal{S}$, it follows that

$$\begin{aligned}
0 &\le \liminf_{\varepsilon \to 0^+} \left(\frac{\mathcal{S}(u_\alpha + \varepsilon h) - \mathcal{S}(u_\alpha)}{\varepsilon} + \alpha \frac{\mathcal{R}(u_\alpha + \varepsilon h) - \mathcal{R}(u_\alpha)}{\varepsilon} \right) \\
&\le \limsup_{\varepsilon \to 0^+} \left(\frac{\mathcal{S}(u_\alpha + \varepsilon h) - \mathcal{S}(u_\alpha)}{\varepsilon} \right) + \alpha \limsup_{\varepsilon \to 0^+} \left(\frac{\mathcal{R}(u_\alpha + \varepsilon h) - \mathcal{R}(u_\alpha)}{\varepsilon} \right) \\
&= \mathcal{S}'(u_\alpha; h) + \alpha \mathcal{R}'(u_\alpha; h), \qquad h \in X,
\end{aligned}$$

showing (4.13).

To prove the converse direction, we note that from the convexity of $\mathcal{S}$ and $\mathcal{R}$, and (4.13) it follows that

$$\big(\mathcal{S}(u+h) - \mathcal{S}(u)\big) + \alpha\big(\mathcal{R}(u+h) - \mathcal{R}(u)\big) \ge \mathcal{S}'(u; h) + \alpha \mathcal{R}'(u; h) \ge 0, \quad h \in X.$$

Thus $u \in \mathcal{D}$ satisfying (4.13) is a global minimizer. $\qquad \square$

Remark 4.12. Assume additionally that $\mathcal{S}'(u; \cdot)$ is positively homogeneous. Because $\mathcal{R}$ is convex, for all $u \in \mathcal{D}$, $h \in X$ we have $\mathcal{R}'(u; h) \le \mathcal{R}(u+h) - \mathcal{R}(u)$. Consequently it follows from (4.13) that

$$-\mathcal{S}'(u; h) \le \alpha\big(\mathcal{R}(u + h) - \mathcal{R}(u)\big), \qquad h \in X. \qquad (4.14)$$

Replacing h by εh with $\varepsilon > 0$, it follows from (4.14) that

$$-\mathcal{S}'(u;h) \le \alpha \limsup_{\varepsilon \to 0^+} \frac{\mathcal{R}(u+\varepsilon h) - \mathcal{R}(u)}{\varepsilon} \le \alpha \mathcal{R}'(u;h), \quad h \in X .$$

Thus (4.13) and (4.14) are equivalent. $\diamondsuit$

The following result is an immediate consequence of Theorem 4.11.

Corollary 4.13. *Let Assumption 4.10 hold. Then*

$$-\mathcal{S}'(0;h) \le \alpha \mathcal{R}'(0;h), \quad h \in X ,$$

if and only if $0 \in \mathcal{D}$ minimizes $\mathcal{T}_\alpha$.

Remark 4.14. Let $\mathcal{R}$ be positively homogeneous. Then the definition of u_α shows that

$$\mathcal{S}(u_\alpha) + \alpha \mathcal{R}(u_\alpha) \le \mathcal{S}\big(u_\alpha + \varepsilon(\pm u_\alpha)\big) + \alpha(1 \pm \varepsilon)\,\mathcal{R}(u_\alpha), \quad 0 < \varepsilon < 1 ,$$

and therefore

$$\mp \alpha \mathcal{R}(u_\alpha) \le \liminf_{\varepsilon \to 0^+} \frac{1}{\varepsilon}\big(\mathcal{S}\big(u_\alpha + \varepsilon(\pm u_\alpha)\big) - \mathcal{S}(u_\alpha)\big) .$$

The passage to the limit gives

$$-\mathcal{S}'(u_\alpha; u_\alpha) \le \alpha \mathcal{R}(u_\alpha) \le \mathcal{S}'(u_\alpha; -u_\alpha) .$$

In particular, if $\mathcal{S}$ is Gâteaux differentiable, then

$$-\mathcal{S}'(u_\alpha)\, u_\alpha = \alpha \mathcal{R}(u_\alpha) . \tag{4.15}$$

More generally, if $\mathcal{R}$ satisfies for some $p \ge 1$

$$\mathcal{R}\big((1 \pm \varepsilon)u_\alpha\big) \le (1 \pm p\varepsilon)\,\mathcal{R}(u_\alpha) + o(\varepsilon) ,$$

then

$$-\mathcal{S}'(u_\alpha; u_\alpha) \le \alpha p\,\mathcal{R}(u_\alpha) \le \mathcal{S}'(u_\alpha; -u_\alpha) .$$

In particular, if $\mathcal{S}$ is Gâteaux differentiable, then

$$-\mathcal{S}'(u_\alpha)u_\alpha = \alpha p \mathcal{R}(u_\alpha) . $$ $\diamondsuit$

Analytical Examples

In the following, we use Theorem 4.11 to characterize minimizers of different regularization functionals. Before that, we summarize derivatives of convex functionals used in this section:

Assume that $p \geq 1$ and $X = L^p(\Omega)$. Let

$$\mathcal{S}_p : X \to \mathbb{R} \cup \{\infty\}, \quad u \mapsto \frac{1}{p} \int_\Omega |u - u^\delta|^p .$$

The directional derivative of $\mathcal{S}_p$ at $u \in X$ in direction $h \in X$ is given by

$$\mathcal{S}_p'(u; h) = \int_\Omega |u - u^\delta|^{p-1} \operatorname{sgn}(u - u^\delta)h \quad \text{if } p > 1 ,$$

$$\mathcal{S}_1'(u; h) = \int_{\{u \neq u^\delta\}} \operatorname{sgn}(u - u^\delta)h + \int_{\{u = u^\delta\}} |h| . \tag{4.16}$$

Let $l \in \mathbb{N}$, then the directional derivative at 0 of $\mathcal{R}_l$ defined in (4.6) satisfies

$$\mathcal{R}_l'(0; h) = \mathcal{R}_l(h), \qquad h \in X .$$

Example 4.15. For this example, we assume that either Ω is bocL and $X = L_\diamond^2(\Omega)$ or $\Omega = \mathbb{R}^n$ and $X = L^2(\mathbb{R}^n)$. We consider the pair $(X, \mathcal{R}_1)$. Let $u^\delta \in X$. Corollary 4.13 implies that $u_\alpha = 0 = \arg\min \mathcal{T}_{\alpha,u^\delta}^{2,1}$ if and only if

$$\int_\Omega u^\delta h = -\mathcal{S}_2'(0; h) \leq \alpha \mathcal{R}_1'(0; h) = \alpha \mathcal{R}_1(h), \qquad h \in X \cap \mathcal{BV}^1 ,$$

which is equivalent to

$$\left| \int_\Omega u^\delta h \right| \leq \alpha \mathcal{R}_1(h), \qquad h \in X \cap \mathcal{BV}^1 . \tag{4.17}$$

Equation (4.17) is equivalent to $\|u^\delta\|_* \leq \alpha$, where $\|\cdot\|_* = \|\cdot\|_{*,L^2(\Omega),\mathcal{R}_1}$.

From (4.15), it follows that

$$\alpha \mathcal{R}_1(u_\alpha) = -\int_\Omega (u_\alpha - u^\delta) u_\alpha . \tag{4.18}$$

Taking into account inequality (4.14) and the triangle inequality, it follows that

$$-\int_\Omega (u_\alpha - u^\delta) h \leq \alpha \big(\mathcal{R}_1(u_\alpha + h) - \mathcal{R}_1(u_\alpha)\big) \leq \alpha \mathcal{R}_1(h), \quad h \in X \cap \mathcal{BV}^1 . \tag{4.19}$$

Equation (4.19) implies that $\|u_\alpha - u^\delta\|_* \leq \alpha$. Conversely, it follows from (4.18) that $\|u_\alpha - u^\delta\|_* \geq \alpha$. In [275], it was shown that (4.19) and the condition $\|u_\alpha - u^\delta\|_G = \alpha$ uniquely characterize the minimizer u_α of the ROF-functional in the case $\|u^\delta\|_G > \alpha$. ◇

The following example concerns L^1-BV minimization. In this case, $T^{1,1}_{\alpha,u^\delta}$ can have multiple minimizers, as the functional is not strictly convex.

Example 4.16. We consider the pair $(X = L^1(\Omega), \mathcal{R}_1)$. Let $u^\delta \in X$. From Theorem 4.11 and (4.16), it follows that $u_\alpha \in \arg\min T^{1,1}_{\alpha,u^\delta}$ if and only if

$$-\int_{\{u_\alpha \neq u^\delta\}} \mathrm{sgn}(u_\alpha - u^\delta)\, h - \int_{\{u_\alpha = u^\delta\}} |h| \leq \alpha \mathcal{R}'_1(u_\alpha; h)\,, \qquad h \in X\,. \quad (4.20)$$

In particular, $u_\alpha = 0$ if and only if

$$\int_{\{0 \neq u^\delta\}} \mathrm{sgn}(u^\delta)\, h - \int_{\{0 = u^\delta\}} |h| \leq \alpha \mathcal{R}_1(h)\,, \qquad h \in X \cap \mathcal{BV}^1\,.$$

Using this estimate both with h and $-h$, it follows that

$$\left(\left| \int_{\{0 \neq u^\delta\}} \mathrm{sgn}(u^\delta)\, h \right| - \int_{\{0 = u^\delta\}} |h| \right)^+ \leq \alpha \mathcal{R}_1(h)\,, \qquad h \in X \cap \mathcal{BV}^1\,.$$

These results have been derived in [350] using a different mathematical methodology.

In [93], minimizers of the functional $T^{1,1}_{\alpha,u^\delta}$ with $u^\delta = \chi_E$, $E \subset \Omega$, have been calculated analytically. Some of the results can be reproduced from the considerations above. From Corollary 4.13, it follows that $0 \in \arg\min T^{1,1}_{\alpha,u^\delta}$ if and only if

$$\left(\left| \int_E h \right| - \int_{\mathbb{R}^n \setminus E} |h| \right)^+ \leq \alpha \mathcal{R}_1(h)\,, \qquad h \in X \cap \mathcal{BV}^1\,. \qquad (4.21)$$

Taking $h = \chi_E$, it follows from (4.21) that in the case $u_\alpha = 0$, we have $\mathcal{L}^n(E)/\mathrm{Per}(E; \Omega) \leq \alpha$.

Using Remark 4.12, it follows from (4.20) that $u_\alpha = u^\delta = \chi_E$ implies that

$$-\int_\Omega |h| \leq \alpha \left(\mathcal{R}_1(u^\delta + h) - \mathcal{R}_1(u^\delta) \right)\,, \qquad h \in X \cap \mathcal{BV}^1\,.$$

Taking $h = -\chi_E$ shows that $\alpha \leq \mathcal{L}^n(E)/\mathrm{Per}(E; \Omega)$. $\Diamond$

The next example concerns an inverse problem.

Example 4.17. Assume that Ω is bocL. We consider the pair $(X = L^2(\Omega), \mathcal{R}_1)$ and assume that L is a bounded linear operator on X. This implies that the functional $\mathcal{S}(u) := \frac{1}{2} \left\| Lu - v^\delta \right\|_2^2$ is convex. We consider minimization of

$$\mathcal{T}_{\alpha,v^\delta}(u) := \mathcal{S}(u) + \alpha \mathcal{R}_1(u) = \frac{1}{2} \left\| Lu - v^\delta \right\|_2^2 + \alpha \mathcal{R}_1(u)\,, \qquad u \in X\,.$$

From Theorem 4.11, it follows that $u_\alpha = 0$ if and only if $\left\| L^* v^\delta \right\|_* \leq \alpha$, where L^* is the adjoint of L on $X = L^2(\Omega)$. If $v^\delta = Lu^\dagger$, then this means that $\left\| L^* L u^\dagger \right\|_* \leq \alpha$.

Now consider the regularization functional

$$\mathcal{T}_{\alpha,v^\delta}(u) := \frac{1}{2} \left\| Lu - v^\delta \right\|_2^2 + \frac{\alpha}{2} \left\| \nabla u \right\|_2^2 .$$

From Theorem 4.11, it follows that 0 is a minimizing element of $\mathcal{T}_{\alpha,v^\delta}$ if and only if $L^*v^\delta = 0$. In addition, if $v^\delta = Lu^\dagger$, then this means that $u^\dagger$ is an element of the null-space of L. Therefore, aside from trivial situations, it is *not* possible to completely remove data as it is the case for total variation regularization. $\diamond$

The following example shows that variational regularization methods with a semi-norm penalization are capable of obtaining zero as a minimizer for non-trivial data.

Example 4.18. Let $\Omega = \mathbb{R}^n$. We consider the pair $(X = L^2(\mathbb{R}^n), \mathcal{R})$ with $\mathcal{R}(u) = \|\nabla u\|_2$, if $u \in \mathcal{W}^{1,2} \cap L^2(\mathbb{R}^n)$, and $\mathcal{R}(u) = \infty$ else. Assume that $L : X \to X$ is a bounded linear operator. For $u \in \mathcal{W}^{1,2} \cap L^2(\mathbb{R}^n)$ and $h \in L^2(\mathbb{R}^n)$, the directional derivative of $\mathcal{R}$ is given by

$$\mathcal{R}'(u; h) = \begin{cases} \|\nabla h\|_2 , & \text{if } h \in \mathcal{W}^{1,2} \text{ and } u = 0 , \\[2mm] \dfrac{1}{\|\nabla u\|_2} \displaystyle\int_\Omega \nabla u \cdot \nabla h , & \text{if } h \in \mathcal{W}^{1,2} \text{ and } u \neq 0 , \\[2mm] \infty , & \text{if } h \notin \mathcal{W}^{1,2} . \end{cases}$$

From Theorem 4.11, it follows that zero is a minimizer of

$$\mathcal{T}_{\alpha,v^\delta}(u) := \frac{1}{2} \left\| Lu - v^\delta \right\|_2^2 + \alpha \mathcal{R}(u), \qquad u \in L^2(\mathbb{R}^n) ,$$

if and only if

$$\int_\Omega L^*v^\delta h \leq \alpha \|\nabla h\|_2 , \qquad h \in \mathcal{W}^{1,2} \cap L^2(\mathbb{R}^n) .$$

This is equivalent to stating that $\left\| L^*v^\delta \right\|_* \leq \alpha$. Applying Theorem 4.7, it follows that zero minimizes $\mathcal{T}_{\alpha,v^\delta}$, if and only if $\left\| i^*(L^*v^\delta) \right\|_{\mathcal{W}^{1,2}} \leq \alpha$, where $i^* : L^2(\mathbb{R}^n) \to \mathcal{W}^{1,2}$ denotes the adjoint of the inclusion $i : \mathcal{W}^{1,2} \cap L^2(\mathbb{R}^n) \to L^2(\mathbb{R}^n)$. $\diamond$

Applications of Duality

Below we relate the $*$-number with the dual functional of $\mathcal{R}_l$ (see Definition 10.9). We show that duality is an alternative concept to the $*$-number, and consequently, by Corollary 4.8, is more general than the G-norm. In the following, we show the relation between the $*$-number and the dual functional in the case of the total variation $\mathcal{R}_l$.

Theorem 4.19. *Assume that* $l \in \mathbb{N}$, $1 \le p < \infty$, *and* $\alpha > 0$. *We consider the pair* $(X = L^p(\Omega), \mathcal{R}_l)$. *Then*

$$(\alpha \mathcal{R}_l)^*(u^*) = \begin{cases} 0 & \text{if } \|u^*\|_* \le \alpha, \\ \infty & \text{else}. \end{cases}$$

Moreover $\|u^*\|_* = \infty$ *if* $\int_\Omega u^* q \ne 0$ *for some polynomial* $q \in L^p(\Omega)$ *of degree at most* $l - 1$.

Proof. From the definition of the ∗-number, it follows that $\|u^*\|_* \le \alpha$ if and only if

$$\int_\Omega u^* u \le \alpha, \qquad u \in X, \ \mathcal{R}_l(u) \le 1.$$

This is equivalent to

$$\int_\Omega u^* u \le \alpha \mathcal{R}_l(u), \qquad u \in X.$$

Now recall that

$$(\alpha \mathcal{R}_l)^*(u^*) = \sup \left\{ \int_\Omega u^* u - \alpha \mathcal{R}_l(u) : u \in X \right\}. \tag{4.22}$$

Thus, if $\|u^*\|_* \le \alpha$, it follows that $\int_\Omega u^* u - \alpha \mathcal{R}_l(u) \le 0$ for all u, and consequently $(\alpha \mathcal{R}_l)^*(u^*) \le 0$. Choosing $u = 0$ in the right-hand side of (4.22) shows that $(\alpha \mathcal{R}_l)^*(u^*) = 0$.

If on the other hand $\|u^*\|_* > \alpha$, then it follows that there exists $u_0 \in X$ with $\int_\Omega u^* u_0 - \alpha \mathcal{R}_l(u_0) > 0$. Consequently,

$$(\alpha \mathcal{R}_l)^*(u^*) \ge \sup \left\{ \int_\Omega t u^* u_0 - \alpha \mathcal{R}_l(t u_0) : t \in \mathbb{R} \right\} = \infty.$$

The remaining part of the assertion follows from Lemma 4.6.   □

Remark 4.20. Assume that $1 \le p < \infty$, $l \in \mathbb{N}$. Consider the pair $(X = L^p(\Omega), \mathcal{R}_l)$. Let u_α and u_α^* be extrema of $T_{\alpha,u^\delta}^{p,l}$, $(T_{\alpha,u^\delta}^{p,l})^*$, where $(T_{\alpha,u^\delta}^{p,l})^*(u^*) := (\mathcal{S}_p)^*(u^*) + (\alpha \mathcal{R}_l)^*(-u^*)$ is the Fenchel transform as defined in Definition 10.19. Then from Theorem 10.22, it follows that

$$\inf_{u \in X} T_{\alpha,u^\delta}^{p,l} = \inf_{u^* \in X^*} (T_{\alpha,u^\delta}^{p,l})^*.$$

Thus, it follows from Theorem 10.21 that u_α and u_α^* satisfy the Kuhn–Tucker condition $-u_\alpha^* \in \partial(\alpha \mathcal{R}_l)(u_\alpha)$. From Theorem 10.18 we therefore obtain that

$$-\alpha \mathcal{R}_l(u_\alpha) = \int_\Omega u_\alpha^* u_\alpha. \tag{4.23}$$

This is a generalization of (4.18) for arbitrary $l \in \mathbb{N}$ and $p \ge 1$.   ◇

4.3 One-dimensional Results

In the following, we consider the case $\Omega = (a,b) \subset \mathbb{R}$.

For $l \in \mathbb{N}$ and $v \in L^1(\Omega)$, we define

$$\rho_v^l(x) := (-1)^{l-1} \int_a^x \left(\cdots \int_a^{t_2} v(t_1) \, dt_1 \cdots \right) dt_l \, , \qquad x \in \Omega \, . \qquad (4.24)$$

Theorem 4.21. *Let* $1 \le p < \infty$, *and* $u^* \in L^{p_*}(\Omega)$. *Then* $(\alpha \mathcal{R}_l)^*(u^*) < \infty$, *if and only if* $\rho_{u^*}^l \in W_0^{l,1}(\Omega)$, *and* $\left\| \rho_{u^*}^l \right\|_\infty \le \alpha$.

Proof. Because $\rho_{u^*}^l$ is defined as the l-fold integral of u^*, it follows that $\rho_{u^*}^l \in W^{l,1}(\Omega)$. Now note that a function $\psi \in W^{l,1}(\Omega)$ is an element of $W_0^{l,1}(\Omega)$ if and only if

$$\psi^{(i)}(a) = \psi^{(i)}(b) = 0 \, , \qquad 1 \le i \le l - 1 \, .$$

In the case of $\psi = \rho_{u^*}^l$, this property follows for the point a directly from the definition of $\rho_{u^*}^l$.

From Theorem 4.19, it follows that $(\alpha \mathcal{R}_l)^*(u^*) < \infty$, if and only if $\|u^*\|_* := \|u^*\|_{*,L^{p_*},\mathcal{R}_l} \le \alpha$. From the definition of $\|u^*\|_*$ in Definition 4.5, it follows that this is the case, if and only if

$$\int_\Omega u^* u \le \alpha \, , \qquad u \in BV^l(\Omega), \ \mathcal{R}_l(u) \le 1 \, . \qquad (4.25)$$

From Lemma 9.92, it follows that for every $u \in BV^l(\Omega)$, there exists a sequence $(u_k) \in C^\infty(\bar{\Omega})$ with $\|u_k - u\|_1 \to 0$, and $\mathcal{R}_l(u_k) \to \mathcal{R}_l(u)$. Consequently (4.25) is equivalent to

$$\int_\Omega u^* u \le \alpha \, , \qquad u \in C^\infty(\bar{\Omega}), \ \mathcal{R}_l(u) \le 1 \, .$$

Inserting the definition of $\rho_{u^*}^l$ and integrating by parts shows that this in turn is equivalent to

$$-\int_\Omega \rho_{u^*}^l \, u^{(l)} + \sum_{i=0}^{l-1} (\rho_{u^*}^l)^{(i)}(b) \, u^{(l-1-i)}(b) \le \alpha, \qquad u \in C^\infty(\bar{\Omega}), \ \left\| u^{(l)} \right\|_1 \le 1 \, . \qquad (4.26)$$

Now assume that $(\alpha \mathcal{R}_l)^*(u^*) < \infty$. Then inequality (4.26) holds in particular for all polynomials of degree at most $l-1$. This implies that $(\rho_{u^*}^l)^{(i)}(b) = 0$ for all $0 \le i \le l - 1$, that is, $\rho_{u^*}^l \in W_0^{l,1}(\Omega)$. Consequently, inequality (4.26) reduces to

$$-\int_\Omega \rho_{u^*}^l \, u^{(l)} \le \alpha, \qquad u \in C^\infty(\bar{\Omega}), \ \left\| u^{(l)} \right\|_1 \le 1 \, .$$

Because $\{u^{(l)} : u \in C^\infty(\bar{\Omega})\}$ is dense in $L^1(\Omega)$, this shows that $\left\| \rho_{u^*}^l \right\|_{1_*} = \left\| \rho_{u^*}^l \right\|_\infty \le \alpha$.

Conversely, if $\rho_{u^*}^l \in W_0^{l,1}(\Omega)$ and $\|\rho_{u^*}^l\|_\infty \leq \alpha$, then (4.26) is satisfied, which proves that $(\alpha \mathcal{R}_l)^*(u^*) < \infty$. $\qquad\qquad\qquad\qquad\qquad\qquad\qquad\square$

In the following, we denote by u_α and u_α^* minimizers of $\mathcal{T}_{\alpha,u^\delta}^{p,l}$ and its Fenchel transform $(\mathcal{T}_{\alpha,u^\delta}^{p,l})^*$, respectively. Note that u_α and u_α^* are related via the Kuhn–Tucker condition $u_\alpha^* \in \partial \mathcal{S}_p(u_\alpha)$. In the case $p > 1$, it follows that we have the relation (cf. (10.6))

$$ u_\alpha^* = \mathcal{J}_p(u_\alpha - u^\delta) = (u_\alpha - u^\delta)\left|u_\alpha - u^\delta\right|^{p-2} . \tag{4.27} $$

We show below that u_α is piecewise either a polynomial of order $l-1$ or equals u^δ.

Theorem 4.22. *Let $1 \leq p < \infty$ and assume that u_α and u_α^* are minimizers of $\mathcal{T}_{\alpha,u^\delta}^{p,l}$ and its Fenchel transform $(\mathcal{T}_{\alpha,u^\delta}^{p,l})^*$, respectively. Then u_α and $\rho_{u_\alpha^*}^l$ satisfy the following relations:*

1. *$\rho_{u_\alpha^*}^l \in W_0^{l,1}(\Omega)$ and $\|\rho_{u_\alpha^*}^l\|_\infty \leq \alpha$.*
2. *The function $u_\alpha^{(l-1)}$ is non-decreasing in a neighborhood of each $x \in (a,b)$ where $\rho_{u_\alpha^*}^l(x) > -\alpha$, and non-increasing in a neighborhood of each $x \in (a,b)$ where $\rho_{u_\alpha^*}^l(x) < \alpha$.*
3. *For almost every $x \in \Omega$ satisfying $\left|\rho_{u_\alpha^*}^l(x)\right| = \alpha$ we have $u_\alpha(x) = u^\delta(x)$.*

Proof. Item 1 follows from Theorem 4.21.

For the proof of Item 2, let $x \in \Omega$ satisfy $\rho_{u_\alpha^*}^l(x) > -\alpha$. Denote $\gamma := \rho_{u_\alpha^*}^l(x) + \alpha$. Let $\eta \in C_0^\infty(\mathbb{R})$ be a mollifier (see Definition 9.51), and denote by η_ε, $\varepsilon > 0$, the rescaled function $\eta_\varepsilon(y) = \eta(y/\varepsilon)/\varepsilon$. Define for $\varepsilon > 0$ the functions

$$ \chi_\varepsilon := \chi_{(a+2\varepsilon, b-2\varepsilon)} * \eta_\varepsilon , \qquad \text{and} \qquad \tilde{\rho}_\varepsilon := (\rho_{u_\alpha^*}^l * \eta_\varepsilon)\,\chi_\varepsilon , $$

where we assume for the definition of $\rho_{u_\alpha^*}^l * \eta_\varepsilon$ that $\rho_{u_\alpha^*}^l$ is continued by zero outside of Ω. It follows from Theorem 9.50 and Lemmas 9.49 and 9.53 that $\tilde{\rho}_\varepsilon \in C^\infty(\Omega)$, $\|\tilde{\rho}_\varepsilon\|_\infty \leq \|\rho_{u_\alpha^*}^l\|_\infty \leq \alpha$, and $\|\tilde{\rho}_\varepsilon - \rho_{u_\alpha^*}^l\|_{l,1} \to 0$ as $\varepsilon \to 0$. Moreover, it follows from Lemma 9.52 that $\operatorname{supp}(\chi_\varepsilon) \subset [-1+\varepsilon, 1-\varepsilon]$. Consequently, $\tilde{\rho}_\varepsilon \in C_0^\infty(\Omega)$.

Because $\rho_{u_\alpha^*}^l$ is continuous, the sequence $\tilde{\rho}_\varepsilon$ converges to $\rho_{u_\alpha^*}^l$ locally uniformly (see Lemma 9.54). In particular, there exists an interval $(a_x, b_x) \subset \Omega$ such that $x \in (a_x, b_x)$ and $\tilde{\rho}_\varepsilon + \alpha > \gamma/2$ on (a_x, b_x) for ε small enough.

Let now $\omega \in C_0^\infty(a_x, b_x)$ satisfy $0 \leq \omega(y) \leq \gamma/2$ for all y, and $\operatorname{supp}(\omega) \subset (a_x, b_x)$. Then $\tilde{\rho}_\varepsilon - \omega \in C_0^\infty(a_x, b_x)$, and $\|\tilde{\rho}_\varepsilon - \omega\|_\infty \leq \alpha$. From the definition of the l-th order total variation $\mathcal{R}_l(u_\alpha)$, it follows that

$$ -\int_\Omega (\tilde{\rho}_\varepsilon - \omega)' u_\alpha^{(l-1)} = (-1)^l \int_\Omega (\tilde{\rho}_\varepsilon - \omega)^{(l)} u_\alpha \leq \alpha \mathcal{R}_l(u_\alpha). \tag{4.28} $$

Using (4.23) and the definition of $\rho_{u_\alpha^*}^l$ in (4.24), we obtain that

$$\alpha \mathcal{R}_l(u_\alpha) = -\int_\Omega u_\alpha^* u_\alpha = (-1)^l \int_\Omega (\rho_{u_\alpha^*}^l)^{(l)} u_\alpha = -\int_\Omega (\rho_{u_\alpha^*}^l)' u_\alpha^{(l-1)} . \quad (4.29)$$

In particular, it follows from (4.28) and (4.29) that

$$\int_\Omega (\tilde{\rho}_\varepsilon - \omega - \rho_{u_\alpha^*}^l)' u_\alpha^{(l-1)} \geq 0 . \quad (4.30)$$

Consequently, we obtain from (4.30) and the fact that $\left\| \tilde{\rho}_\varepsilon - \rho_{u_\alpha^*}^l \right\|_{l,1} \to 0$ that

$$-\int_\Omega \omega' u_\alpha^{(l-1)}$$
$$\geq \liminf_{\varepsilon \to 0} \left[\int_\Omega (\tilde{\rho}_\varepsilon - \omega - \rho_{u_\alpha^*}^l)' u_\alpha^{(l-1)} - \left\| (\tilde{\rho}_\varepsilon - \rho_{u_\alpha^*}^l)' \right\|_1 \left\| u_\alpha^{(l-1)} \right\|_\infty \right] \geq 0 . \quad (4.31)$$

Because (4.31) holds for every $\omega \in C_0^\infty(a_x, b_x)$ with $\omega \geq 0$, it follows from Corollary 9.91 that $u_\alpha^{(l-1)}|_{(a_x,b_x)}$ is non-decreasing.

The second part of Item 2 follows by regarding $-u^\delta$, $-u_\alpha$, and $-u_\alpha^*$ instead of u^δ, u_α, and u_α^*.

In order to show Item 3, we use the Kuhn–Tucker condition $u_\alpha^* \in \partial \mathcal{S}_p(u_\alpha)$, which in our case is equivalent to

$$u_\alpha^* \in \operatorname{sgn}(u_\alpha(x) - u^\delta(x)) |u_\alpha(x) - u^\delta(x)|^{p-1} , \quad \text{a.e. } x \in \Omega .$$

Note that we define the sign function set valued (cf. (3.53)). Because $u_\alpha^*(x) = 0$ for almost every x with $|\rho_{u_\alpha^*}^l(x)| = \alpha$, it follows that in this case $u_\alpha(x) = u^\delta(x)$. $\quad \square$

Remark 4.23. From Item 2 in Theorem 4.22, it follows that $u_\alpha^{(l-1)}$ is constant in a neighborhood (a_x, b_x) of every point x with $|\rho_{u_\alpha^*}^l(x)| < \alpha$. This shows that u_α is a polynomial of order $l-1$ in (a_x, b_x). $\quad \diamond$

Remark 4.24. Assume that $u^\delta \in BV(\Omega)$, and consider minimization of $\mathcal{T}_{\alpha,u^\delta}^{2,1}$. If u_α has a positive jump at $x_0 \in \Omega$, that is, if $u(x_0^+) - u(x_0^-) = Du_\alpha(x_0) > 0$, then there exists no neighborhood of x_0 on which u_α is non-increasing. Consequently, it follows from Item 2 in Theorem 4.22 that $\rho_{u_\alpha^*}^1(x_0) = \alpha$. From Item 1, it follows that $\left\| \rho_{u_\alpha^*}^1 \right\|_\infty \leq \alpha$, which implies that

$$\alpha \geq \rho_{u_\alpha^*}^1(x) = \rho_{u_\alpha^*}^1(x_0) + \int_{x_0}^x (u_\alpha - u^\delta) = \alpha + \int_{x_0}^x (u_\alpha - u^\delta) .$$

Consequently,

$$\lim_{x \to x_0^+} u_\alpha(x) - u^\delta(x) \leq 0, \qquad \lim_{x \to x_0^-} u_\alpha(x) - u^\delta(x) \geq 0,$$

which implies that

$$u^\delta(x_0^-) \leq u_\alpha(x_0^-) < u_\alpha(x_0^+) \leq u^\delta(x_0^+) \,.$$

Similarly, if $Du_\alpha(x) < 0$, then also $Du^\delta(x) < 0$. This shows that minimization of $\mathcal{T}_{\alpha,u^\delta}^{2,1}$ creates no new discontinuities in a function and smoothes all existing jumps. Note that in higher dimensions, an analogous result has been shown in [81]. $\diamond$

Corollary 4.25. *Assume that u^δ is non-decreasing, non-increasing, respectively, in a neighborhood of some $x \in \Omega$, then so is $u_\alpha = \arg\min \mathcal{T}_{\alpha,u^\delta}^{2,1}$.*

Proof. Assume that u^δ is non-decreasing in a neighborhood of $x \in \Omega$. If $\rho_{u_\alpha^*}^1(x) > -\alpha$, then it follows from Item 2 in Theorem 4.22 that u_α is non-decreasing in a neighborhood of x. Thus, in order to prove the assertion, we may restrict our attention to the case $\rho_{u_\alpha^*}^1(x) = -\alpha$.

From the continuity of $\rho_{u_\alpha^*}^1$, it follows that there exists $\varepsilon > 0$ such that $\rho_{u_\alpha^*}^1 < \alpha$ in $(x - \varepsilon, x + \varepsilon)$. Consequently u_α is non-increasing in $(x - \varepsilon, x + \varepsilon)$. Because for sufficiently small $\varepsilon > 0$ the function u^δ is non-decreasing in $(x - \varepsilon, x + \varepsilon)$, this implies that $u_\alpha - u^\delta$ is non-increasing in $(x - \varepsilon, x + \varepsilon)$. Thus it follows from the definition of $\rho_{u_\alpha^*}^1$ that $-\rho_{u_\alpha^*}^1$ is convex in $(x - \varepsilon, x + \varepsilon)$. Consequently,

$$-\alpha = \rho_{u_\alpha^*}^1(x) \geq \frac{1}{2}\left(\rho_{u_\alpha^*}^1(x - \gamma) + \rho_{u_\alpha^*}^1(x + \gamma)\right), \qquad 0 < \gamma < \varepsilon \,.$$

Because $\rho_{u_\alpha^*}^1(x \pm \gamma) \geq -\alpha$, this implies that $\rho_{u_\alpha^*}^1 = -\alpha$ in $(x - \varepsilon, x + \varepsilon)$, which in turn implies that $u_\alpha = u^\delta$ in $(x - \varepsilon, x + \varepsilon)$. Thus u_α is non-decreasing in $(x - \varepsilon, x + \varepsilon)$. $\square$

The next result states that the conditions obtained in Theorem 4.22 already uniquely determine u_α in the case $p > 1$. For the sake of simplicity of notation, we denote

$$\rho_u^* := \rho_{\mathcal{J}_p(u-u^\delta)}^l \,, \qquad u \in L^p(\Omega), \tag{4.32}$$

where $\mathcal{J}_p : L^p(\Omega) \to L^{p*}(\Omega)$ is the p-duality mapping defined in (10.6).

Theorem 4.26. *Let $p > 1$ and $l \in \mathbb{N}$. Then there exists a unique function $u \in L^p(\Omega)$ such that $\rho_u^* \in W_0^{l,1}(\Omega)$, $\|\rho_u^*\|_\infty \leq \alpha$, $u^{(l-1)}$ is non-decreasing in a neighborhood of every point $x \in \Omega$ with $\rho_u^*(x) > -\alpha$ and non-increasing in a neighborhood of every point $x \in \Omega$ with $\rho_u^*(x) < \alpha$.*

Proof. Let v be another function satisfying the assumptions of the theorem.

Assume that $\rho_u^*(x) > \rho_v^*(x)$ for some $x \in \Omega$. Then there exists a neighborhood (a_x, b_x) of x such that $\rho_u^* > \rho_v^*$ in (a_x, b_x). Because by assumption $\|\rho_u^*\|_\infty \leq \alpha$ and $\|\rho_v^*\|_\infty \leq \alpha$, we have

$$\alpha \geq \rho_u^*(t) > \rho_v^*(t) \geq -\alpha \,, \qquad t \in (a_x, b_x) \,.$$

Consequently, it follows that $u^{(l-1)}$ is non-decreasing and $v^{(l-1)}$ is non-increasing in (a_x, b_x). From Lemma 9.90, it follows that this is equivalent to stating that $D^l u \llcorner (a_x, b_x)$ and $-D^l v \llcorner (a_x, b_x)$ are positive Radon measures. Because $\rho_u^* > \rho_v^*$ in (a_x, b_x), this implies that

$$\int_{a_x}^{b_x} (\rho_u^* - \rho_v^*)\, \mathrm{d}D^l(u - v) \geq 0 .$$

By exchanging the roles of u and v, we find that the same holds true whenever $\rho_v^*(x) > \rho_u^*(x)$. Thus

$$\int_{\Omega} (\rho_u^* - \rho_v^*)\, \mathrm{d}D^l(u - v) \geq 0 .$$

With integration by parts, it follows that

$$(-1)^l \int_{\Omega} (\rho_u^* - \rho_v^*)^{(l)}(u - v) \geq 0 .$$

Because by definition of ρ_u^* and ρ_v^* (cf. (4.32) and (4.24)) we have $(\rho_u^*)^{(l)} = \mathcal{J}_p(u - u^\delta)$ and $(\rho_v^*)^{(l)} = \mathcal{J}_p(v - u^\delta)$, this shows that

$$-\int_{\Omega} (\mathcal{J}_p(u - u^\delta) - \mathcal{J}_p(v - u^\delta))(u - v) \geq 0 . \qquad (4.33)$$

Because by (10.6) we have $\mathcal{J}_p(w) = |w|^{p-2} w$, and the function $t \to |t|^{p-2} t$ is strictly increasing, it follows that $\mathcal{J}_p(u - u^\delta) > \mathcal{J}_p(v - u^\delta)$, if and only if $u > v$. Consequently, the integrand in (4.33) is non-negative and equals zero if and only if $u = v$. This proves that $u = v$ almost everywhere.   □

Corollary 4.27. Let $1 < p < \infty$. Then $u \in L^p(\Omega)$ is a minimizer of $T_{\alpha,u^\delta}^{p,l}$ if and only if u and $\rho_{\mathcal{J}_p(u-u^\delta)}^l$ satisfy Items 1 and 2 in Theorem 4.22.

Proof. This directly follows from Theorems 4.22 and 4.26, the equality $u_\alpha^* = \mathcal{J}_p(u_\alpha - u^\delta)$ (cf. (4.27)), and the existence of a minimizer of $T_{\alpha,u^\delta}^{p,l}$.   □

Analytical Examples

In the following, we present exact results for the cases $p = 1, 2$, $l = 1, 2$, $\Omega = (-1, 1)$, and $u^\delta = \chi_{[-1/2,1/2]} - 1/2$.
 We define

$$\Psi_\alpha^{l,p} := \{u^* \in L^{p^*}(\Omega) : (\alpha \mathcal{R}_l)^*(u^*) = 0\} .$$

Then

$$(T_{\alpha,u^\delta}^{p,l})^*(u^*) = \begin{cases} (\mathcal{S}_p)^*(u^*) & \text{if } u^* \in \Psi_\alpha^{l,p}, \\ \infty & \text{else .} \end{cases}$$

We refer to Example 10.13, where $(\mathcal{S}_p)^*$ is analytically calculated.

From Theorem 4.21, it follows that

$$\Psi_\alpha^{l,p} = \left\{ u^* \in L^{p_*}(\Omega) : \rho_{u^*}^l \in W_0^{1,1}(\Omega), \ \|\rho_{u^*}^l\|_\infty \le \alpha \right\}.$$

For a detailed analysis of the following examples we refer to [323]. There the dual formulations have been used for the analytical calculation of the minimizers in the following examples.

Example 4.28 (L^1-BV regularization). Let $X = L^1(\Omega)$. The dual problem consists in minimizing

$$(\mathcal{T}_{\alpha,u^\delta}^{1,1})^*(u^*) = \int_{-1}^{1} u^\delta u^*, \qquad \text{for } u^* \in \Psi_\alpha^{1,1} \text{ and } \|u^*\|_\infty \le 1.$$

We have three possibilities:

- $\alpha > 1/2$. Here the minimizers are the constant functions $u_\alpha = c$ with $c \in [-1/2, 1/2]$.
- $\alpha = 1/2$. The minimizers u_α have the form

$$u_\alpha = \begin{cases} c_1 & \text{in } (-1, -1/2), \text{ with } -1/2 \le c_1, \\ c_2 & \text{in } (-1/2, 1/2), \text{ with } c_1 \le c_2 \le 1/2, \\ c_3 & \text{in } (1/2, 1), \text{ with } -1/2 \le c_3 \le c_2. \end{cases}$$

- $\alpha < 1/2$. The unique minimizer is $u_\alpha = u^\delta$.

See Figs. 4.2–4.4. Note that in Figs. 4.3 and 4.4, the function $\rho_{u^*}^1/\alpha$ touches the α-tube at the points where u_α is discontinuous. $\diamond$

Example 4.29 (L^2-BV regularization). The dual problem consists in minimizing

$$(\mathcal{T}_{\alpha,u^\delta}^{2,1})^*(u^*) = \int_\Omega \frac{1}{2}(u^*)^2 + u^\delta u^*, \qquad \text{for } u^* \in \Psi_\alpha^{1,2}.$$

It can be shown that the minimizer u_α of $\mathcal{T}_{\alpha,u^\delta}^{2,1}$ is

$$u_\alpha = u^\delta + u_\alpha^* = \begin{cases} 0 & \text{if } \alpha \ge 1/4, \\ (1 - 4\alpha)u^\delta & \text{if } 0 \le \alpha \le 1/4. \end{cases}$$

See also Figs. 4.5 and 4.6. Again, the points where $\rho_{u^*}^1/\alpha$ touches the α-tube coincide with the discontinuities of u_α. $\diamond$

Example 4.30 (L^1-BV^2 regularization). The dual problem consists in minimizing

$$(\mathcal{T}_{\alpha,u^\delta}^{1,2})^*(u^*) = \int_\Omega u^\delta u^*, \qquad \text{for } u^* \in \Psi_\alpha^{2,1} \text{ and } \|u^*\|_\infty \le 1.$$

Examples of minimizers for different parameters are shown in Figs. 4.7–4.9. Note that the points where $\rho_{u^*}^2$ touches the α-tube coincide with the points where u_α bends. $\diamond$

L^1-BV regularization

(a)   **(b)**   **(c)**

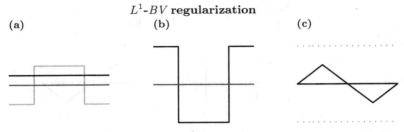

Fig. 4.2. $\alpha > 1/2$: (a) u_α, u^δ (*gray*); (b) u_α^*; (c) $\rho_{u_\alpha^*}^1/\alpha$.

(a)   **(b)**   **(c)**

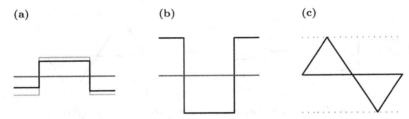

Fig. 4.3. $\alpha = 1/2$: (a) u_α, u^δ (*gray*); (b) u_α^*; (c) $\rho_{u_\alpha^*}^1/\alpha$.

(a)   **(b)**   **(c)**

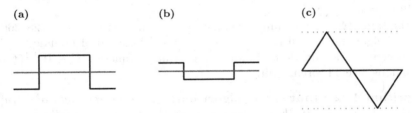

Fig. 4.4. $\alpha < 1/2$: (a) $u_\alpha = u^\delta$; (b) u_α^*; (c) $\rho_{u_\alpha^*}^1/\alpha$. Note that $\rho_{u_\alpha^*}^1/\alpha$ is not unique.

Example 4.31 (L^2-BV^2 regularization). The dual problem consists in minimizing

$$(\mathcal{T}_{\alpha,u^\delta}^{2,2})^*(u^*) = \int_\Omega \frac{1}{2}(u^*)^2 + u^* u^\delta, \qquad \text{for } u^* \in \Psi_\alpha^{2,1}.$$

Examples of minimizers for different parameters are shown in Figs. 4.10–4.12.

$\diamond$

4.4 Taut String Algorithm

In this section, we review various equivalent formulations of the total variation regularization functional for functions defined on the one-dimensional domain $\Omega = (0,1)$. Moreover, we discuss possible generalizations to higher dimensions.

L^2-BV **regularization**

(a)   **(b)**   **(c)**

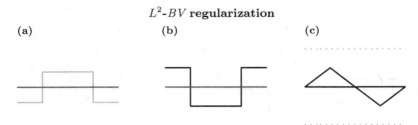

Fig. 4.5. $\alpha \geq \frac{1}{4}$: (a) $u_\alpha = 0$, u^δ (gray); (b) u_α^*; (c) $\rho_{u_\alpha^*}^1/\alpha$.

(a)   **(b)**   **(c)**

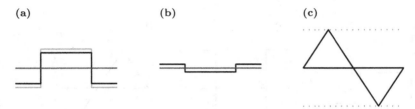

Fig. 4.6. $\alpha < \frac{1}{4}$: (a) u_α, u^δ (gray); (b) u_α^*; (c) $\rho_{u_\alpha^*}^1/\alpha$.

These formulations are based on the so-called taut string algorithm, which is a highly efficient method for the minimization of a certain discretization of the functional $\mathcal{T}_{\alpha,u^\delta}^{2,1}$.

The taut string algorithm is commonly used in statistics (see [128, 266]). For this algorithm, recall that a one-dimensional function of bounded variation is continuous outside its jump set, and that a function $U \in W^{1,1}(\Omega)$ is continuous (see Theorem 9.89).

Algorithm 4.32 (Taut string algorithm) *Given discrete data* $\mathbf{u}^\delta = (u_i^\delta)$, $i = 1, \ldots, s$, *and* $\alpha > 0$, *the taut string algorithm is defined as follows:*

- *Let* $U_0^\delta = 0$ *and* $U_i^\delta = \frac{1}{s} \sum_{j=1}^i u_j^\delta$, $i = 1, \ldots, s$. *We denote by* U^δ *the linear spline with nodal points* $x_i = i/s$, $i = 0, \ldots, s$, *and function values* U_i^δ *at* x_i.
- *Define the* α-*tube*

$$\mathcal{Y}_\alpha := \big\{ U \in W^{1,1}(0,1) : U^\delta(0) = U(0), \ U^\delta(1) = U(1),$$
$$\text{and } \big|U^\delta(t) - U(t)\big| \leq \alpha \text{ for } t \in (0,1) \big\} \, .$$

- *We calculate the function* $U_\alpha \in \mathcal{Y}_\alpha$ *which minimizes the graph length, that is,*

$$U_\alpha = \operatorname*{arg\,min}_{U \in \mathcal{Y}_\alpha} \int_0^1 \sqrt{1 + (U')^2} \, .$$

- $u_\alpha := U_\alpha'$ *is the outcome of the taut string algorithm.*

Lemma 4.33. *The taut string algorithm 4.32 has a unique solution* u_α.

L^1-BV^2 **regularization**

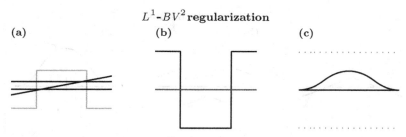

Fig. 4.7. $\alpha > \frac{1}{4}$: (a) u_α (*bold*), u^δ (*gray*). Note that u_α is not unique. (b) u_α^*; (c) $\rho_{u_\alpha^*}^2/\alpha$.

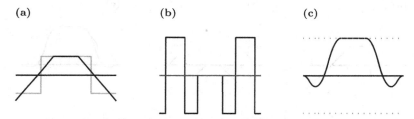

Fig. 4.8. (a) u_α bends at $x = \pm x_{1,\alpha}$, u^δ (*gray*); (b) u_α^*; (c) $\rho_{u_\alpha^*}^2/\alpha$.

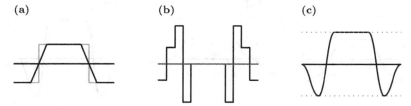

Fig. 4.9. $\alpha < \frac{3}{8} - \frac{1}{4}\sqrt{2}$: (a) u_α bends at $x = \pm\left(1/2 \pm \sqrt{2\alpha}\right)$, u^δ (*gray*); (b) $u^* = -(\rho_\alpha^*)''$; (c) here ρ_α^* touches the α-tube at $x = \pm\left(1/2 \pm \sqrt{2\alpha}\right)$, where u_α bends.

Proof. See [266]. □

Moreover, it is shown in [266] that the taut string algorithm is equivalent to minimizing the *discrete total variation regularization functional*

$$\mathcal{T}_{\alpha,\mathbf{u}^\delta}(u) := \frac{1}{2s}\sum_{i=1}^{s}\left(u_i^\delta - u\left(\frac{x_i + x_{i-1}}{2}\right)\right)^2 + \alpha\mathcal{R}_1(u)$$

over the space of piecewise constant splines with nodes $x_i = i/s$, $0 \le i \le s$.

We also consider data u_i^δ at irregularly spaced sampling points $0 \le x_{i-1} < x_i \le 1$, $1 \le i \le s$. Setting $h_i = x_i - x_{i-1}$, we define the *irregularly sampled discrete total variation regularization functional*

$$\mathcal{T}_{\alpha,\mathbf{u}^\delta}(u) := \frac{1}{2}\sum_{i=1}^{s} h_i\left(u_i^\delta - u\left(\frac{x_i + x_{i-1}}{2}\right)\right)^2 + \alpha\mathcal{R}_1(u)$$

L^2-BV^2regularization

(a)   **(b)**   **(c)**

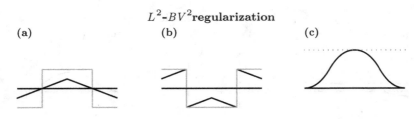

Fig. 4.10. (a) u_α bends at $x = 0$, gray: u^δ; (b) u_α^*; (c) $\rho_{u_\alpha^*}^2$.

(a)   **(b)**   **(c)**

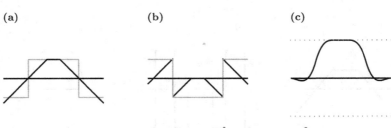

Fig. 4.11. (a) u_α, gray: u^δ; (b) u_α^*; (c) $\rho_{u_\alpha^*}^2$.

(a)   **(b)**   **(c)**

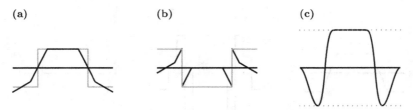

Fig. 4.12. (a) u_α, gray: u^δ; (b) u_α^*; (c) $\rho_{u_\alpha^*}^2$.

over the space

$$\mathcal{P} := \{u : u \text{ is constant in } (x_{i-1}, x_i), 1 \leq i \leq s\} \ .$$

In what follows, we associate with $\mathbf{u}^\delta \in \mathbb{R}^s$ a function $u^\delta \in \mathcal{P}$ with value u_i^δ on (x_{i-1}, x_i), $1 \leq i \leq s$.

Lemma 4.34. *Let $u^\delta \in \mathcal{P}$ be the piecewise constant function associated with* $\mathbf{u}^\delta$. *Then*

$$\underset{u \in L^2(\Omega)}{\arg\min} \mathcal{T}_{\alpha,u^\delta}^{2,1}(u) = \underset{u \in \mathcal{P}}{\arg\min} \mathcal{T}_{\alpha,\mathbf{u}^\delta}(u) \ .$$

Proof. In order to show that

$$\underset{u \in \mathcal{P}}{\arg\min} \mathcal{T}_{\alpha,u^\delta}^{2,1}(u) = \underset{u \in \mathcal{P}}{\arg\min} \mathcal{T}_{\alpha,\mathbf{u}^\delta}(u), \tag{4.34}$$

note that the first part of $\mathcal{T}_{\alpha,\mathbf{u}^\delta}$ is a quadrature formula for $\frac{1}{2}\int_0^1 (u - u^\delta)^2$ that is exact on $\mathcal{P}$. This proves that actually

$$\mathcal{T}_{\alpha,u^\delta}^{2,1}(u) = \mathcal{T}_{\alpha,\mathbf{u}^\delta}(u)\,, \qquad u \in \mathcal{P}\,,$$

which in particular shows (4.34).

The next step is to show that

$$\underset{u\in L^2(\Omega)}{\arg\min}\, \mathcal{T}_{\alpha,u^\delta}^{2,1}(u) = \underset{u\in\mathcal{P}}{\arg\min}\, \mathcal{T}_{\alpha,u^\delta}^{2,1}(u)\,. \tag{4.35}$$

Denote by u_α the minimizer of $\mathcal{T}_{\alpha,u^\delta}^{2,1}(u)$ in $L^2(\Omega)$. In order to show (4.35), it is enough to prove that $u_\alpha \in \mathcal{P}$. This is, however, a direct consequence of Corollary 4.25. $\qquad\square$

Above we have seen that the taut string algorithm and total variation regularization are equivalent. In fact, this equivalence can be generalized to a by far larger class of functionals:

Theorem 4.35. *Let* $c : \mathbb{R} \to \mathbb{R}$ *be strictly convex. Then* U_α *as defined in Algorithm 4.32 is the unique minimizer of the functional*

$$\mathcal{C}(U) = \int_0^1 c(U')\,, \qquad U \in \mathcal{Y}_\alpha\,.$$

Proof. We refer to Theorem 4.46, where the result is shown for arbitrary dimensions. Note that $U \in \mathcal{Y}_\alpha$ if and only if $\left\| U_\alpha' - u^\delta \right\|_* \le \alpha$, where $\|\cdot\|_*$ denotes the $*$-number with respect to $(L^2(\Omega), \mathcal{R}_1)$. $\qquad\square$

Remark 4.36. We have proven that the solution of discrete total variation regularization, that is, minimization of $\mathcal{T}_{\alpha,\mathbf{u}^\delta}$, equals the solution of the continuous total variation regularization, if the data $\mathbf{u}^\delta$ are identified with a piecewise constant spline u^δ. Moreover, discrete total variation regularization is equivalent to the taut string problem. In particular, it follows from these equivalence relations that the primitive of the solution of continuous total variation regularization minimizes the graph length in $\mathcal{Y}_\alpha$. $\qquad\diamond$

Remark 4.37. In [363], it has been shown that the minimizer of $\mathcal{T}_{\alpha,\mathbf{u}^\delta}$ coincides with the solution of the *space discrete total variation flow* equation at time $t = \alpha$

$$\frac{\partial u_1}{\partial t} \in \operatorname{sgn}(u_2 - u_1)\,,$$

$$\frac{\partial u_i}{\partial t} \in \operatorname{sgn}(u_{i+1} - u_i) - \operatorname{sgn}(u_i - u_{i-1})\,, \qquad i = 2,\ldots,s-1\,,$$

$$\frac{\partial u_s}{\partial t} \in -\operatorname{sgn}(u_s - u_{s-1})\,,$$

$$\mathbf{u}(0) = \mathbf{u}^\delta\,. \tag{4.36}$$

In Chapter 6, the solution of the total variation flow equation (see Example 6.19)

$$\frac{\partial u}{\partial t} \in -\partial \mathcal{R}_1(u), \qquad u(0) = u^\delta,$$

at time t is defined as $u(t) = \lim_{N\to\infty} u_N^N$, where $u_0^N = u^\delta$ and $u_k^N = \arg\min \mathcal{T}_{t/N, u_{k-1}^N}^{2,1}$, $1 \le k \le N$. The following result shows that $u_N^N = \arg\min \mathcal{T}_{t, u^\delta}^{2,1}$ for all $N \in \mathbb{N}$, which implies that the minimizer u_α of $\mathcal{T}_{\alpha, u^\delta}^{2,1}$ coincides with the solution of the total variation flow equation at time $t = \alpha$. This generalizes the according result for the space discrete total variation flow (see Remark 4.37).

Theorem 4.38. *For $v \in L^2(\Omega)$ and $\alpha > 0$ denote*

$$S_\alpha(v) := \arg\min_{u \in L^2(\Omega)} \mathcal{T}_{\alpha, v}^{2,1}(u).$$

Then

$$S_{\alpha+\beta}(u^\delta) = S_\beta\big(S_\alpha(u^\delta)\big), \qquad \alpha, \beta > 0, \ u^\delta \in L^2(\Omega).$$

Proof. Define for $\gamma > 0$ and $v \in L^2(\Omega)$

$$\rho_{\gamma, v}(x) := \int_0^x \big(S_\gamma(v)(t) - v(t)\big) \, \mathrm{d}t, \qquad x \in \Omega.$$

For simplicity, denote $\tilde{u} := S_\beta\big(S_\alpha(u^\delta)\big)$. Define moreover

$$\tilde{\rho}(x) := \int_0^x \big(\tilde{u}(t) - u^\delta(t)\big) \, \mathrm{d}t, \qquad x \in \Omega.$$

From Corollary 4.27, it follows that $\tilde{u} = S_{\alpha+\beta}(u^\delta)$, if and only if $\tilde{\rho}$ satisfies Items 1 and 2 in Theorem 4.22. We therefore have to show that $\tilde{\rho} \in W_0^{1,1}(\Omega)$, $\|\tilde{\rho}\|_\infty \le \alpha + \beta$, and that $\tilde{u}$ is non-decreasing in a neighborhood of every point x with $\tilde{\rho}(x) > -\alpha - \beta$, and non-increasing in a neighborhood of every point x with $\tilde{\rho}(x) < \alpha + \beta$.

From Theorem 4.22, it follows that $\rho_{\alpha, u^\delta}, \rho_{\beta, S_\alpha(u^\delta)} \in W_0^{1,1}(\Omega)$,

$$\|\rho_{\alpha, u^\delta}\|_\infty \le \alpha, \qquad \|\rho_{\beta, S_\alpha(u^\delta)}\|_\infty \le \beta.$$

Because $\tilde{\rho} = \rho_{\beta, S_\alpha(u^\delta)} + \rho_{\alpha, u^\delta}$, it follows that also $\tilde{\rho} \in W_0^{1,1}(\Omega)$ and

$$\|\tilde{\rho}\|_\infty \le \|\rho_{\beta, S_\alpha(u^\delta)}\|_\infty + \|\rho_{\alpha, u^\delta}\|_\infty \le \beta + \alpha.$$

This shows that $\tilde{\rho}$ satisfies Item 1 in Theorem 4.22 with α replaced by $\alpha + \beta$.

In order to show Item 2, let $x \in \Omega$ be such that $\tilde{\rho}(x) > -\alpha - \beta$. Because $\tilde{\rho} = \rho_{\beta, S_\alpha(u^\delta)} + \rho_{\alpha, u^\delta}$, it follows that at least one of the inequalities

$\rho_{\beta,S_\alpha(u^\delta)}(x) > -\beta$ or $\rho_{\alpha,u^\delta}(x) > -\alpha$ holds. We show now that either inequality implies that $\tilde{u}$ is non-decreasing near x.

Assume first that $\rho_{\beta,S_\alpha(u^\delta)}(x) > -\beta$. Because $\tilde{u}$ is a minimizer of $\mathcal{T}_{\beta,S_\alpha(u^\delta)}$, it follows from Item 2 in Theorem 4.22 that $\tilde{u}$ is non-decreasing in a neighborhood of x.

Now assume that $\rho_{\alpha,u^\delta}(x) > -\alpha$. Because $S_\alpha(u^\delta)$ minimizes $\mathcal{T}^{2,1}_{\alpha,u^\delta}$, it follows from Item 2 in Theorem 4.22 that $S_\alpha(u^\delta)$ is non-decreasing in a neighborhood of x. Then it follows from Corollary 4.25 that $\tilde{u} = S_\beta(S_\alpha(u^\delta))$ is non-decreasing in a neighborhood of x.

In a similar manner, it follows that $\tilde{u}$ is non-increasing in a neighborhood of every point $x \in \Omega$ with $\tilde{\rho}(x) < \alpha + \beta$. Consequently, the function $\tilde{\rho}$ satisfies Item 2 in Theorem 4.22.

Thus it follows from Corollary 4.27 that $\tilde{u}$ is the unique minimizer of $\mathcal{T}^{2,1}_{\alpha+\beta,u^\delta}$, that is, $\tilde{u} = S_{\alpha+\beta}(u^\delta)$. □

The first step in the taut string algorithm is the integration of the data. Therefore, less regularity of the data is needed than in the case of total variation regularization. Essentially, it is enough that the data can be integrated, which means that they are a finite Radon measure.

In this case, the taut string algorithm reads as follows:

Algorithm 4.39 (Generalized taut string algorithm). *Let μ^δ be a finite Radon measure on $\Omega = (0,1)$ and $\alpha > 0$.*

- *Define the integrated data $U^\delta(x) := \mu^\delta\big((0,x)\big)$.*
- *Construct the α-tube around U^δ setting*

$$\mathcal{Y}_\alpha := \big\{ U \in BV(\Omega) : \big\|U - U^\delta\big\|_\infty \leq \alpha,\ U^{(r)}(0) = 0,\ U^{(l)}(1) = U^\delta(1) \big\},$$

where $U^{(r)}(0)$, $U^{(l)}(1)$ denote the right and left limits of U at 0 and 1, respectively.
- *Define*

$$U_\alpha := \underset{U \in \mathcal{Y}_\alpha}{\arg\min} \int_0^1 \sqrt{1 + (DU)^2} := \underset{U \in \mathcal{Y}_\alpha}{\arg\min} \int_0^1 \sqrt{1 + (U')^2} + |D^s U|\,(0,1),$$

where $DU := U'\mathcal{L}^1 + D^s U$ is the Lebesgue decomposition of DU (see Theorem 9.19).
- *$\mu_\alpha := DU_\alpha$ is the outcome of the generalized taut string algorithm.*

Lemma 4.40. *The generalized taut string algorithm 4.39 has a unique solution μ_α. Denote $\Sigma_\alpha^+(\mu^\delta) := \{x : \mu^\delta(\{x\}) > 2\alpha\}$, and $\Sigma_\alpha^-(\mu^\delta) := \{x : \mu^\delta(\{x\}) < -2\alpha\}$. Then there exists a function $u_\alpha \in L^1(\Omega)$ such that*

$$\mu_\alpha = u_\alpha \mathcal{L}^1 + \sum_{x \in \Sigma_\alpha^+(\mu^\delta)} (\mu^\delta(\{x\}) - 2\alpha)\delta_x + \sum_{x \in \Sigma_\alpha^-(\mu^\delta)} (\mu^\delta(\{x\}) + 2\alpha)\delta_x,$$

where δ_x denotes the Dirac measure centered at x (see Example 9.22).

Proof. See [188].   □

In particular, if $\left|\mu^\delta(\{x\})\right| \leq 2\alpha$ for all $x \in \Omega$, then the result of the algorithm can be identified with the function u_α.

Multi-dimensional Taut String

For the sake of simplicity of notation, we consider data $u^\delta : \Omega = (0,1)^n \subset \mathbb{R}^n \to \mathbb{R}$.

Table 4.3, which summarizes the equivalences shown above for one-dimensional total variation regularization, indicates several possibilities of formulating the taut string algorithm in higher dimensions:

1. Minimization of $\mathcal{T}_{\alpha,u^\delta}^{2,1}(u) = \frac{1}{2}\int_\Omega (u - u^\delta)^2 + \alpha\mathcal{R}_1(u)$.
2. Discrete total variation minimization:

    For $\mathbf{i} \in \{0,\ldots,s\}^n$ define $\mathbf{x_i} := \mathbf{i}/s \in \Omega$. Define for $\mathbf{i} \in \mathcal{I} := \{1,\ldots,s\}^n$

    $$u_{\mathbf{i}}^\delta := u^\delta\left(\frac{\mathbf{x_i} + \mathbf{x_{i-1}}}{2}\right),$$

    where $\mathbf{1} := (1,\ldots,1)$. Discrete total variation minimization consists in minimization of

    $$\mathcal{T}_{\alpha,\mathbf{u}^\delta}(\mathbf{u}) := \frac{1}{2s^n} \sum_{\mathbf{i}\in\{1,\ldots,s\}^n} \left(u_{\mathbf{i}} - u_{\mathbf{i}}^\delta\right)^2 +$$

    $$+ \frac{\alpha}{s^{n-1}} \sum_{\mathbf{i}\in\{1,\ldots,s-1\}^n} \left(\sum_{j=1}^n (u_{\mathbf{i}+\mathbf{e}_j} - u_{\mathbf{i}})^2\right)^{1/2}$$

    over $\mathbb{R}^\mathcal{I}$, where $\mathbf{e}_j$ denotes the j-th unit vector.

Table 4.3. Equivalent methods for total variation minimization in space dimension one.

Total variation minimization	$u_\alpha = \arg\min \mathcal{T}_{\alpha,u^\delta}^{2,1}$
Discrete total variation minimization	$u_\alpha = \arg\min \mathcal{T}_{\alpha,\mathbf{u}^\delta}$
Discrete total variation flow	$u(\alpha)$ solves (4.36)
Taut string algorithm	Algorithm 4.32
Contact problem with strictly convex energy minimization	Theorem 4.35

3. Solution of the *total variation flow equation*

$$\frac{\partial u}{\partial t} \in -\partial \mathcal{R}_1(u), \qquad u(0) = u^\delta,$$

at time α.

4. In [211], we have generalized the taut string algorithm to the following method:

Given data $u^\delta \in L^2_\diamond(\Omega)$, a tube is constructed by first solving Poisson's equation

$$\Delta \tilde{u}^\delta = u^\delta \text{ on } \Omega \text{ and } \frac{\partial \tilde{u}^\delta}{\partial \mathbf{n}} = 0 \text{ on } \partial\Omega,$$

and then defining the high-dimensional α-tube around $\mathbf{u}^\delta := \nabla \tilde{u}^\delta$ as

$$\mathcal{Y}_\alpha := \left\{ \mathbf{u} : \Omega \to \mathbb{R}^n : \left\| \mathbf{u} - \mathbf{u}^\delta \right\|_\infty \leq \alpha \text{ and } \mathbf{u} \cdot \mathbf{n} = 0 \text{ on } \partial\Omega \right\}.$$

The approximation u_α of u^δ is $\nabla \cdot (\mathbf{v}_\alpha)$ with

$$\mathbf{v}_\alpha := \arg\min_{\mathbf{v} \in \mathcal{Y}_\alpha} \int_\Omega \sqrt{1 + |\nabla \mathbf{v}|^2}.$$

5. Solution of the constrained minimization problem

$$\mathcal{C}(u) := \int_\Omega c(u) \to \min, \qquad \left\| u - u^\delta \right\|_* \leq \alpha,$$

where $c : \mathbb{R} \to \mathbb{R}$ is any strictly convex function and $\|\cdot\|_*$ denotes the $*$-number with respect to $(L^2(\Omega), \mathcal{R}_1)$.

Of the five possibilities of extending the taut string algorithm to higher dimensions, only the first and the last are known to be equivalent. Before we prove this, we need additional results concerning the subdifferential of the total variation:

Theorem 4.41. *Let $\Omega \subset \mathbb{R}^n$ be bocL and $u \in BV(\Omega)$. Then $u^* \in \partial \mathcal{R}_1(u)$ if and only if $u^* \in L^{p_*}(\Omega)$ satisfies*

$$\int_U u^* \leq \operatorname{Per}(U; \Omega), \qquad U \subset \Omega \text{ measurable}, \qquad (4.37)$$

and

$$\int_{\{u \geq t\}} u^* = \operatorname{Per}(\{u \geq t\}; \Omega), \qquad a.e.\ t \in \mathbb{R}. \qquad (4.38)$$

Proof. The inclusion $u^* \in \partial \mathcal{R}_1(u)$ is equivalent to

$$\int_\Omega u^*(v - u) \leq \mathcal{R}_1(v) - \mathcal{R}_1(u), \qquad v \in BV(\Omega). \qquad (4.39)$$

We first show that $u^* \in \partial \mathcal{R}_1(u)$ implies (4.37) and (4.38). Assume therefore that (4.39) holds. Let $U \subset \Omega$. If U is no set of finite perimeter in Ω, then (4.37) trivially holds, because the right-hand side is infinite. If, on the other hand, U is a set of finite perimeter, then $\mathcal{R}_1(\chi_U) = \mathrm{Per}(U; \Omega)$, and consequently, $\mathcal{R}_1(u + \chi_U) \leq \mathcal{R}_1(u) + \mathrm{Per}(U; \Omega)$. Thus, (4.37) follows from (4.39) by choosing there $v = u + \chi_U$.

Now define

$$v_{\varepsilon,t}(\mathbf{x}) := \begin{cases} u(\mathbf{x}), & \text{if } u(\mathbf{x}) \leq t, \\ t, & \text{if } t \leq u(\mathbf{x}) \leq t + \varepsilon, \\ u(\mathbf{x}) - \varepsilon, & \text{if } u(\mathbf{x}) \geq t + \varepsilon. \end{cases}$$

Then we have for almost every $t \in \mathbb{R}$ and every $\varepsilon > 0$ that

$$\int_\Omega u^*(v_{\varepsilon,t} - u) = \int_{\{u \geq t+\varepsilon\}} u^*(u - \varepsilon - u) + \int_{\{t < u < t+\varepsilon\}} u^*(t - u)$$

$$\geq -\varepsilon \int_{\{u \geq t+\varepsilon\}} u^* - \varepsilon \int_{\{t < u < t+\varepsilon\}} |u^*| . \quad (4.40)$$

Note that $\{v_{\varepsilon,t} \geq s\} = \{u \geq s\}$ for $s \leq t$, and $\{v_{\varepsilon,t} \geq s\} = \{u \geq s + \varepsilon\}$ for $s > t$. Thus it follows from the coarea formula, Theorem 9.75, that for almost every $t \in \mathbb{R}$

$$\mathcal{R}_1(v_{\varepsilon,t}) = \int_{-\infty}^\infty \mathrm{Per}(\{v_{\varepsilon,t} \geq s\}; \Omega) \, ds$$

$$= \int_{-\infty}^t \mathrm{Per}(\{u \geq s\}; \Omega) \, ds + \int_{t+\varepsilon}^\infty \mathrm{Per}(\{u \geq s\}; \Omega) \, ds$$

$$= \mathcal{R}_1(u) - \int_t^{t+\varepsilon} \mathrm{Per}(\{u \geq s\}; \Omega) \, ds .$$

Consequently, it follows from (4.40) and (4.39) that for almost every $t \in \mathbb{R}$

$$-\int_{\{u \geq t+\varepsilon\}} u^* \leq \frac{1}{\varepsilon} \int_\Omega u^*(v_{\varepsilon,t} - u) + \int_{\{t < u < t+\varepsilon\}} |u^*|$$

$$\leq \frac{1}{\varepsilon}(\mathcal{R}_1(v_{\varepsilon,t}) - \mathcal{R}_1(u)) + \int_{\{t < u < t+\varepsilon\}} |u^*| \quad (4.41)$$

$$= -\frac{1}{\varepsilon} \int_t^{t+\varepsilon} \mathrm{Per}(\{u \geq s\}; \Omega) \, ds + \int_{\{t < u < t+\varepsilon\}} |u^*| .$$

Because $u \in BV(\Omega)$, we have for almost every $t \in \mathbb{R}$ that

$$\lim_{\varepsilon \to 0} \frac{1}{\varepsilon} \int_t^{t+\varepsilon} \mathrm{Per}(\{u \geq s\}; \Omega) \, ds = \mathrm{Per}(\{u \geq t\}; \Omega),$$

$$\lim_{\varepsilon \to 0} \mathcal{L}^n(\{t < u < t + \varepsilon\}) = 0 .$$

Because $u^* \in L^{p_*}(\Omega) \subset L^1(\Omega)$, this implies that also

$$\lim_{\varepsilon \to 0} \int_{\{t<u<t+\varepsilon\}} |u^*| = 0 .$$

Thus the passage to limit $\varepsilon \to 0$ in (4.41) yields that for almost every $t \in \mathbb{R}$

$$\int_{\{u \geq t\}} u^* = \lim_{\varepsilon \to 0} \int_{\{u \geq t+\varepsilon\}} u^* \geq \mathrm{Per}(\{u \geq t\}; \Omega) .$$

The converse inequality follows from (4.37), which proves (4.38).

Now assume that (4.37) and (4.38) hold. From the coarea formula, Theorem 9.75, it follows that

$$\int_{-\infty}^{+\infty} \mathrm{Per}(\{u \geq t\}; \Omega) = \mathcal{R}_1(u) < \infty .$$

In particular, there exists a sequence $(t_k) \subset \mathbb{R}$ with $\lim_k t_k = -\infty$, such that (4.38) holds for every t_k and $\lim_k \mathrm{Per}(\{u \geq t_k\}; \Omega) = 0$. Consequently, it follows from (4.38) that

$$\int_{\Omega} u^* = \lim_k \int_{\{u \geq t_k\}} u^* = \lim_k \mathrm{Per}(\{u \geq t_k\}; \Omega) = 0 .$$

Now let $v \in BV(\Omega) \cap L^{p_*}(\Omega)$. In order to show that $u^* \in \partial \mathcal{R}_1(u)$, we have to verify (4.39). Because $\int_{\Omega} u^* = 0$, it follows from Corollary 9.16 applied to $u^* v$ and $u^* u$ that

$$\int_{\Omega} u^*(v - u) = \int_{-\infty}^{\infty} \left(\int_{\{v \geq t\}} u^* - \int_{\{u \geq t\}} u^* \right) dt .$$

This equation together with (4.37) applied to the sets $\{v \geq t\}$, (4.38) applied to $\{u \geq t\}$, and the coarea formula, Theorem 9.75, implies that

$$\int_{\Omega} u^*(v - u) = \int_{-\infty}^{\infty} \left(\int_{\{v \geq t\}} u^* - \int_{\{u \geq t\}} u^* \right) dt \leq$$

$$\leq \int_{-\infty}^{\infty} \left(\mathrm{Per}(\{v \geq t\}; \Omega) - \mathrm{Per}(\{u \geq t\}; \Omega) \right) dt = \mathcal{R}_1(v) - \mathcal{R}_1(u) ,$$

which proves the inequality (4.39).   □

Definition 4.42. A *measurable function* $\phi : \mathbb{R} \to \mathbb{R}$ *is an N-function, if* $\mathcal{L}^1(\phi(E)) = 0$ *whenever* $\mathcal{L}^1(E) = 0$ *(see [210, Def. 18.24]).*

Remark 4.43. Every absolutely continuous function $\phi : \mathbb{R} \to \mathbb{R}$ is an N-function. In particular, every Lipschitz function is an N-function (see [210, Thm. 18.25]).   ◇

Corollary 4.44. *Let* $\phi : \mathbb{R} \to \mathbb{R}$ *be a non-decreasing N-function. If* $u \in BV(\Omega)$ *is such that* $\phi(u) \in BV(\Omega)$, *then* $\partial \mathcal{R}_1(u) \subset \partial \mathcal{R}_1(\phi(u))$.

Proof. Let $u^* \in \partial \mathcal{R}_1(u)$. Define

$$
E := \left\{ t \in \mathbb{R} : \int_{\{u \geq t\}} u^* \neq \mathrm{Per}(\{u \geq t\}; \Omega) \right\}.
$$

From Theorem 4.41, it follows that $\int_U u^* \leq \mathrm{Per}(U; \Omega)$ for every measurable $U \subset \Omega$, and $\mathcal{L}^1(E) = 0$. Now note that

$$
\phi(E) = \left\{ s \in \mathbb{R} : \int_{\{\phi(u) \geq s\}} u^* \neq \mathrm{Per}(\{\phi(u) \geq s\}; \Omega) \right\}.
$$

Because ϕ is an N-function, it follows from $\mathcal{L}^1(E) = 0$ that $\mathcal{L}^1(\phi(E)) = 0$. Consequently, we have for almost every $s \in \mathbb{R}$ that

$$
\int_{\{\phi(u) \geq s\}} u^* = \mathrm{Per}(\{\phi(u) \geq s\}; \Omega).
$$

Thus it follows from Theorem 4.41 that $u^* \in \partial \mathcal{R}_1(\phi(u))$, which shows that $\partial \mathcal{R}_1(u) \subset \partial \mathcal{R}_1(\phi(u))$.   □

Remark 4.45. Let $\phi : \mathbb{R} \to \mathbb{R}$ be non-decreasing and Lipschitz continuous, and let $u \in BV(\Omega)$. From the coarea formula, it follows that

$$
\begin{aligned}
\mathcal{R}_1(\phi(u)) &= \int_{-\infty}^{\infty} \mathrm{Per}(\{\phi(u) \geq s\}; \Omega) \, \mathrm{d}s \\
&= \int_{-\infty}^{\infty} \mathrm{Per}(\{\phi(u) \geq \phi(t)\}; \Omega) \, \phi'(t) \, \mathrm{d}t \\
&\leq \mathrm{Lip}(\phi) \int_{-\infty}^{\infty} \mathrm{Per}(\{u \geq t\}; \Omega) \, \mathrm{d}t \\
&= \mathrm{Lip}(\phi) \mathcal{R}_1(u) < \infty.
\end{aligned}
$$

Consequently, $\phi(u) \in BV(\Omega)$, which implies that Corollary 4.44 applies to this situation.   ◇

Theorem 4.46. *Let* $c : \mathbb{R} \to \mathbb{R}$ *be convex and denote* $u_\alpha := \arg\min \mathcal{T}_{\alpha, u^\delta}^{2,1}$ *(cf. (4.6)). If* $\int_\Omega c(u_\alpha) < \infty$, *then* u_α *is a solution of*

$$
\mathcal{C}(u) := \int_\Omega c(u) \to \min, \qquad \|u - u^\delta\|_* \leq \alpha, \tag{4.42}
$$

where $\|v\|_*$ *denotes the* *-number of* v *with respect to* $(L^2(\Omega), \mathcal{R}_1)$ *(see Definition 4.5). If* c *is strictly convex, then* u_α *is the unique minimizer of (4.42).*

Proof. Assume first that $c \in C^1(\mathbb{R})$ is such that $\phi := c'$ is Lipschitz continuous. Because c is convex, it follows that $\phi : \mathbb{R} \to \mathbb{R}$ is non-decreasing. From Theorems 10.21 and 10.22, it follows that there exists $u_\alpha^* \in L^2(\Omega)$ satisfying the Kuhn–Tucker conditions

$$u_\alpha^* \in \partial \mathcal{S}_2(u), \qquad -u_\alpha^* \in \partial(\alpha \mathcal{R}_1)(u) .$$

Because $\partial \mathcal{S}_2(u) = u - u^\delta$ (see Example 10.40), it follows that $u_\alpha^* = u - u^\delta$. Denote $w := \phi(u_\alpha)$. Because $\mathcal{R}_1$ is symmetric, that is, $\mathcal{R}_1(v) = \mathcal{R}_1(-v)$, it follows that $\partial \mathcal{R}_1(-v) = -\partial \mathcal{R}_1(v)$ for all v. From Corollary 4.44 and Remark 4.45, it follows that $-u_\alpha^* \in \partial(\alpha \mathcal{R}_1)(w) = -\partial(\alpha \mathcal{R}_1)(-w)$, which implies that $-w \in \partial(\alpha \mathcal{R}_1)^*(u_\alpha^*) = \partial(\alpha \mathcal{R}_1)^*(u_\alpha - u^\delta)$ (see Theorem 10.18).

From Theorem 10.39, it follows that $\partial \mathcal{C}(v) = \phi(v)$ for all v. In particular, $w = \phi(u_\alpha) \in \partial \mathcal{C}(u_\alpha)$. Thus, w satisfies the Kuhn–Tucker conditions

$$w \in \partial \mathcal{C}(u_\alpha), \qquad -w \in \partial(\alpha \mathcal{R}_1)^*(u_\alpha - u^\delta) .$$

Consequently, it follows from Theorem 10.21 that

$$u_\alpha = \arg\min\left(\mathcal{C}(u) + (\alpha \mathcal{R}_1)^*(u - u^\delta)\right) .$$

From Theorem 4.19, it follows that

$$(\alpha \mathcal{R}_1)^*(v) = \begin{cases} 0, & \text{if } \|v\|_* \leq \alpha, \\ \infty, & \text{else.} \end{cases}$$

This proves the assertion for $c \in C^1(\mathbb{R})$ with c' Lipschitz.

Now let $c : \mathbb{R} \to \mathbb{R}$ be an arbitrary convex function. From Lemma 10.32, it follows that c is differentiable almost everywhere. Denote $\phi := c'$. Let ρ be a mollifier and denote by ρ_ε, $\varepsilon > 0$, the rescaled function $\rho_\varepsilon(x) = \rho(x/\varepsilon)/\varepsilon$ (see Definition 9.51). Define moreover for $\varepsilon > 0$ the function

$$\tilde{\phi}_\varepsilon(x) := \begin{cases} \phi\big((x - \varepsilon)/(1 + \varepsilon x)\big), & \text{if } x > \varepsilon, \\ \phi(0), & \text{if } |x| \leq \varepsilon, \\ \phi\big((x + \varepsilon)/(1 - \varepsilon x)\big), & \text{if } x < -\varepsilon . \end{cases}$$

Because ϕ is non-decreasing, it follows that $\tilde{\phi}_\varepsilon$ is a non-decreasing function for every $\varepsilon > 0$, and $(\tilde{\phi}_\varepsilon)_{\varepsilon > 0}$ pointwise converges to ϕ as $\varepsilon \to 0$ from below for almost every $x > 0$ and from above for almost every $x < 0$. Moreover we have $\lim_{x \to \pm\infty} \tilde{\phi}_\varepsilon(x) = \phi(1/\varepsilon^\pm)$.

Now denote

$$\phi_\varepsilon := \rho_\varepsilon * \tilde{\phi}_\varepsilon .$$

Then also $(\phi_\varepsilon)_{\varepsilon > 0}$ pointwise converges to ϕ as $\varepsilon \to 0$, and $\phi_\varepsilon(x) \leq \phi(x)$ for $x > 0$ and $\phi_\varepsilon(x) \geq \phi(x)$ for $x < 0$. Moreover, $\phi_\varepsilon \in C^\infty(\mathbb{R})$ is bounded for every $\varepsilon > 0$, and ϕ_ε is non-decreasing. In particular, the functions ϕ_ε are Lipschitz.

Now define

$$c_\varepsilon(x) := c(0) + \int_0^x \phi_\varepsilon .$$

Then $c_\varepsilon \in C^\infty(\mathbb{R})$ and $c'_\varepsilon = \phi_\varepsilon$ is Lipschitz. Because ϕ_ε is non-decreasing, it follows that c_ε is convex. Moreover, the properties of ϕ_ε imply that for every $x \in \mathbb{R}$, the sequence (c_ε) pointwise converges to c and $c_\varepsilon(x) \leq c(x)$ for all $\varepsilon > 0$ and $x \in \mathbb{R}$. Thus Fatou's Lemma 9.8 implies that

$$\mathcal{C}(u) \geq \limsup_{\varepsilon \to 0} \int_\Omega c_\varepsilon(u) \geq \int_\Omega \liminf_{\varepsilon \to 0} c_\varepsilon(u) = \int_\Omega c(u) = \mathcal{C}(u), \quad u \in L^1(\Omega) . \tag{4.43}$$

From the first part of the proof, it follows that

$$\int_\Omega c_\varepsilon(u_\alpha) \leq \int_\Omega c_\varepsilon(u), \quad u \in BV(\Omega), \ \|u - u^\delta\|_* \leq \alpha .$$

Thus (4.43) implies that u_α is a solution of the constrained minimization problem (4.42).

Finally note that, in the case c is strictly convex, also $\mathcal{C}$ is strictly convex, which shows that its minimizer is unique. This proves the last part of the assertion.   □

Remark 4.47. Theorem 4.46 states that in the dual formulation of total variation regularization, the actual choice of the functional to be minimized does not matter (as long as it remains convex and proper). From a computational point of view, the choice $c(t) = t^2/2$ is natural, as solving the corresponding optimality condition becomes a linear problem.

There is, however, an interesting implication when using a different choice of c. First note that from the density result Theorem 9.71, it follows that for $u^* \in L^2(\Omega)$ we have

$$\|u^*\|_* = \sup\left\{ \int_\Omega u^* u : u \in L^2(\Omega) \cap BV(\Omega), \ \mathcal{R}_1(u) \leq 1 \right\}$$

$$= \sup\left\{ \int_\Omega u^* u : u \in C^\infty(\Omega), \ \mathcal{R}_1(u) \leq 1 \right\} . \tag{4.44}$$

Because the integral in the second line of (4.44) is defined for every $u^* \in L^1(\Omega)$, the last term in (4.44) can be used as a generalization of $\|\cdot\|_*$ to $L^1(\Omega)$. Moreover the functional

$$\mathcal{C}(u) = \int_\Omega c(u), \quad u \in L^1(\Omega),$$

is well-defined and finite if there exist $C_1 \in \mathbb{R}$ and $C_2 > 0$ such that

$$c(t) \le C_1 + C_2 \left| t \right|, \qquad t \in \mathbb{R},$$

for instance if $c(t) = \sqrt{1 + t^2}$. As a consequence, it is possible to generalize total variation regularization to data $u^\delta \in L^1(\Omega)$ by solving

$$\mathcal{C}(u) = \int_\Omega c(u) \to \min, \qquad u \in L^1(\Omega), \quad \left\| u - u^\delta \right\|_* \le \alpha.$$

From Theorem 4.46, it follows that this denoising method is consistent with BV regularization in that it yields the same results for $u^\delta \in L^2(\Omega)$.   ◇

4.5 Mumford–Shah Regularization

One of the most frequently cited papers on variational methods in computer vision is [284]. The functional proposed therein is derived from the following model of image formation: Real-world images are projections of objects in three-dimensional space onto the two-dimensional image plane (see [298]). Assuming that object surfaces are "homogeneous" up to some degree, each object gives rise to a smooth image region that is bordered by the object's projected silhouette. In general, the projected silhouette will coincide with a discontinuity in the image function. This model suggests the functional

$$\boxed{\mathcal{T}^{\mathrm{MS}}_{\alpha,\beta,u^\delta}(u,K) = \frac{1}{2} \int_\Omega (u - u^\delta)^2 + \alpha \int_{\Omega \setminus K} |\nabla u|^2 + \beta \mathcal{H}^1(K)} \qquad (4.45)$$

with parameters α, $\beta > 0$. Here $\Omega \subset \mathbb{R}^2$ denotes the image domain, u^δ is the recorded image, and K is a set of piecewise smooth curves that divide Ω into finitely many disjoint open sets Ω_i, such that $\bar{\Omega}$ coincides with the closure of $\Omega_1 \cup \Omega_2 \cup \ldots \cup \Omega_N$. The Hausdorff measure $\mathcal{H}^1(K)$ denotes the "size" of the curve set K.

A minimizing pair (u, K) of the Mumford–Shah functional consists of a piecewise smooth function u with discontinuities along the curve set K, which coincides with the object boundaries. The term $\beta \mathcal{H}^1(K)$ prevents the discontinuity set from becoming too large, and thereby the segmentation (the partitioning) of Ω from becoming exceedingly fine. Although the primary intention of the Mumford–Shah functional has originally been image segmentation, it may be used for image denoising as well. A detailed mathematical study of the Mumford–Shah approach can be found in [276].

In [284], two other functionals are considered, which can be viewed as limit cases of (4.45): If the set of admissible functions u is restricted to

$$\{u : u = a_i \text{ on } \Omega_i, \quad a_i \in \mathbb{R}, \quad 1 \le i \le N\},$$

that is, functions that are constant on each Ω_i, then it is easy to see that for a minimizer u, the values a_i are the mean values of u^δ on Ω_i. In this case, (4.45) can be rewritten as

$$\mathcal{T}_{\beta,u^\delta}^{MS,\infty}(K) = \frac{1}{2}\sum_i \int_{\Omega_i} \left(u^\delta - \text{mean}_{\Omega_i}\left(u^\delta\right)\right)^2 + \beta\mathcal{H}^1(K), \qquad (4.46)$$

where $\text{mean}_{\Omega_i}(u^\delta) := \int_{\Omega_i} u^\delta$. When K is fixed in (4.45), then for a sequence $\alpha_k \to \infty$ the sequence of minimizers u_k of $\mathcal{T}_{\alpha_k,\beta,u^\delta}^{MS}$ tends to a piecewise constant function. Therefore, (4.46) can be considered as a limit functional of (4.45) as $\alpha_k \to \infty$. Note that in the right-hand side of (4.46) the sets Ω_i are defined by K, and that there is no gradient operator in the functional. Further, (4.46) is the basis for the image segmentation model proposed in [100].

The third functional considered in [284] is

$$\mathcal{T}_{\beta_0,u^\delta}^{MS,0}(K) = \int_K \left(\beta_0 - \left(\frac{\partial u^\delta}{\partial \nu}\right)^2\right) \, d\mathcal{H}^1, \qquad (4.47)$$

for some constant $\beta_0 > 0$, where ν is a unit normal vector to K. The functional (4.47) can be viewed as a limit functional of (4.45) as $\alpha \to 0$.

The Mumford–Shah functional has the form of a free discontinuity problem. In its numerical solution, the necessity to compute geometric properties of the curve set K, as well as topological considerations (formation of junctions and crack-tips), provide serious difficulties. Therefore, some authors propose to approximate (4.45) by elliptic functionals. For example, the Ambrosio–Tortorelli approximation [13] is given by

$$\mathcal{T}_{\alpha,\beta,u^\delta,k}^{AT}(u,z) = \frac{1}{2}\int_\Omega (u-u^\delta)^2 + \alpha \int_\Omega \left(|\nabla u|^2 + |\nabla z|^2\right)(1-z^2)^{2k} + \beta^2 \int_\Omega \frac{k^2 z^2}{4}$$
$$(4.48)$$

with $u, z \in W^{1,2}(\Omega)$, and $0 \le z \le 1$ almost everywhere in Ω. The function z characterizes the set K. That is, z is approximately 1 near points of K and close to 0 away from K. If k increases, the region where z is close to 1 shrinks. To analyze the limit of a sequence of functionals $(\mathcal{T}_k)$, the concept of Γ-convergence is frequently used:

Definition 4.48 (Γ-convergence). *Let $(\mathcal{T}_k)$ be a sequence of functionals on a metric space X. If there exists a functional $\mathcal{T}$ on X, such that*

1. for all sequences $(u_k) \to u$ one has $\liminf_k \mathcal{T}_k(u_k) \ge \mathcal{T}(u)$,

2. for each u there exists a sequence $(u_k) \to u$ such that $\limsup_k \mathcal{T}_k(u_k) \le \mathcal{T}(u)$,

then $(\mathcal{T}_k)$ is said to Γ-converge to the Γ-limit $\mathcal{T}$, denoted by

$$\mathcal{T} = \Gamma\text{-}\lim_k \mathcal{T}_k .$$

Note that for a constant sequence $(\mathcal{T}_0)$, the Γ-limit only coincides with $\mathcal{T}_0$, if $\mathcal{T}_0$ is lower semi-continuous. Otherwise the Γ-limit of $\mathcal{T}_0$ is the relaxation of $\mathcal{T}_0$ (to be defined in the following chapter).

Proposition 4.49 (Properties of the Γ-limit). *Let $(\mathcal{T}_k)$ be a sequence of functionals on a metric space X, which Γ-converges to a functional $\mathcal{T}$. Then $\mathcal{T}$ is unique and lower semi-continuous. Let further $(\mathcal{T}_k)$ be* equi-coercive, *that is, for each $t \in \mathbb{R}$ there exists a compact set $K_t \subset X$ such that* $\mathrm{level}_t(\mathcal{T}_k) \subset K_t$ *for all k. Let moreover u_k be a minimizer of $\mathcal{T}_k$, $k \in \mathbb{N}$. Then every cluster point of (u_k) is a minimizer of $\mathcal{T}$.*

The proof of the proposition and further information on Γ-convergence can be found in [124].

In [13], it is shown that for $k \to \infty$, the functional (4.48) Γ-converges to the Mumford–Shah functional. Therefore, if (u_k, z_k) is a sequence of pairs minimizing $\mathcal{T}_k$, then the limit $u = \lim_k u_k$ (if it exists) is a minimizer of the Mumford–Shah functional. The sequence (z_k) converges to 0 strongly in $L^2(\Omega)$.

Different choices for $(\mathcal{T}_k)$ are possible, for example the sequence

$$
\mathcal{T}^{\mathrm{AT}'}_{\alpha,\beta,u^\delta,k}(u,z) = \frac{1}{2} \int_\Omega (u - u^\delta)^2 + \alpha \int_\Omega \left(z^2 \, |\nabla u|^2 + \frac{1}{k} \, |\nabla z|^2 \right) + \beta^2 \int_\Omega \frac{k(z-1)^2}{4}
$$
(4.49)

also Γ-converges to the Mumford–Shah functional for $k \to \infty$ (see [14]). Note that, contrary to the Ambrosio–Tortorelli approximation, here $\{z \approx 0\}$ characterizes the set K, and $z_k \to 1$ almost everywhere.

In the Mumford–Shah functional, only the size of the discontinuity set K is measured by $\mathcal{H}^1(K)$, but not its smoothness. Therefore in a minimizing pair (u, K), the set K can – and in general will – have junctions, corners, and crack-tips. If this is not desired, one can also penalize the curvature of K. The modified Mumford–Shah functional then is

$$
\mathcal{T}^{\mathrm{MSE}}_{\alpha,\beta,\gamma,u^\delta}(u,K) = \frac{1}{2} \int_\Omega (u - u^\delta)^2 + \alpha \int_{\Omega \setminus K} |\nabla u|^2 + \int_K \left(\beta + \gamma \kappa(s)^2 \right) \, \mathrm{d}s \,. \tag{4.50}
$$

Here K denotes a parameterized curve with arc length element $\mathrm{d}s$ and curvature $\kappa(s)$. One possible approximation (in the sense of Γ-convergence) of (4.50), suggested in [270], is

$$
\mathcal{T}^{\mathrm{MSE}}_{\alpha,\beta,\gamma,u^\delta}(u,z) = \frac{1}{2} \int_\Omega (u - u^\delta)^2 + \alpha \int_\Omega z^2 \, |\nabla u|^2
$$
$$
+ \beta \int_\Omega \left(\frac{1}{k} \, |\nabla z|^2 + kW(z) \right) + \gamma k \int_\Omega \left(2\frac{\Delta z}{k} - kW'(z) \right)^2 \,. \tag{4.51}
$$

Here $W(z) = \left(1 - z^2\right)^2$ is a so-called double-well potential due to its two minima at $z = \pm 1$. For $k \to \infty$, minimizers z_k of (4.51) converge to a function z that is $+1$ or -1 almost everywhere. The zero level line of z represents the curve K.

In all cases presented above, to numerically compute a minimizer of $\mathcal{T}_k$, one has to solve the corresponding optimality conditions. Those are given by two coupled non-linear second-order PDEs (fourth order in case of (4.51)), which can be solved using a finite difference or finite element approach. Thereby no topological considerations about the curve set K, like for example splitting or merging of curves, have to be taken into account.

An example for denoising with the Mumford–Shah functional is shown in Fig. 4.13. Its bottom row shows a minimizing pair (u, z) of (4.49), with u^δ given by the image in the top row. Recall that the set $\{z \approx 0\}$, that is, the dark regions in the bottom right image, correspond to the discontinuity set (the edges) of the image u, resp., u^δ.

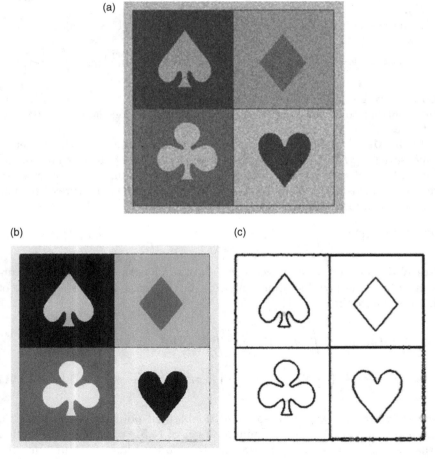

(a)

(b)   (c)

Fig. 4.13. Mumford–Shah regularization. (a) The *cards* image with 10% Gaussian noise. (b) Image denoised using (4.49) as approximation for the Mumford–Shah functional. (c) Corresponding edge signature function z.

4.6 Recent Topics on Denoising with Variational Methods

The idea of image decomposition goes back to Y. Meyer [275] who rewrote denoising models as constrained optimization problems

$$\mathcal{T}^{\mathrm{d}}_{\alpha,u^\delta}(u,v) = \rho(v) + \alpha\mathcal{R}(u) \quad \text{subject to} \quad u + v = u^\delta\,.$$

Meyer called v the *noise component* and u the *image component*.

In [28], a regularization for constrained decomposition is proposed. It consists in minimization of

$$\mathcal{T}^{\mathrm{cd}}_{\alpha,u^\delta}(u,w) = \frac{1}{2}\left\|u^\delta - (u+w)\right\|_2^2 + \alpha_1\mathcal{R}_1(u) \quad \text{subject to} \quad \|w\|_* \le \mu\,,$$

where, as usual in this book, $\mathcal{R}_1$ denotes the total variation semi-norm. The superscript (cd) stands for *constrained decomposition*. In the decomposition model, u is referred to as image component, w is referred to as *texture component*, and $v = u^\delta - u - w$ is the noise component. This approach is based on ideas in [377], where unconstrained regularization models of the form

$$\mathcal{T}^{\mathrm{d}}_{\alpha,u^\delta}(u,w) = \frac{1}{2}\left\|u^\delta - u - w\right\|_2^2 + \alpha_1\Re_1(u) + \alpha_2\Re_2(w)\,,$$

are considered, where $\Re_i$, $i = 1, 2$, are two penalization functionals. The original approach in [377] uses the regularization terms $\Re_1(\cdot) = \mathcal{R}_1(\cdot)$ and $\Re_2(\cdot) = \|\cdot\|_*$. The choice of the $*$-number for regularization is motivated by the model assumption that texture has finite $*$-number. In [377], instead of the $*$-number, an approximation is considered, where $w = \nabla(\mathbf{w})$ and $\Re_2(w) = \|\mathbf{w}\|_p$. For $p \to \infty$, this term approaches the $*$-number. To implement the ideas, the following optimization problem is considered:

$$\mathcal{T}^{\mathrm{d}}_{\alpha,u^\delta}(u,\mathbf{w}) = \frac{1}{2}\left\|u^\delta - u - \nabla\cdot(\mathbf{w})\right\|_2^2 + \alpha_1\mathcal{R}_1(u) + \alpha_2\Re_2(\nabla\cdot(\mathbf{w}))\,.$$

In [312], they also proposed functionals of the form

$$\mathcal{T}_{\alpha,u^\delta}(u) = \frac{1}{2}\left\|-\nabla\Delta^{-1}(u^\delta - u)\right\|_2^2 + \alpha\mathcal{R}_1(u)\,,$$

where $-\Delta^{-1}$ is the solution of the Laplace equation with homogeneous Neumann boundary data, that is, $v = -\Delta^{-1}\rho$ solves

$$\begin{aligned}
-\Delta v &= \rho \quad \text{in } \Omega\,,\\
\frac{\partial v}{\partial \mathbf{n}} &= 0 \quad \text{in } \partial\Omega\,.
\end{aligned} \tag{4.52}$$

Let Ω have C^1-boundary and $u^\delta \in L^2(\Omega)$, then from [195, Ex. 7.4.8, Thm. 9.1.16] it follows that, for $\rho \in L^2(\Omega)$, (4.52) has a unique solution $v \in W^{2,2}(\Omega)$ and

$$\|v\|_{2,2} \le C \|\rho\|_2 \ .$$

Consequently,

$$\left\|-\nabla\Delta^{-1}(u^\delta - u)\right\|_2 \le \left\|-\nabla\Delta^{-1}(u^\delta - u)\right\|_{1,2} \le C \left\|u^\delta - u\right\|_2 \ .$$

This shows that $\left\|-\nabla\Delta^{-1}(\cdot)\right\|_2$ is weaker than $\|\cdot\|_2$ and penalizes less for textured data.

The use of such variational methods is motivated similarly as the regularization models proposed by Meyer [275, p. 41], which consist in minimization of

$$\mathcal{T}_{\alpha,u^\delta}(u) = \left\|u^\delta - u\right\|_{\dot{B}_\infty^{-1,\infty}} + \alpha\mathcal{R}_1(u) \, ,$$

where $\left\|u^\delta - u\right\|_{\dot{B}_\infty^{-1,\infty}}$ is the norm on the Besov space $\dot{B}_\infty^{-1,\infty}(\Omega)$. The difficulty associated with such a functional is that it is not strictly convex, and thus *a priori* there may be multiple minimizers.

In general, *texture decomposition models* for two energy functionals J and G consist in solving the constraint optimization problem

$$\inf\{J(u) + G(v)\} \, , \qquad \text{subject to} \quad u + v = u^\delta \ . \tag{4.53}$$

Typical choices are $J(u) = \alpha\mathcal{R}_1(u)$ and $G(v) = \frac{1}{2}\|v\|_2^2$, in which case (4.53) reduces to original ROF-model [339]. Decomposition models have been extended to more than two components, decomposing an image into *Cartoon*, *Noise*, and *Texture* (see [31]).

Y. Meyer's decomposition model uses $J(u) = \alpha\mathcal{R}_1(u)$ and $G(v) = \|v\|_*$. This problem has been considered in [24]; in [196], it has been shown independently with different methods that the decomposition is not unique. Another reference to decomposition models is [147]. Curvelets decomposition has been presented in [225]. Moreover, in [400] it has been shown that Bregman iteration for image decomposition is in fact an *augmented Lagrangian method*. For a general introduction to augmented Lagrangian methods, we refer to [183], and for a detailed mathematical analysis concerning the relation between the augmented Lagrangian method and iterative Bregman distance regularization, we refer to [171]; for the usage in the context of image processing and inverse problems, we refer for instance to [221].

Duality formulations for minimization of convex variational problems have been widely used, see for instance [29, 87], and [212] for the predual setting.

Recent publications on decomposition concern for instance *BV-Gabor* models [30]. This work is based on [312, 377].

Quadratic higher-order variation regularization models have been widely discussed in the splines literature. We mention the fundamental works by Reinsch [328] and Schoenberg [352]. For more background on splines theory, we refer to [353]. An elementary exposition of the relation between approximating splines and variational methods has been given in [206]. In [374, 375], *rational splines* have been developed, and the relation to quadratic regularization with rational derivatives has been discussed. For the statistical context on higher-order regularization, we refer to [177, 250]. Higher order models also appear in variational level set formulations when the curvature κ is penalized by $\int_\Omega |\kappa|^2$ (see [139]). This energy formulation is associated with the *Willmore flow*. Higher-order regularization is used in [45] to support anisotropic regularization in an ROF model with angular dependence of the level sets.

In image processing, non-linear variational methods of higher order have been introduced by Chambolle and Lions [90]. They suggested the decomposition model of minimizing

$$\mathcal{T}_{\alpha,u^\delta}(u,w) = \frac{1}{2} \left\| u^\delta - u \right\|_2^2 + \alpha_1 \mathcal{R}_1(u-w) + \alpha_2 \mathcal{R}_2(u),$$

where $\mathcal{R}_2(u) = |D^2 u|$ is the total variation of the gradient of u.

Without the middle regularization term, that is, for $\alpha_1 = 0$, the functional has been considered in [344] with an application for material testing. Related fourth-order PDEs can be found for instance in [190, 264]. Discretized partial differential equations have been considered in [362], and numerical methods for their solution can be found in [95]. Dual formulations in the continuous setting have been considered for instance in [301].

Besov space norm regularization has become an active field for image analysis, see for instance [127, 176].

Considering discontinuous functions as continuous graphs has been proposed in [292]. The advantage of this approach is that it allows one to consider the regularization method in a Hilbert space setting. The work has been extended to higher dimension in [237–240]. Similar ideas of interpreting images as embedded maps and minimal surfaces have been considered in [235, 342].

Reconstruction of discontinuous functions for ill-posed problems with equivalent $W^{s,2}$ norm, $s < \frac{1}{2}$, has been studied in [291]. Also there, wavelet techniques have been used for numerical minimization. Wavelet-Galerkin methods have been proposed in [132].

Maximum entropy regularization in imaging has been considered in many papers concerned with imaging and statistical applications, see for instance [10, 121, 142, 154, 222, 253]. One reason why this ME regularization is successful is that it respects positivity of the solution. Kullback–Leibler minimization for the solution of inverse problems has been considered for instance in [331]. In the analysis of these methods, the Bregman distance defined in [59] plays an important role.

Regularization models for filtering Poisson noise have attracted much attention; we refer to only a few papers, especially to the work by M. Nikolova et al. [92, 293, 294].

To analyze statistical Poisson data, we have suggested to use a Delaunay triangulation (tetrahedrization) (for more background on Delaunay triangulation, we refer to [140]), and use one over the area of the triangles as an approximation of the density on the triangles (see [302]). The piecewise constant initial data are then smoothed by total variation regularization. It has been shown in [188] that for one-dimensional data, this approach is equivalent to the taut string algorithm (see also [128]). Instead of using total variation regularization, we also have considered in [302] minimization of the functional

$$\mathcal{T}_{\text{Fisher}}(u) := \frac{1}{2} \int_{\Omega} (u - u^{\delta})^2 + \frac{\alpha}{2} \int_{\Omega} \frac{|\nabla u|^2}{|u|},$$

which pronounces high peaks in u^{δ}. Following [12], we called this approach *Fisher information regularization*.

An important problem in denoising with variational methods is the choice of the regularization parameter. There have been numerous approaches in the statistical framework. We mention for instance *generalized cross evaluation* [379]. For more background on statistics and inverse problems, we refer to [378]. A survey on numerous statistical parameter choice strategies, such as *variance tuning*, *minimizing estimated mean square error*, and *marginal likelihood estimation*, has been given in [250]. In the deterministic setting, parameter choice strategies have been presented in Chapter 3. There mostly information on δ, which estimates the data error $\|v^{\delta} - v\|$, is used. We mention again Morozov's discrepancy principle [277]. For the solution of linear ill-posed problems, order optimal strategies for choosing the regularization parameter have been proposed in [150] – a similar strategy has been developed in [325, 326]. The strategy of [150] has been generalized to non-linear ill-posed problems in [348]. For inverse problems, L-curve criteria have been suggested by Hansen [205]. More heuristic based type stopping criteria have been suggested for instance in [31, 181, 282], to mention a few recent publications.

There exist several articles on total variation denoising and deblurring, see for example [98, 99]. It is interesting to see that the equivalent constraint formulation of the ROF functional (see (4.7)) can also be solved with algorithms from convex analysis (see for example [115], where imaging problems have been considered as applications of the abstract theory). Multiplicative noise models have been considered, for instance, in [24, 337, 346].

Piecewise constant function recovery and segmentation with variational and PDE methods has been proposed in [100]; thereby adapting the Mumford–Shah regularization model to piecewise constant functions. Many references followed this approach.

A very recent approach on total variation regularization for data with high-dimensional range is [355].

5

Variational Calculus for Non-convex Regularization

In Chapter 4, we have studied regularization methods for denoising, consisting in minimization of convex variational functionals. In this chapter, we turn to the study of first-order *non-convex* variational regularization techniques. Here we call a regularization functional of the type

$$\rho(u, u^\delta) + \alpha \mathcal{R}(u) := \int_\Omega \phi(\mathbf{x}, u, \nabla u, u^\delta) + \alpha \int_\Omega \psi(\mathbf{x}, u, \nabla u)$$

non-convex if the sum of the integrands $\phi + \alpha\psi$ is non-convex with respect to ∇u. We use this notation paying tribute to the fact that *standard* results from the calculus of variations require convexity in the ∇u variable.

Note that the term "non-convex regularization" is not used consistently in the literature. Mostly, the term non-convex regularization is used in the field of discrete regularization methods, see, e.g., [177, 178, 180, 189, 250, 257, 283, 295].

The main motivation for developing this theory are problems that consist in minimization of the functionals $\mathcal{F}^{(p)} : W^{1,p}(\Omega) \to \mathbb{R} \cup \{\infty\}$ defined by

$$\mathcal{F}^{(p)}(u) := \int_\Omega \frac{(u - u^\delta)^2}{2 |\nabla u|^p} + \alpha |\nabla u|^p , \qquad (5.1)$$

where $u^\delta \in L^\infty(\Omega)$ and $1 \leq p < \infty$ (see (2.33)). Here and in the following, $\Omega \subset \mathbb{R}^n$ is always bocL.

There are several theoretical questions concerning the functional $\mathcal{F}^{(p)}$. First note that $\mathcal{F}^{(p)}(u)$ is not well-defined, if there exists a set U of positive measure such that $u = u^\delta$ and $\nabla u = 0$ on U, as in this case both the numerator and the denominator of the first term in the integral become zero. It is, however, necessary to define the integral in such situations; for instance, in the trivial case $u^\delta = 0$, one would expect $u = 0$ to be a minimizer of $\mathcal{F}^{(p)}$. Therefore, we need a meaningful way to extend $\mathcal{F}^{(p)}$ to the whole space $W^{1,p}(\Omega)$.

A second question is the existence of a minimizer of $\mathcal{F}^{(p)}$. One method for proving existence of minimizers is the usage of direct methods (cf. Sect. 5.1

below). Here it is essential that the regarded functional is coercive and lower semi-continuous with respect to a suitable topology. In case of integral functionals, the weak topology is suited, as weak coercivity translates to a growth condition for the integrand, which is usually satisfied in applications. The weak lower semi-continuity, however, is basically equivalent to the convexity of the integrand with respect to ∇u. Indeed, one can easily construct non-convex examples where no minimizer exists. Thus, instead of minimizing $\mathcal{F}^{(p)}$, one computes minimizers of a relaxed functional $\mathcal{RF}^{(p)}$, which is defined as the largest weakly lower semi-continuous functional below $\mathcal{F}^{(p)}$. It turns out that in many cases, this functional can be obtained by computing the convex hull of the integrand of $\mathcal{F}^{(p)}$ with respect to ∇u.

In the case $p = 1$, even the convexification is not enough to guarantee the existence of a minimizer in $W^{1,1}(\Omega)$. In fact, the natural space of definition for functionals with linear growth in ∇u is the space $BV(\Omega)$. Thus, we compute a suitable extension of $\mathcal{RF}^{(1)}$ to $BV(\Omega)$.

5.1 Direct Methods

Let X be a topological space. A functional $\mathcal{F} : X \to \mathbb{R} \cup \{\infty\}$ is *sequentially coercive*, if every level set $\mathrm{level}_\alpha(\mathcal{F})$ is sequentially pre-compact. In other words, $\mathcal{F}$ is sequentially coercive, if and only if every sequence $(u_k) \subset X$ with $\sup_k \mathcal{F}(u_k) < \infty$ has a convergent subsequence.

The notion of sequential coercivity strongly depends on the topology on X. In the case that X is a subset of a locally convex space, we say that $\mathcal{F}$ is weakly (weakly*) coercive, if it is coercive with respect to the restriction of the weak (weak*) topology to X.

Theorem 5.1. *Let $\mathcal{F} : X \to \mathbb{R} \cup \{\infty\}$ be sequentially coercive, sequentially lower semi-continuous, and proper. Then $\mathcal{F}$ attains a minimizer in X.*

Proof. Let $(u_k) \subset \mathcal{D}(\mathcal{F})$ be a minimizing sequence, that is,

$$\lim_k \mathcal{F}(u_k) = \inf\{\mathcal{F}(v) : v \in X\}.$$

From the sequential coercivity of $\mathcal{F}$, it follows that (u_k) has a subsequence $(u_{k'})$ converging to $u \in X$. The sequential lower semi-continuity implies that

$$\mathcal{F}(u) \leq \liminf_{k'} \mathcal{F}(u_{k'}) = \inf\{\mathcal{F}(v) : v \in X\}.$$

Thus, u is a minimizer of $\mathcal{F}$, which proves the assertion. □

In the following, we apply direct methods to integral functionals $\mathcal{F} : W^{1,p}(\Omega) \to \mathbb{R} \cup \{\infty\}$ of the form

$$\mathcal{F}(u) := \int_\Omega f(\mathbf{x}, u, \nabla u), \tag{5.2}$$

where $f : \Omega \times (\mathbb{R} \times \mathbb{R}^n) \to \mathbb{R} \cup \{\infty\}$ is a normal integrand (see Definition 10.36).

Because for $u \in W^{1,p}(\Omega)$ the function $\mathbf{x} \mapsto (u(\mathbf{x}), \nabla u(\mathbf{x}))$ is measurable, it follows from Lemma 10.38 that the functional $\mathcal{F}(u)$ is well-defined.

We say that $f : \Omega \times \mathbb{R} \times \mathbb{R}^n \to \mathbb{R} \cup \{\infty\}$ is a *convex integrand*, if for every $(\mathbf{x}, \xi) \in \Omega \times \mathbb{R}$ the function $\mathbf{t} \mapsto f(\mathbf{x}, \xi, \mathbf{t})$ is convex, that is, f is convex in the last component.

In what follows, we always assume that the functional $\mathcal{F}$ is proper.

Theorem 5.2. *Let $f : \Omega \times \mathbb{R} \times \mathbb{R}^n \to \mathbb{R} \cup \{\infty\}$ be a normal and convex integrand. Assume that*

$$f(\mathbf{x}, \xi, \mathbf{t}) \geq -c\left(1 + |\xi|^q + |\mathbf{t}|^r\right)$$

for some $c \geq 0$, $q \geq 1$, and either $1 \leq r < p$ or $r = p = 1$. Then for all sequences $(u_k) \subset L^q(\Omega)$ strongly converging to u and $(\mathbf{v}_k) \subset L^r(\Omega; \mathbb{R}^n)$ weakly converging to $\mathbf{v}$, we have

$$\liminf_k \int_\Omega f(\mathbf{x}, u_k, \mathbf{v}_k) \geq \int_\Omega f(\mathbf{x}, u, \mathbf{v}) \ .$$

In particular, if $1 \leq q < np/(n-p)$, the functional $\mathcal{F}$ defined in (5.2) is weakly sequentially lower semi-continuous in $W^{1,p}(\Omega)$.

Proof. See for instance [182, Thm. 4.4] in the case that f is continuous. For the case of a normal integrand we refer to [220], where, additionally, a collection of by far more general lower semi-continuity results of the same type is presented. □

Corollary 5.3. *Let $p > 1$. Assume that $f : \Omega \times \mathbb{R} \times \mathbb{R}^n \to \mathbb{R} \cup \{\infty\}$ is a normal and convex integrand satisfying*

$$f(\mathbf{x}, \xi, \mathbf{t}) \geq c_1 + c_2\left(|\xi|^p + |\mathbf{t}|^p\right) \tag{5.3}$$

for some $c_1 \in \mathbb{R}$ and $c_2 > 0$. Let $\mathcal{F} : W^{1,p}(\Omega) \to \mathbb{R} \cup \{\infty\}$ be as in (5.2), and let $X \subset W^{1,p}(\Omega)$ be a closed and convex subset. If there exists $u \in X$ with $\mathcal{F}(u) < \infty$, then $\mathcal{F}|_X$ attains a minimizer in X.

Proof. We first show that $\mathcal{F}|_X$ is weakly sequentially coercive on $X \subset W^{1,p}(\Omega)$. To that end, we have to show that every level set $\text{level}_\alpha(\mathcal{F}|_X)$ is weakly sequentially pre-compact in X. From (5.3), it follows that

$$\mathcal{F}(u) \geq c_1 \mathcal{L}^n(\Omega) + c_2 \int_\Omega \left(|u|^p + |\nabla u|^p\right) = c_1 \mathcal{L}^n(\Omega) + c_2 \|u\|_{1,p}^p \ .$$

Consequently,

$$\text{level}_\alpha(\mathcal{F}|_X) \subset X \cap \left\{u \in W^{1,p}(\Omega) : \|u\|_{1,p}^p \leq (\alpha - c_1 \mathcal{L}^n(\Omega))/c_2\right\} \ .$$

Because X is a convex and closed subset of $W^{1,p}(\Omega)$, it follows that X is weakly closed (see Lemma 8.50). On the other hand, because by assumption $p > 1$, the space $W^{1,p}(\Omega)$ is a reflexive and separable Banach space, which implies that the unit ball in $W^{1,p}(\Omega)$ is weakly sequentially compact (see Theorem 8.51). Thus $\mathrm{level}_\alpha(\mathcal{F}|_X)$ is contained in the intersection of a weakly sequentially compact set and a weakly closed set. Consequently, $\mathrm{level}_\alpha(\mathcal{F}|_X)$ is weakly sequentially pre-compact. This shows that $\mathcal{F}|_X$ is weakly sequentially coercive.

From Theorem 5.2, it follows that $\mathcal{F}$ is weakly sequentially lower semi-continuous. Using Theorem 5.1, the existence of a minimizer of $\mathcal{F}|_X$ in X follows. $\square$

5.2 Relaxation on Sobolev Spaces

As we have shown above, the main ingredient for proving the existence of minimizers of integral functionals of the type

$$\mathcal{F}(u) = \int_\Omega f(\mathbf{x}, u, \nabla u)$$

is the convexity of f with respect to ∇u. In case this convexity does not hold, the function $\mathcal{F}$ need not be weakly sequentially lower semi-continuous. As a consequence, minimizers may not exist. If, however, $\mathcal{F}$ is weakly sequentially coercive, then there exist weakly converging sequences (u_k) every one of which satisfies

$$\lim_k \mathcal{F}(u_k) = \inf\{\mathcal{F}(u) : u \in W^{1,p}(\Omega)\}.$$

All the limits of such sequences can be regarded as *generalized minimizers* of $\mathcal{F}$. It is convenient to define a functional whose minimizers are exactly the generalized minimizers of $\mathcal{F}$.

We define the relaxation $\mathcal{RF}$ of $\mathcal{F} : X \subset W^{1,p}(\Omega) \to \mathbb{R} \cup \{\infty\}$ by

$$\boxed{\mathcal{RF}(u) := \inf\left\{\liminf_k \mathcal{F}(u_k) : (u_k) \subset X \text{ and } u_k \rightharpoonup u \text{ in } W^{1,p}(\Omega)\right\}.}$$

Here we set $\mathcal{RF}(u) := \infty$, if there exists no sequence $(u_k) \subset X$ weakly converging to u; in this case, u is not contained in the weak closure of X in $W^{1,p}(\Omega)$.

In general, the construction of $\mathcal{RF}$ does not ensure that it is weakly sequentially lower semi-continuous. However, an additional growth assumption on the integrand f is sufficient to guarantee weak sequential lower semi-continuity of $\mathcal{RF}$.

Lemma 5.4. *Let $p > 1$. Assume that $f : \Omega \times \mathbb{R} \times \mathbb{R}^n \to \mathbb{R} \cup \{\infty\}$ is normal and satisfies*

$$f(\mathbf{x}, \xi, \mathbf{t}) \geq c_1 + c_2 |\mathbf{t}|^p , \qquad (\mathbf{x}, \xi, \mathbf{t}) \in \Omega \times \mathbb{R} \times \mathbb{R}^n , \qquad (5.4)$$

for some $c_1 \in \mathbb{R}$ and $c_2 > 0$. Then $\mathcal{RF}$ is weakly sequentially lower semi-continuous in $W^{1,p}(\Omega)$.

Proof. Let $u \in W^{1,p}(\Omega)$ and $(u_k) \rightharpoonup u$. We have to show that

$$d := \liminf_k \mathcal{RF}(u_k) \geq \mathcal{RF}(u) .$$

Without loss of generality, we may assume that $\liminf_k \mathcal{RF}(u_k) < \infty$, else the assertion is trivial.

There exists a subsequence $(u_{k'})$ of (u_k) such that $d = \lim_{k'} \mathcal{RF}(u_{k'})$. From the definition of $\mathcal{RF}$, it follows that for every $\varepsilon > 0$ and k' there exists a sequence $(u_{k',l})$ weakly converging to $u_{k'}$ such that $\lim_l \mathcal{F}(u_{k',l}) \leq \mathcal{RF}(u_{k'}) + \varepsilon$. After possibly passing to a subsequence, we may assume that $\|u_{k'} - u_{k',l}\|_p \leq 1/l$, and $\mathcal{F}(u_{k',l}) \leq \mathcal{RF}(u_{k'}) + \varepsilon + 1/l$.

Now define $\tilde{u}_{k'} = u_{k',k'}$. Then

$$\|\tilde{u}_{k'} - u\|_p \leq \|\tilde{u}_{k'} - u_{k'}\|_p + \|u_{k'} - u\|_p \leq \|u_{k'} - u\|_p + 1/k' .$$

Because the sequence $(u_{k'})$ weakly converges to u in $W^{1,p}(\Omega)$, it follows from the Rellich–Kondrašov Theorem 9.39 (see also Remark 9.40) that $(u_{k'})$ strongly converges to u in $L^p(\Omega)$. This proves that $(\tilde{u}_{k'})$ converges to u in $L^p(\Omega)$. Because $f(\mathbf{x}, \xi, \mathbf{t}) \geq c_1 + c_2 |\mathbf{t}|^p$ (see (5.4)), it follows that

$$\limsup_{k'} \left(c_1 \mathcal{L}^n(\Omega) + c_2 \|\nabla \tilde{u}_{k'}\|_p^p \right) \leq \limsup_{k'} \mathcal{F}(\tilde{u}_{k'}) \leq \lim_{k'} \mathcal{RF}(u_{k'}) + \varepsilon = d + \varepsilon .$$

In particular, the sequence $(\nabla \tilde{u}_{k'})$ is bounded in $L^p(\Omega; \mathbb{R}^n)$, which proves that $(\tilde{u}_{k'})$ weakly converges to u in $W^{1,p}(\Omega)$. Now the definition of $\mathcal{RF}(u)$ implies that

$$\mathcal{RF}(u) \leq \liminf_{k'} \mathcal{F}(\tilde{u}_{k'}) \leq \lim_{k'} \mathcal{RF}(u_{k'}) + \varepsilon = d + \varepsilon .$$

Because ε was arbitrary, this proves the weak sequential lower semi-continuity of $\mathcal{RF}$. □

In Theorem 5.2 above, we have seen that weak sequential lower semi-continuity of an integral functional is strongly tied with the convexity of the integrand. In the following, we show that the relaxation of a large class of functionals can be obtained by convexification of the integrand $f : \Omega \times \mathbb{R} \times \mathbb{R}^n \to \mathbb{R} \cup \{\infty\}$. The convexification $\mathrm{co}\, f$ with respect to the last variable is defined as the largest convex integrand below f. Using Carathéodory's theorem (see [334, Cor. 17.1.5]), it follows that

$$\mathrm{co}\, f(\mathbf{x}, \xi, \mathbf{t}) = \inf\left\{ \sum_{k=1}^{n+1} \lambda_k f(\mathbf{x}, \xi, \mathbf{t}_k) : 0 \leq \lambda_k \leq 1, \ \sum_{k=1}^{n+1} \lambda_k \mathbf{t}_k = \mathbf{t} \right\} . \qquad (5.5)$$

Theorem 5.5. *Let $p > n$ and $f : \Omega \times \mathbb{R} \times \mathbb{R}^n \to \mathbb{R} \cup \{\infty\}$ be Carathéodory. Assume that for almost every $\mathbf{x} \in \Omega$, the integrand f is bounded in a neighborhood of each point $(\mathbf{x}, \xi, \mathbf{t})$ where $f(\mathbf{x}, \xi, \mathbf{t})$ is finite. Moreover, assume that*

$$f(\mathbf{x}, \xi, \mathbf{t}) \geq c_1 + c_2 |\mathbf{t}|^p$$

for some $c_1 \in \mathbb{R}$ and $c_2 > 0$. Then

$$\mathcal{RF}(u) = \int_\Omega \mathrm{co}\, f(\mathbf{x}, u, \nabla u), \qquad u \in W^{1,1}(\Omega).$$

Proof. See [365, Thm. 1.1]. □

The result is quite general in that it assumes only a very mild form of boundedness of f. It is, however, only applicable if the integrand is Carathéodory and if $p > n$. Both conditions are not satisfied by the integrand in (5.1).

Theorem 5.6. *Let $p \geq 1$. Assume that there exists a decreasing sequence $f_k : \Omega \times \mathbb{R} \times \mathbb{R}^n \to \mathbb{R} \cup \{\infty\}$ of non-negative Carathéodory integrands pointwise converging to f satisfying*

$$c_k |\mathbf{t}|^q \leq f_k(\mathbf{x}, \xi, \mathbf{t})$$

for some $q > n$ and $c_k > 0$, such that for almost every $\mathbf{x} \in \Omega$ and $k \in \mathbb{N}$, the integrand f_k is bounded in a neighborhood of each point $(\mathbf{x}, \xi, \mathbf{t})$ where $f_k(\mathbf{x}, \xi, \mathbf{t})$ is finite. Assume moreover that

$$\mathrm{ess\,sup}\{\mathrm{co}\, f_k(\mathbf{x}, \xi, \mathbf{t}) : \mathbf{x} \in \Omega, |\xi| < r, |\mathbf{t}| < r\} < \infty, \qquad r > 0, \ k \in \mathbb{N}, \tag{5.6}$$

and that $\mathrm{co}\, f$ is a Carathéodory integrand satisfying

$$0 \leq \mathrm{co}\, f(\mathbf{x}, \xi, \mathbf{t}) \leq c_1 + c_2\big(|\xi|^p + |\mathbf{t}|^p\big)$$

for some $c_1 \in \mathbb{R}$ and $c_2 > 0$.
    Then

$$\mathcal{RF}(u) = \mathcal{F}_c(u) := \int_\Omega \mathrm{co}\, f(\mathbf{x}, u, \nabla u), \qquad u \in W^{1,p}(\Omega).$$

Proof. By definition, $\mathrm{co}\, f$ is a convex integrand. Moreover, it is a non-negative Carathéodory function by assumption. Thus, it follows from Theorem 5.2 that $\mathcal{F}_c$ is weakly sequentially lower semi-continuous in $W^{1,s}(\Omega)$ for every $1 \leq s < \infty$, which in particular implies that $\mathcal{RF}_c = \mathcal{F}_c$. Because $\mathcal{F}_c(u) \leq \mathcal{F}(u)$ for every u, this implies that $\mathcal{F}_c(u) \leq \mathcal{RF}(u)$ for every $u \in W^{1,1}(\Omega)$.

Now (see (5.5))

$$\inf_{k} \operatorname{co} f_k(\mathbf{x}, \xi, \mathbf{t}) = \inf_{k} \inf \Big\{ \sum_{j=1}^{n+1} \lambda_j f_k(\mathbf{x}, \xi, \mathbf{t}_j) : 0 \le \lambda_j \le 1,\ \sum_{j=1}^{n+1} \lambda_j \mathbf{t}_j = \mathbf{t} \Big\}$$

$$= \inf \Big\{ \inf_{k} \sum_{j=1}^{n+1} \lambda_j f_k(\mathbf{x}, \xi, \mathbf{t}_j) : 0 \le \lambda_j \le 1,\ \sum_{j=1}^{n+1} \lambda_j \mathbf{t}_j = \mathbf{t} \Big\}$$

$$= \inf \Big\{ \sum_{j=1}^{n+1} \lambda_j f(\mathbf{x}, \xi, \mathbf{t}_j) : 0 \le \lambda_j \le 1,\ \sum_{j=1}^{n+1} \lambda_j \mathbf{t}_j = \mathbf{t} \Big\}$$

$$= \operatorname{co} f(\mathbf{x}, \xi, \mathbf{t}) .$$

Denote by

$$\mathcal{F}_k(u) := \int_{\Omega} f_k(\mathbf{x}, u, \nabla u) .$$

Then it follows from Theorem 5.5 that

$$\mathcal{R}\mathcal{F}_k(u) = \int_{\Omega} \operatorname{co} f_k(\mathbf{x}, u, \nabla u) , \qquad u \in W^{1,1}(\Omega) .$$

From (5.6), it follows that $\mathcal{R}\mathcal{F}_k(u) < \infty$ for every $u \in W^{1,\infty}(\Omega)$. Using the dominated convergence theorem (see Theorem 9.9), it follows that for every $u \in W^{1,\infty}(\Omega)$

$$\inf_{k} \mathcal{R}\mathcal{F}_k(u) = \lim_{k} \int_{\Omega} \operatorname{co} f_k(\mathbf{x}, u, \nabla u) =$$

$$= \int_{\Omega} \lim_{k} \operatorname{co} f_k(\mathbf{x}, u, \nabla u) = \int_{\Omega} \operatorname{co} f(\mathbf{x}, u, \nabla u) = \mathcal{F}_c(u) .$$

Consequently, because $f \le f_k$ for all k,

$$\mathcal{R}\mathcal{F}(u) \le \inf_{k} \mathcal{R}\mathcal{F}_k(u) = \mathcal{F}_c(u) , \qquad u \in W^{1,\infty}(\Omega) .$$

Now let $u \in W^{1,p}(\Omega)$ be arbitrary. From Theorem 9.37, it follows that there exists a sequence $(u_k) \subset W^{1,\infty}(\Omega)$ strongly converging to u with respect to the $W^{1,p}$ norm. After possibly passing to a subsequence, we may assume without loss of generality that both (u_k) and (∇u_k) converge to u and ∇u, respectively, pointwise almost everywhere (see Lemma 9.6). Because $\operatorname{co} f$ by assumption is Carathéodory, it follows that $\operatorname{co} f(\mathbf{x}, u_k, \nabla u_k)$ converges to $\operatorname{co} f(\mathbf{x}, u, \nabla u)$ pointwise almost everywhere. Using Fatou's lemma (see Theorem 9.8) we obtain that

$$\liminf_k \big(\mathcal{F}_c(u_k) - c_2 \mathcal{L}^n(\Omega) - c_3 \|u_k\|_{1,p}^p \big) =$$

$$= -\limsup_k \int_\Omega \big(c_2 + c_3(|u_k|^p + |\nabla u_k|^p) - \mathrm{co}\, f(\mathbf{x}, u_k, \nabla u_k) \big)$$

$$\leq -\liminf_k \int_\Omega \big(c_2 + c_3(|u_k|^p + |\nabla u_k|^p) - \mathrm{co}\, f(\mathbf{x}, u_k, \nabla u_k) \big)$$

$$\leq -\int_\Omega \big(c_2 + c_3(|u|^p + |\nabla u|^p) - \mathrm{co}\, f(\mathbf{x}, u, \nabla u) \big)$$

$$= \mathcal{F}_c(u) - c_2 \mathcal{L}^n(\Omega) - c_3 \|u\|_{1,p}^p .$$

This shows that

$$\mathcal{RF}(u) \leq \liminf_k \mathcal{RF}(u_k) = \liminf_k \mathcal{F}_c(u_k) \leq \mathcal{F}_c(u) ,$$

which proves the assertion.   □

Corollary 5.7. *Let* $p \geq 1$, $u^\delta \in L^\infty(\Omega)$, *and*

$$f^{(p)}(\mathbf{x}, \xi, \mathbf{t}) := \frac{\big(\xi - u^\delta(\mathbf{x}) \big)^2}{2 |\mathbf{t}|^p} + \alpha |\mathbf{t}|^p ,$$

where we use the convention $f^{(p)}(\mathbf{x}, \xi, \mathbf{t}) := 0$, *if* $\xi = u^\delta(\mathbf{x})$ *and* $\mathbf{t} = 0$. *Then*

$$\mathcal{RF}^{(p)}(u) = \mathcal{F}_c^{(p)}(u) , \qquad u \in W^{1,p}(\Omega) .$$

Proof. In order to apply Theorem 5.6, we define

$$f_k^{(p)}(\mathbf{x}, \xi, \mathbf{t}) := \begin{cases} \dfrac{\big(\xi - u^\delta(\mathbf{x}) \big)^2 + 1/k}{2 |\mathbf{t}|^p - 1/k} + \alpha |\mathbf{t}|^p + \dfrac{|\mathbf{t}|^{n+1}}{k}, & \text{if } 2 |\mathbf{t}|^p > 1/k , \\ \infty, & \text{else} . \end{cases}$$

Then $f_k^{(p)}$ pointwise converges from above to the function

$$\hat{f}^{(p)}(\mathbf{x}, \xi, \mathbf{t}) := \begin{cases} f^{(p)}(\mathbf{x}, \xi, \mathbf{t}), & \text{if } \mathbf{t} \neq 0 , \\ \infty, & \text{if } \mathbf{t} = 0 . \end{cases}$$

Define

$$\hat{\mathcal{F}}^{(p)}(u) := \int_\Omega \hat{f}^{(p)}(\mathbf{x}, u, \nabla u) .$$

Then it follows from Theorem 5.6 that

$$\mathcal{R}\hat{\mathcal{F}}^{(p)}(u) = \int_\Omega \mathrm{co}\, \hat{f}^{(p)}(\mathbf{x}, u, \nabla u) , \qquad u \in W^{1,p}(\Omega) .$$

It is easy to show that $\mathrm{co}\, \hat{f}^{(p)} = \mathrm{co}\, f^{(p)}$ and thus

$$\mathcal{R}\hat{\mathcal{F}}^{(p)}(u) = \mathcal{F}_c^{(p)}(u) , \qquad u \in W^{1,p}(\Omega) .$$

Thus, as by definition $\hat{f}^{(p)} \geq f^{(p)}$ and $\mathcal{F}_c$ is sequentially lower semi-continuous, it follows that

$$\mathcal{F}_c^{(p)}(u) \leq \mathcal{R}\mathcal{F}^{(p)}(u) \leq \mathcal{R}\hat{\mathcal{F}}^{(p)}(u) = \mathcal{F}_c^{(p)}(u) , \qquad u \in W^{1,p}(\Omega) .$$

This proves the assertion. □

5.3 Relaxation on BV

In Section 5.2, we have treated the relaxation of integral functionals on $W^{1,p}(\Omega)$. In the case $p = 1$, the relaxation results still hold, but in general we cannot prove the existence of minimizers of $\mathcal{R}\mathcal{F}$, because $W^{1,1}(\Omega)$ is not reflexive and thus bounded sets need not be weakly pre-compact.

Therefore, instead of considering $\mathcal{F}$ on $W^{1,1}(\Omega)$, we extend it to $BV(\Omega)$ by

$$\mathcal{F}(u) = \begin{cases} \mathcal{F}(u), & \text{if } u \in W^{1,1}(\Omega) , \\ \infty, & \text{if } u \in BV(\Omega) \setminus W^{1,1}(\Omega) . \end{cases}$$

Similarly as in the case of non-convex functionals on Sobolev spaces, we define the relaxation of $\mathcal{F}$ on $BV(\Omega)$ by

$$\mathcal{R}_{BV}\mathcal{F}(u) := \inf \left\{ \liminf_{k \to \infty} \mathcal{F}(u_k) : (u_k) \subset W^{1,1}(\Omega) \text{ and } u_k \overset{*}{\rightharpoonup} u \text{ in } BV(\Omega) \right\} .$$

Note that in many reference works (see, for instance, [55]), instead of weak* convergence, the convergence of the approximating sequences in the L^1 norm is considered. Given an appropriate growth condition, which is also needed in all relaxation results in $BV(\Omega)$, both definitions are equivalent.

Similar to the Sobolev case, a suitable growth of f with respect to the last variable implies the weak* sequential lower semi-continuity of the relaxed functional $\mathcal{R}_{BV}\mathcal{F}$. Moreover, we have the following relation between relaxation on $W^{1,1}(\Omega)$ and $BV(\Omega)$:

Theorem 5.8. *Assume that $f : \Omega \times \mathbb{R} \times \mathbb{R}^n \to \mathbb{R} \cup \{\infty\}$ is normal and satisfies the growth condition*

$$f(\mathbf{x}, \xi, \mathbf{t}) \geq c_1 + c_2 |\mathbf{t}|$$

for some $c_1 \in \mathbb{R}$ and $c_2 > 0$. Then $\mathcal{R}_{BV}\mathcal{F}$ is weakly sequentially lower semi-continuous. Moreover*

$$\mathcal{R}_{BV}\mathcal{F}(u) = \mathcal{R}_{BV}\mathcal{R}\mathcal{F}(u) , \qquad u \in BV(\Omega) .$$

Proof. The proof is similar to the proof of Lemma 5.4. □

Theorem 5.8 shows that $\mathcal{R}_{BV}\mathcal{F}$ can be computed in two steps, by first computing the relaxation of $\mathcal{F}$ on $W^{1,1}(\Omega)$ and then the relaxation of $\mathcal{R}\mathcal{F}$ on $BV(\Omega)$. Recalling the results of the previous section, this implies that for relaxation on $BV(\Omega)$, it is essentially enough to consider the relaxation of convex integrands.

The main problem in the relaxation on $BV(\Omega)$ of integrals with convex integrands concerns the jump part and Cantor part of a function $u \in BV(\Omega)$. If $(u_k) \subset W^{1,1}(\Omega)$ is a sequence converging to u with respect to the weak* topology on $BV(\Omega)$, then the absolute values of the gradients of u_k tend to infinity near points in the jump and Cantor part of u. Therefore, we have to determine the asymptotic behavior of the integrand f as $|\nabla u| \to \infty$.

Definition 5.9. *Let* $f : \Omega \times \mathbb{R} \times \mathbb{R}^n \to \mathbb{R} \cup \{\infty\}$. *The* recession function $f^\infty : \Omega \times \mathbb{R} \times \mathbb{R}^n \to \mathbb{R} \cup \{\infty\}$ *is defined by* $f^\infty(\mathbf{x}, \xi, 0) := 0$ *and*

$$f^\infty(\mathbf{x}, \xi, \mathbf{t}) := \liminf_{\lambda \to \infty} \frac{f(\mathbf{x}, \xi, \lambda \mathbf{t})}{\lambda}, \qquad \mathbf{t} \in \mathbb{R}^n \setminus \{0\} . \qquad (5.7)$$

In particular, the function f^∞ satisfies

$$f^\infty(\mathbf{x}, \xi, \lambda \mathbf{t}) = \lambda \, f^\infty(\mathbf{x}, \xi, \mathbf{t}), \qquad \lambda > 0 .$$

If f is a convex integrand, then the lower limit in (5.7) is in fact the limit. Moreover, f^∞ is a convex integrand as well. Indeed,

$$\begin{aligned}
f^\infty\big(\mathbf{x}, \xi, \mu\mathbf{t} + (1-\mu)\hat{\mathbf{t}}\big) &= \liminf_{\lambda \to \infty} \frac{f\big(\mathbf{x}, \xi, \mu\lambda\mathbf{t} + (1-\mu)\lambda\hat{\mathbf{t}}\big)}{\lambda} \\
&\leq \lim_{\lambda \to \infty} \frac{f(\mathbf{x}, \xi, \mu\lambda\mathbf{t})}{\lambda} + \lim_{\lambda \to \infty} \frac{f(\mathbf{x}, \xi, (1-\mu)\lambda\hat{\mathbf{t}})}{\lambda} \\
&= f^\infty(\mathbf{x}, \xi, \mu\mathbf{t}) + f^\infty\big(\mathbf{x}, \xi, (1-\mu)\hat{\mathbf{t}}\big) \\
&= \mu f^\infty(\mathbf{x}, \xi, \mathbf{t}) + (1-\mu)f^\infty(\mathbf{x}, \xi, \hat{\mathbf{t}}) .
\end{aligned}$$

For the next results, we recall that the distributional derivative Du of $u \in BV(\Omega)$ can be decomposed as

$$Du = \nabla u \, \mathcal{L}^n + D^j u + D^c u = \nabla u \, \mathcal{L}^n + (u_+ - u_-)\mathcal{H}^{n-1} \, \llcorner \, \Sigma(u) + D^c u ,$$

where $D^j u$ is the jump part, $D^c u$ is the Cantor part of Du, the set $\Sigma(u)$ is the jump set of u, and $u_+(\mathbf{x})$, $u_-(\mathbf{x})$, denote the approximative upper and lower limits of u at $\mathbf{x} \in \Omega$ (see Lemma 9.72 and Definition 9.73).

In case the integrand f is convex, only depends on $\mathbf{t}$, and satisfies certain growth conditions, it has been shown in [130] that

$$\mathcal{R}_{BV}\mathcal{F}(u) = \int_\Omega f(\nabla u) + \int_\Omega f^\infty\Big(\frac{\mathrm{d}D^s u}{\mathrm{d}\,|D^s u|}\Big) \, \mathrm{d}\,|D^s u| , \qquad u \in BV(\Omega) ,$$

where $D^s u = D^j u + D^c u$ denotes the singular part of the Radon measure Du. If f also depends on the $\mathbf{x}$ and ξ variable, then the situation is more complicated, especially if f is discontinuous in the first component and f^∞ depends on ξ.

Theorem 5.10 (Bouchitté, Fonseca, Mascarenhas). *Assume that* $f :$ $\Omega \times \mathbb{R} \times \mathbb{R}^n \to \mathbb{R}$ *is a convex integrand and Borel function such that the following hold:*

1. *There exists $C > 1$ such that*

$$C^{-1}|\mathbf{t}| \le f(\mathbf{x}, \xi, \mathbf{t}) \le C(1 + |\mathbf{t}|), \qquad (\mathbf{x}, \xi, \mathbf{t}) \in \Omega \times \mathbb{R} \times \mathbb{R}^n . \quad (5.8)$$

2. *For every $\varepsilon > 0$, there exists $\delta > 0$ such that*

$$|f(\mathbf{x}, \xi, \mathbf{t}) - f(\mathbf{x}, \zeta, \mathbf{t})| \le C\varepsilon(1 + |\mathbf{t}|)$$

whenever $(\mathbf{x}, \xi, \mathbf{t}) \in \Omega \times \mathbb{R} \times \mathbb{R}^n$ and $\zeta \in \mathbb{R}$ satisfy $|\xi - \zeta| < \delta$.

3. *There exist $0 < m < 1$ and $L > 0$ such that*

$$\left| f^\infty(\mathbf{x}, \xi, \mathbf{t}) - \frac{f(\mathbf{x}, \xi, \lambda \mathbf{t})}{\lambda} \right| \le \frac{C}{\lambda^m}$$

whenever $\mathbf{t} \in \mathbb{R}^n$ with $|\mathbf{t}| = 1$, $\lambda > L$, and $(\mathbf{x}, \xi) \in \Omega \times \mathbb{R}$.

Then

$$\mathcal{R}_{BV}\mathcal{F}(u) = \int_\Omega f(\mathbf{x}, u, \nabla u) + \int_{\Sigma(u)} g\left(\mathbf{x}, u_+, u_-, \frac{\mathrm{d}Du}{\mathrm{d}|Du|}\right) \mathrm{d}\mathcal{H}^{n-1}$$

$$+ \int_\Omega h\left(\mathbf{x}, u, \frac{\mathrm{d}Du}{\mathrm{d}|Du|}\right) \mathrm{d}|D^c u| .$$

Here,

$$g(\mathbf{x}, \xi, \zeta, \boldsymbol{\nu}) := \limsup_{\varepsilon \to 0^+} \inf_{\substack{v \in W^{1,1}(Q_{\boldsymbol{\nu}}), \\ v(\mathbf{y}) = \xi \text{ on } \partial Q_{\boldsymbol{\nu}} \cap Q_{\boldsymbol{\nu}}^+, \\ v(\mathbf{y}) = \zeta \text{ on } \partial Q_{\boldsymbol{\nu}} \cap Q_{\boldsymbol{\nu}}^-}} \left\{ \int_{Q_{\boldsymbol{\nu}}} f^\infty(\mathbf{x} + \varepsilon \mathbf{y}, v(\mathbf{y}), \nabla v(\mathbf{y})) \, \mathrm{d}\mathbf{y} \right\},$$

$$(5.9)$$

$$h(\mathbf{x}, \xi, \boldsymbol{\nu}) := \limsup_k \limsup_{\varepsilon \to 0^+}$$

$$\inf_{\substack{v \in W^{1,1}(Q_{\boldsymbol{\nu}}^{(k)}), \\ v(\mathbf{y}) = \boldsymbol{\nu} \cdot \mathbf{y} \text{ on } \partial Q_{\boldsymbol{\nu}}^{(k)}}} \left\{ k^{1-n} \int_{Q_{\boldsymbol{\nu}}^{(k)}} f^\infty(\mathbf{x} + \varepsilon \mathbf{y}, \xi, \nabla v(\mathbf{y})) \, \mathrm{d}\mathbf{y} \right\},$$

$$(5.10)$$

where

$$Q_{\boldsymbol{\nu}} := R_{\boldsymbol{\nu}}([-1/2, 1/2]^n),$$

$$Q_{\boldsymbol{\nu}}^+ := R_{\boldsymbol{\nu}}([-1/2, 1/2]^{n-1} \times [0, 1/2]),$$

$$Q_{\boldsymbol{\nu}}^- := R_{\boldsymbol{\nu}}([-1/2, 1/2]^{n-1} \times [-1/2, 0]),$$

$$Q_{\boldsymbol{\nu}}^{(k)} := R_{\boldsymbol{\nu}}([-k/2, k/2]^{n-1} \times [-1/2, 1/2]),$$

with $R_{\boldsymbol{\nu}}$ being a rotation such that $R_{\boldsymbol{\nu}}(\mathbf{e}_n) = \boldsymbol{\nu}$.

Proof. See [55, Thm. 4.1.4].   □

The next result concerns the case where the recession function f^∞ has a very simple form, which implies that the functions g and h defined in Theorem 5.10 coincide with f^∞.

Corollary 5.11. *Let the assumptions of Theorem 5.10 be satisfied. Moreover, assume that there exist continuous functions $\beta : \Omega \to \mathbb{R}$ and $\gamma : \mathbb{R}^n \to \mathbb{R}$ satisfying*

$$\gamma(\lambda \mathbf{t}) = \lambda \gamma(\mathbf{t}), \qquad \mathbf{t} \in \mathbb{R}^n, \ \lambda \geq 0, \tag{5.11}$$

such that

$$f^\infty(\mathbf{x}, \xi, \mathbf{t}) = \beta(\mathbf{x})\gamma(\mathbf{t}), \qquad (\mathbf{x}, \xi, \mathbf{t}) \in \Omega \times \mathbb{R} \times \mathbb{R}^n .$$

Then

$$\mathcal{R}_{BV}\mathcal{F}(u) = \int_\Omega f(\mathbf{x}, u, \nabla u) + \int_\Omega \beta(\mathbf{x})\gamma\Big(\frac{\mathrm{d}D^s u}{\mathrm{d}\,|D^s u|}\Big)\,\mathrm{d}\,|D^s u| , \tag{5.12}$$

where $D^s u = D^j u + D^c u$ denotes the singular part of Du with respect to $\mathcal{L}^n$.

Proof. Because $D^j u$ and $D^c u$ are mutually singular (see Definition 9.73), it follows that

$$\int_\Omega \beta(\mathbf{x})\gamma\Big(\frac{\mathrm{d}D^s u}{\mathrm{d}\,|D^s u|}\Big)\,\mathrm{d}\,|D^s u| =$$
$$\int_\Omega \beta(\mathbf{x})\gamma\Big(\frac{\mathrm{d}D^s u}{\mathrm{d}\,|D^s u|}\Big)\,\mathrm{d}\,|D^c u| + \int_\Omega \beta(\mathbf{x})\gamma\Big(\frac{\mathrm{d}D^s u}{\mathrm{d}\,|D^s u|}\Big)\,\mathrm{d}\,|D^j u| . \tag{5.13}$$

Moreover, from Lemma 9.72 and (5.11), it follows that

$$\int_\Omega \beta(\mathbf{x})\gamma\Big(\frac{\mathrm{d}D^s u}{\mathrm{d}\,|D^s u|}\Big)\,\mathrm{d}\,|D^j u| = \int_{\Sigma(u)} \beta(\mathbf{x})\gamma\big((u^+ - u^-)\boldsymbol{\nu}_u\big)\,\mathrm{d}\mathcal{H}^{n-1} . \tag{5.14}$$

Let $g : \Omega \times \mathbb{R} \times \mathbb{R} \times S^{n-1} \to \mathbb{R}$ and $h : \Omega \times \mathbb{R} \times S^{n-1} \to \mathbb{R}$ be as in (5.9) and (5.10). From (5.13) and (5.14), it follows that in order to prove (5.12), we have to show that

$$g(\mathbf{x}, \xi, \zeta, \boldsymbol{\nu}) = \beta(\mathbf{x})\gamma\big((\xi - \zeta)\boldsymbol{\nu}\big), \qquad$$
$$h(\mathbf{x}, \xi, \boldsymbol{\nu}) = \beta(\mathbf{x})\gamma(\boldsymbol{\nu}), \qquad (\mathbf{x}, \xi, \zeta, \boldsymbol{\nu}) \in \Omega \times \mathbb{R} \times \mathbb{R} \times S^{n-1} . \tag{5.15}$$

Denote

$$V := \big\{v \in W^{1,1}(Q_{\boldsymbol{\nu}}) : v(\mathbf{y}) = \xi \text{ on } \partial Q_{\boldsymbol{\nu}} \cap Q_{\boldsymbol{\nu}}^+, \ v(\mathbf{y}) = \zeta \text{ on } \partial Q_{\boldsymbol{\nu}} \cap Q_{\boldsymbol{\nu}}^-\big\} .$$

From the definition of g in (5.9) and the continuity of β, it follows that

$$g(\mathbf{x}, \xi, \zeta, \boldsymbol{\nu}) = \limsup_{\varepsilon \to 0^+} \inf_{v \in V} \left\{ \int_{Q_{\boldsymbol{\nu}}} \beta(\mathbf{x} + \varepsilon \mathbf{y}) \gamma(\nabla v(\mathbf{y})) \, \mathrm{d}\mathbf{y} \right\}$$

$$\geq \limsup_{\varepsilon \to 0^+} \inf_{\tilde{\mathbf{x}} \in \mathbf{x} + \varepsilon Q_{\boldsymbol{\nu}}} \left\{ \beta(\tilde{\mathbf{x}}) \inf_{v \in V} \int_{Q_{\boldsymbol{\nu}}} \gamma(\nabla v) \right\}$$

$$= \beta(\mathbf{x}) \inf_{v \in V} \left\{ \int_{Q_{\boldsymbol{\nu}}} \gamma(\nabla v) \right\} .$$

Similarly,

$$g(\mathbf{x}, \xi, \zeta, \boldsymbol{\nu}) \leq \limsup_{\varepsilon \to 0^+} \sup_{\tilde{\mathbf{x}} \in \mathbf{x} + \varepsilon Q_{\boldsymbol{\nu}}} \left\{ \beta(\tilde{\mathbf{x}}) \inf_{v \in V} \int_{Q_{\boldsymbol{\nu}}} \gamma(\nabla v) \right\}$$

$$= \beta(\mathbf{x}) \inf_{v \in V} \left\{ \int_{Q_{\boldsymbol{\nu}}} \gamma(\nabla v) \right\} .$$

This shows that

$$g(\mathbf{x}, \xi, \zeta, \boldsymbol{\nu}) = \beta(\mathbf{x}) \inf_{v \in V} \left\{ \int_{Q_{\boldsymbol{\nu}}} \gamma(\nabla v) \right\} .$$

It remains to prove that

$$\inf_{v \in V} \left\{ \int_{Q_{\boldsymbol{\nu}}} \gamma(\nabla v) \right\} = \gamma((\xi - \zeta)\boldsymbol{\nu}) . \tag{5.16}$$

For simplicity of notation, we only consider the case $\boldsymbol{\nu} = \mathbf{e}_n$. Let $v \in V \cap W^{1,\infty}(Q_{\mathbf{e}_n})$. Then we can continue v to $\mathbb{R}^n$ by first continuing v periodically to the strip $Z = \{(\mathbf{y}', y_n) \in \mathbb{R}^n : |y_n| \leq 1/2\}$, and then defining $v(k\mathbf{e}_n + \mathbf{y}) := v(\mathbf{y}) + k(\xi - \zeta)$ for $k \in \mathbb{Z}$ and $\mathbf{y} \in Z$.

Define now $v_k(\mathbf{y}) := v(k\mathbf{y})/k$ for $\mathbf{y} \in Q_{\mathbf{e}_n}$. Then (v_k) converges in the L^∞ norm to the function $\hat{v}(\mathbf{y}) = ((\xi - \zeta)\boldsymbol{\nu})\mathbf{y}$. Moreover the sequence $(\|\nabla v_k\|_\infty)$ is bounded. This implies that (v_k) weakly converges to $\hat{v}$ in $W^{1,p}(Q_{\mathbf{e}_n})$ for all $1 < p < \infty$. Because f is a convex integrand, it follows that f^∞ is a convex integrand, too. Thus the definition of γ implies that γ is convex. Consequently, the functional $v \mapsto \int_{Q_{\mathbf{e}_n}} \gamma(\nabla v)$ is weakly sequentially lower semi-continuous. Thus

$$\gamma((\xi - \zeta)\boldsymbol{\nu}) \leq \liminf_k \int_{Q_{\mathbf{e}_n}} \gamma(\nabla v_k) = \liminf_k \int_{k Q_{\mathbf{e}_n}} k^{-n} \gamma(\nabla v) = \int_{Q_{\mathbf{e}_n}} \gamma(\nabla v) .$$

Now note that $V \cap W^{1,\infty}(Q_{\mathbf{e}_n})$ is dense in V and the functional $v \mapsto \int_{Q_{\mathbf{e}_n}} \gamma(\nabla v)$ is continuous in the $W^{1,1}$ norm. Consequently,

$$\gamma((\xi - \zeta)\boldsymbol{\nu}) \leq \int_{Q_{\mathbf{e}_n}} \gamma(\nabla v), \qquad v \in V .$$

In order to prove the converse inequality, set

$$v_k(\mathbf{y}) := \begin{cases} \xi, & \text{if } y_n > \dfrac{1 - 2\left|\mathbf{y}'\right|}{2k}, \\[2ex] \zeta + (\xi - \zeta)\dfrac{2ky_n}{1 - 2\left|\mathbf{y}'\right|}, & \text{if } 0 < y_n < \dfrac{1 - 2\left|\mathbf{y}'\right|}{2k}, \\[2ex] \zeta, & \text{if } y_n < 0. \end{cases}$$

Then $v_k \in V$. Moreover, because γ is continuous and satisfies (5.11), it follows that

$$\lim_k \int_{Q_{\varrho_n}} \gamma(\nabla v_k) = \gamma\big((\xi - \zeta)\boldsymbol{\nu}\big).$$

This shows (5.16). Thus, the representation of g follows. The representation of h in (5.15) can be shown in a similar manner.   □

5.4 Applications in Non-convex Regularization

In the following, we apply the results of the preceding sections to the non-convex regularization functionals

$$\mathcal{F}^{(p)}(u) = \int_\Omega f^{(p)}\big(\mathbf{x}, u(\mathbf{x}), \nabla u(\mathbf{x})\big)\, d\mathbf{x}$$

with

$$f^{(p)}(\mathbf{x}, \xi, \mathbf{t}) := \frac{\big(\xi - u^\delta(\mathbf{x})\big)^2}{2\left|\mathbf{t}\right|^p} + \alpha\left|\mathbf{t}\right|^p$$

for $1 \le p < \infty$. In particular, we study below the cases $p = 1$ (NCBV functional) and $p = 2$.

According to Corollary 5.7, for the computation of $\mathcal{R}\mathcal{F}^{(p)}$ we need the convex hull of $f^{(p)}$ with respect to the last variable:

Lemma 5.12. *Let $f^{(p)} : \Omega \times \mathbb{R} \times \mathbb{R}^n \to \mathbb{R} \cup \{\infty\}$ be as above. Then the convex hull of $f^{(p)}$ with respect to the last variable is*

$$f_c^{(p)}(\mathbf{x}, \xi, \mathbf{t}) := \begin{cases} \dfrac{\big(\xi - u^\delta(\mathbf{x})\big)^2}{2\left|\mathbf{t}\right|^p} + \alpha\left|\mathbf{t}\right|^p, & \text{if } \sqrt{2\alpha}\left|\mathbf{t}\right|^p > \left|\xi - u^\delta(\mathbf{x})\right|, \\[2ex] \sqrt{2\alpha}\left|\xi - u^\delta(\mathbf{x})\right|, & \text{if } \sqrt{2\alpha}\left|\mathbf{t}\right|^p \le \left|\xi - u^\delta(\mathbf{x})\right|. \end{cases} \quad (5.17)$$

It turns out that the function $f_c^{(p)}$ is not only convex with respect to the last variable $\mathbf{t}$, but in fact with respect to $(\xi, \mathbf{t})$.

Lemma 5.13. *For almost every $\mathbf{x} \in \Omega$, the function $(\xi, \mathbf{t}) \mapsto f_c^{(p)}(\mathbf{x}, \xi, \mathbf{t})$ is convex. Moreover, it is continuously differentiable on $\mathbb{R} \times \mathbb{R}^n \setminus \{(u^\delta(\mathbf{x}), 0)\}$.*

Proof. For $\mathbf{x} \in \Omega$ denote

$$U_1 := \left\{ (\xi, \mathbf{t}) \in \mathbb{R} \times \mathbb{R}^n : \sqrt{2\alpha}\, |\mathbf{t}|^p < \left| \xi - u^\delta(\mathbf{x}) \right| \right\},$$
$$U_2 := \left\{ (\xi, \mathbf{t}) \in \mathbb{R} \times \mathbb{R}^n : \sqrt{2\alpha}\, |\mathbf{t}|^p > \left| \xi - u^\delta(\mathbf{x}) \right| \right\}.$$

In particular, $\left| \xi - u^\delta(\mathbf{x}) \right|$ is strictly greater than zero for every $(\xi, \mathbf{t}) \in U_1$.

In the following, we show that $(\xi, \mathbf{t}) \mapsto f_c^{(p)}(\mathbf{x}, \xi, \mathbf{t})$ is continuously differentiable on $\mathbb{R} \times \mathbb{R}^n \setminus \{(u^\delta(\mathbf{x}), 0)\}$.

For $(\xi, \mathbf{t}) \in U_1$, we have

$$\nabla f_c^{(p)}(\mathbf{x}, \xi, \mathbf{t})^T := \nabla_{\xi, \mathbf{t}} f_c^{(p)}(\mathbf{x}, \xi, \mathbf{t})^T = \left(\sqrt{2\alpha}\, \mathrm{sgn}(\xi - u^\delta(\mathbf{x})), 0 \right),$$

and for $(\xi, \mathbf{t}) \in U_2$ we have

$$\nabla f_c^{(p)}(\mathbf{x}, \xi, \mathbf{t})^T = \left(\frac{\xi - u^\delta(\mathbf{x})}{|\mathbf{t}|^p}, \; p \left(\alpha |\mathbf{t}|^{p-1} - \frac{(\xi - u^\delta(\mathbf{x}))^2}{2|\mathbf{t}|^{p+1}} \right) \frac{\mathbf{t}}{|\mathbf{t}|} \right).$$

Now let $(\xi_0, \mathbf{t}_0) \in \mathbb{R} \times \mathbb{R}^n$ be such that $0 \neq \left| \xi_0 - u^\delta \right| = \sqrt{2\alpha}\, |\mathbf{t}_0|^p$. Let $(\xi_k, \mathbf{t}_k) \subset U_1$ be a sequence converging to $(\xi_0, \mathbf{t}_0)$. Then,

$$\lim_k \nabla f_c^{(p)}(\mathbf{x}, \xi_k, \mathbf{t}_k)^T = \left(\sqrt{2\alpha}\, \mathrm{sgn}(\xi_0 - u^\delta(\mathbf{x})), 0 \right).$$

Let now $(\xi_k, \mathbf{t}_k) \subset U_2$ converge to $(\xi_0, \mathbf{t}_0)$. Then in particular,

$$\lim_k \frac{\xi_k - u^\delta(\mathbf{x})}{|\mathbf{t}_k|^p} = \frac{\xi_0 - u^\delta(\mathbf{x})}{|\mathbf{t}_0|^p} = \sqrt{2\alpha}\, \mathrm{sgn}(\xi_0 - u^\delta(\mathbf{x})).$$

Thus

$$\lim_k \nabla f_c^{(p)}(\mathbf{x}, \xi_k, \mathbf{t}_k)^T =$$

$$= \lim_k \left(\frac{\xi_k - u^\delta(\mathbf{x})}{|\mathbf{t}_k|^p}, \; p \left(\alpha |\mathbf{t}|^{p-1} - \frac{(\xi_k - u^\delta(\mathbf{x}))^2}{2|\mathbf{t}_k|^{p+1}} \right) \frac{\mathbf{t}_k}{|\mathbf{t}_k|} \right)$$

$$= \left(\sqrt{2\alpha}\, \mathrm{sgn}(\xi_0 - u^\delta(\mathbf{x})), \; p \left(\alpha |\mathbf{t}|^{p-1} - \frac{2\alpha}{2} |\mathbf{t}|^{p-1} \right) \frac{\mathbf{t}_0}{|\mathbf{t}_0|} \right)$$

$$= \left(\sqrt{2\alpha}\, \mathrm{sgn}(\xi_0 - u^\delta(\mathbf{x})), 0 \right).$$

This shows that at $(\mathbf{x}, \xi_0, \mathbf{t}_0)$, the function $f_c^{(p)}$ is continuously differentiable in direction $(\xi, \mathbf{t})$.

Now we show that the function $(\xi, \mathbf{t}) \mapsto f_c^{(p)}(\mathbf{x}, \xi, \mathbf{t})$ is convex. Obviously, it is convex on U_1. Because the Hessian of the function $f^{(p)}$ is positive semi-definite on U_2, the mapping $(\xi, \mathbf{t}) \mapsto f_c^{(p)}(\mathbf{x}, \xi, \mathbf{t})$ is convex on U_2.

In order to show that $f_c^{(p)}$ is convex as a whole, we prove that it is convex on each line

$$L = \{(\xi, \mathbf{t}) + \lambda(\zeta, \hat{\mathbf{t}}) : \lambda \in \mathbb{R}\}$$

(see Remark 10.3). Define

$$g_L(\lambda) := f_c^{(p)}(\mathbf{x}, \xi + \lambda\zeta, \mathbf{t} + \lambda\hat{\mathbf{t}}) \ .$$

Assume first that $(u^\delta(\mathbf{x}), 0) \notin L$. Then there exist at most two numbers $\lambda_0 < \lambda_1$ such that $\sqrt{2\alpha} |\mathbf{t} + \lambda_i \hat{\mathbf{t}}| = |\xi + \lambda\zeta - u^\delta(\mathbf{x})|$. In particular, for all $\lambda \notin \{\lambda_0, \lambda_1\}$ we have $(\xi, \mathbf{t}) + \lambda(\zeta, \hat{\mathbf{t}}) \in U_1 \cup U_2$. In order to show the convexity of g_L, we prove that its derivative g_L' is non-decreasing. Because $f_c^{(p)}$ is convex on U_1 and on U_2, it follows that g_L' is non-decreasing in the intervals $(-\infty, t_0)$, (λ_0, λ_1), and $(\lambda_1, +\infty)$. Because $f_c^{(p)}$ is continuously differentiable outside of $(u^\delta(\mathbf{x}), 0)$, it follows that g_L' is continuous on $\mathbb{R}$. Thus, we find that g_L' is non-decreasing on the whole real line.

Now assume that $(u^\delta(\mathbf{x}), 0) \in L$. Then L can be parameterized by

$$L = \{(u^\delta(\mathbf{x}), 0) + \lambda(\zeta, \hat{\mathbf{t}}) : \lambda \in \mathbb{R}\} \ .$$

Consequently,

$$g(\lambda) = \begin{cases} \sqrt{2\alpha} |\lambda\zeta|, & \text{if } \sqrt{2\alpha} |\hat{\mathbf{t}}| \leq |\zeta| \ , \\ |\lambda| \dfrac{\zeta^2}{2 |\mathbf{t}|^p} + \alpha |\lambda\mathbf{t}|^p, & \text{if } \sqrt{2\alpha} |\hat{\mathbf{t}}| > |\zeta| \ . \end{cases}$$

In both cases, the function g is convex. This proves the assertion.   □

Theorem 5.14. *Assume that $u^\delta \in L^\infty(\Omega)$. Then the relaxation of $\mathcal{F}^{(p)}$ is*

$$\mathcal{RF}^{(p)}(u) = \mathcal{F}_c^{(p)}(u) := \int_\Omega f_c^{(p)}(\mathbf{x}, u, \nabla u) \ .$$

Proof. See Corollary 5.7.   □

Lemma 5.15. *Assume that $u^\delta \in L^\infty(\Omega)$ and let $u \in W^{1,p}(\Omega)$. Let $r \geq \operatorname{ess\,sup} u^\delta$. Then $\mathcal{F}_c^{(p)}(\min\{u, r\}) \leq \mathcal{F}_c^{(p)}(u)$. Similarly, if $s \leq \operatorname{ess\,inf} u^\delta$, then $\mathcal{F}_c^{(p)}(\max\{u, s\}) \leq \mathcal{F}_c^{(p)}(u)$.*

The inequalities are strict if $r < \operatorname{ess\,sup} u$ or $s > \operatorname{ess\,inf} u$.

Proof. We only show the first assertion, the second then follows from the first by considering $-u$, $-u^\delta$. Denote $\tilde{u} := \min\{u, r\}$. Then

$$\int_\Omega f_c^{(p)}(\mathbf{x}, \tilde{u}, \nabla\tilde{u}) = \int_{\{u \leq r\}} f_c^{(p)}(\mathbf{x}, u, \nabla u) + \int_{\{u > r\}} \sqrt{2\alpha} |r - u^\delta|$$

$$\leq \int_{\{u \leq r\}} f_c^{(p)}(\mathbf{x}, u, \nabla u) + \int_{\{u > r\}} \sqrt{2\alpha} |u - u^\delta| \qquad (5.18)$$

$$\leq \int_\Omega f_c^{(p)}(\mathbf{x}, u, \nabla u) \ .$$

If moreover $r < \operatorname{ess\,sup} u$, then $\mathcal{L}^n(\{u > r\}) > 0$, which implies that the first inequality in (5.18) is strict. This shows the assertion.   □

Remark 5.16. Denote $M := \{u \in W^{1,p}(\Omega) : \|u\|_\infty \leq \|u^\delta\|_\infty\}$. It follows from Lemma 5.15 that every minimizer of $\mathcal{F}_c^{(p)}$ over $W^{1,p}(\Omega)$ already lies in M. Thus minimizing of $\mathcal{F}_c^{(p)}$ over $W^{1,p}(\Omega)$ is equivalent to minimizing $\mathcal{F}_c^{(p)}$ over M. $\diamond$

Corollary 5.17. *If $p > 1$ and $u^\delta \in L^\infty(\Omega)$, then the functional $\mathcal{F}_c^{(p)}$ attains a minimizer.*

Proof. From Lemma 5.4, it follows that $\mathcal{F}_c^{(p)}$ is weakly sequentially lower semi-continuous on $W^{1,p}(\Omega)$. Now denote $M := \{u \in W^{1,p}(\Omega) : \|u\|_\infty \leq \|u^\delta\|_\infty\}$. From Remark 5.16, it follows that it is sufficient to show that $\mathcal{F}_c^{(p)}|_M$ attains a minimizer.

Now note that $\mathcal{F}_c^{(p)}(u) \geq \alpha \|\nabla u\|_p^p$ for every $u \in W^{1,p}(\Omega)$. Consequently, for every $t \in \mathbb{R}$ we have

$$\text{level}_t(\mathcal{F}_c^{(p)}|_M) \subset M \cap \{u \in W^{1,p}(\Omega) : \|\nabla u\|_p^p \leq t/\alpha\} .$$

This shows that $\text{level}_t(\mathcal{F}_c^{(p)}|_M)$ is sequentially pre-compact, and thus $\mathcal{F}_c^{(p)}|_M$ is weakly sequentially coercive. Using Theorem 5.1, the existence of a minimizer follows. $\square$

In the case $p = 1$, the situation is more complicated, because we have to compute the relaxation on $BV(\Omega)$. This is achieved in the following result:

Theorem 5.18. *Assume that $u^\delta \in L^\infty(\Omega)$. Then the relaxation of $\mathcal{F}^{(1)}$ on $BV(\Omega)$ is*

$$\mathcal{R}_{BV}\mathcal{F}^{(1)}(u) = \mathcal{F}_c^{(1)}(u) := \int_\Omega f_c^{(1)}(\mathbf{x}, u, \nabla u) + \alpha |D^s u| (\Omega) .$$

Proof. From Theorem 5.8, it follows that

$$\mathcal{R}_{BV}\mathcal{F}^{(1)} = \mathcal{R}_{BV}\mathcal{R}\mathcal{F}^{(1)} = \mathcal{R}_{BV}\hat{\mathcal{F}}_c^{(1)} ,$$

where

$$\hat{\mathcal{F}}_c^{(1)}(u) = \int_\Omega f_c^{(1)}(\mathbf{x}, u, \nabla u)$$

is the relaxation of $\mathcal{F}_c^{(1)}$ on $W^{1,1}(\Omega)$ (cf. Theorem 5.6).

For the relaxation of $\hat{\mathcal{F}}_c^{(1)}$ on $BV(\Omega)$, we cannot directly apply Corollary 5.11, because $f_c^{(1)}$ does not satisfy the required growth condition (5.8). Therefore, we define bounded functions $g^{(r)}$, $r > 0$, approximating $f_c^{(1)}$ from below as $r \to \infty$.

For $r > 0$ and $u \in W^{1,\infty}(\Omega)$ let

$$g^{(r)}(\mathbf{x}, \xi, \mathbf{t})$$

$$:= \begin{cases} \dfrac{\min\left\{\left(\xi - u^\delta(\mathbf{x})\right)^2, r^2\right\}}{2\,|\mathbf{t}|} + \alpha\,|\mathbf{t}|, & \text{if } \sqrt{2\alpha}\,|\mathbf{t}| > \min\left\{\left|\xi - u^\delta(\mathbf{x})\right|, r\right\}, \\ \sqrt{2\alpha}\,\min\left\{\left|\xi - u^\delta(\mathbf{x})\right|, r\right\}, & \text{if } \sqrt{2\alpha}\,|\mathbf{t}| \le \min\left\{\left|\xi - u^\delta(\mathbf{x})\right|, r\right\}, \end{cases}$$

and

$$\mathcal{G}^{(r)}(u) := \int_\Omega g^{(r)}(\mathbf{x}, u, \nabla u)\,.$$

Now we compute the relaxation of $\mathcal{G}^{(r)}$ on $BV(\Omega)$. To this end, we have to compute the recession function $g^{(r,\infty)}$ of $g^{(r)}$. For large $\mathbf{t}$ we have $g^{(r)}(\mathbf{x}, \xi, \mathbf{t}) = f^{(1)}(\mathbf{x}, \xi, \mathbf{t})$. Because the recession function is defined by taking the limit $|\mathbf{t}| \to \infty$, this implies that $g^{(r,\infty)} = f^{(1,\infty)}$. Consequently,

$$g^{(r,\infty)}(\mathbf{x}, \xi, \mathbf{t}) = f^{(1,\infty)}(\mathbf{x}, \xi, \mathbf{t}) = \lim_{\lambda \to \infty} \frac{1}{\lambda}\left(\frac{\left(\xi - u^\delta(\mathbf{x})\right)^2}{2\,|\lambda \mathbf{t}|} + \alpha\,|\lambda \mathbf{t}|\right) = \alpha\,|\mathbf{t}|\,.$$

Using Corollary 5.11, it follows that for all $u \in BV(\Omega)$, the equality

$$\mathcal{R}_{BV}\mathcal{G}^{(r)}(u) = \int_\Omega g^{(r)}(\mathbf{x}, u, \nabla u) + \alpha\,|D^s u|\,(\Omega) \tag{5.19}$$

holds.

Now let $u \in BV(\Omega) \cap L^\infty(\Omega)$ and let $r > \|u\|_{L^\infty} + \|u^\delta\|_{L^\infty}$. Then

$$\int_\Omega g^{(r)}(\mathbf{x}, u, \nabla u) = \int_\Omega f_c^{(1)}(\mathbf{x}, u, \nabla u)\,. \tag{5.20}$$

From (5.19) and (5.20), it follows that

$$\mathcal{R}_{BV}\mathcal{G}^{(r)}(u) = \mathcal{F}_c^{(1)}(u), \qquad \|u\|_{L^\infty} + \|u^\delta\|_{L^\infty} < r\,. \tag{5.21}$$

By definition of $\mathcal{R}_{BV}\mathcal{G}^{(r)}$, for every $\varepsilon > 0$ there exists a sequence $(u_k) \subset W^{1,1}(\Omega)$ converging to u with respect to the L^1 norm, such that

$$\lim_k \mathcal{G}^{(2r)}(u_k) \le \mathcal{R}_{BV}\mathcal{G}^{(2r)}(u) + \varepsilon\,.$$

Now define

$$\tilde{u}_k(\mathbf{x}) := \max\left\{\min\{u_k(\mathbf{x}), r\}, -r\right\}\,.$$

Then $(\tilde{u}_k)$ converges to u with respect to the L^1 norm, and it follows from (5.21) that

$$\mathcal{G}^{(2r)}(u_k) \ge \mathcal{G}^{(2r)}(\tilde{u}_k) = \mathcal{F}_c^{(1)}(\tilde{u}_k)\,,$$

which shows that

$$\mathcal{R}_{BV}\hat{\mathcal{F}}_c^{(1)}(u) \le \lim_k \mathcal{F}_c^{(1)}(\tilde{u}_k) \le \mathcal{R}_{BV}\mathcal{G}^{(2r)}(u) + \varepsilon\,.$$

Because ε was arbitrary, and $\mathcal{G}^{(2r)}(v) \leq \mathcal{F}^{(1)}(v)$ for all $v \in BV(\Omega)$, this shows that

$$\mathcal{R}_{BV}\mathcal{F}^{(1)}(u) = \int_\Omega f_c^{(1)}(\mathbf{x}, u, \nabla u) + \alpha \left| D^s u \right|(\Omega) = \mathcal{F}_c^{(1)}(u) .$$

Using [74, Prop. 2.4], it follows that for every $u \in BV(\Omega)$

$$\mathcal{R}_{BV}\mathcal{F}^{(1)}(u) = \lim_{r \to \infty} \mathcal{R}_{BV}\mathcal{F}^{(1)}(\max\{\min\{u, r\}, -r\}) =$$

$$= \lim_{r \to \infty} \int_\Omega g^{(r)}(\mathbf{x}, u, \nabla u) + \alpha \left| D^s(\max\{\min\{u, r\}, -r\}) \right|(\Omega) .$$

From this and the monotone convergence theorem (see Theorem 9.7), the assertion follows. □

Lemma 5.19. *Assume that $u^\delta \in L^\infty(\Omega)$ and let $u \in W^{1,p}(\Omega)$. Let $r > \operatorname{ess\,sup} u^\delta$. Then $\mathcal{F}_c^{(1)}(\min\{u, r\}) \leq \mathcal{F}_c^{(1)}(u)$, and the inequality is strict, if $r < \operatorname{ess\,sup} u$. Similarly, if $s \leq \operatorname{ess\,inf}\{u^\delta(\mathbf{x}) : \mathbf{x} \in \Omega\}$, then $\mathcal{F}_c^{(1)}(\max\{u, s\}) \leq \mathcal{F}_c^{(1)}(u)$, and the inequality is strict, if $s > \operatorname{ess\,inf} u$.*

Proof. The proof is similar to the proof of Lemma 5.15. □

Lemma 5.20. *The functional $\mathcal{F}_c^{(1)}$ attains a minimizer in $BV(\Omega)$.*

Proof. From Theorem 5.8, it follows that $\mathcal{F}_c^{(1)}$ is weak* sequentially lower semi-continuous. Moreover,

$$f_c^{(1)}(\mathbf{x}, \xi, \mathbf{t}) \geq \sqrt{\alpha}/2 \left| \xi - u^\delta(\mathbf{x}) \right| + \alpha/2 \left| \mathbf{t} \right| , \qquad (\mathbf{x}, \xi, \mathbf{t}) \in \Omega \times \mathbb{R} \times \mathbb{R}^n .$$

Consequently, the functional $\mathcal{F}_c^{(1)}$ is weak* sequentially coercive. Thus, using Theorem 5.1, the assertion follows. □

Lemma 5.21. *For every $(\mathbf{x}, \xi, \mathbf{t}) \in \Omega \times \mathbb{R} \times \mathbb{R}^n$ and $(\zeta, \hat{\mathbf{t}}) \in \mathbb{R} \times \mathbb{R}^n$, we have*

$$\left| f_c^{(p)}(\mathbf{x}, \xi, \mathbf{t}) - f_c^{(p)}(\mathbf{x}, \zeta, \mathbf{t}) \right| \leq \sqrt{2\alpha} \left| \xi - \zeta \right| .$$

Moreover, in the case $p = 1$, we have

$$\left| f_c^{(1)}(\mathbf{x}, \xi, \mathbf{t}) - f_c^{(1)}(\mathbf{x}, \xi, \hat{\mathbf{t}}) \right| \leq \alpha \left| \mathbf{t} - \hat{\mathbf{t}} \right| .$$

Proof. Let $(\mathbf{x}, \mathbf{t}) \in \Omega \times \mathbb{R}^n$. From Lemma 5.13, it follows that the function $g : \mathbb{R} \to \mathbb{R}$, $g(\xi) := f_c^{(p)}(\mathbf{x}, \xi, \mathbf{t})$ is convex. Denote by g^∞ the recession function of g, then

$$g^\infty(\xi) = \lim_{\lambda \to \infty} \frac{g(\lambda \xi)}{\lambda} = \lim_{\lambda \to \infty} \frac{\sqrt{2\alpha} \left| \lambda \xi - u^\delta(\mathbf{x}) \right|}{\lambda} = \sqrt{2\alpha} \left| \xi \right| , \qquad \xi \in \mathbb{R} .$$

From [334, Cor. 8.5.1] and the definition of g, it follows that

$$f_c^{(p)}(\mathbf{x}, \xi, \mathbf{t}) - f_c^{(p)}(\mathbf{x}, \zeta, \mathbf{t}) = g(\xi) - g(\zeta) \leq g^\infty(\xi - \zeta) = \sqrt{2\alpha} \left| \xi - \zeta \right| .$$

Thus the first part of the assertion follows.

The second part of the assertion can be shown in an analogous manner.

□

5.5 One-dimensional Results

In the following, we consider the case $n = 1$, that is, $\Omega \subset \mathbb{R}$. We denote the absolutely continuous part of the weak derivative of u by u' instead of ∇u.

Let u be a minimizer of the functional $\mathcal{F}_c^{(p)}$. Assume that $\sqrt{2\alpha} \, |u'(x)|^p \leq |u(x) - u^\delta(x)|$ for some $x \in \Omega$. Then the convexified integrand $f_c^{(p)}$ evaluated at x reads as

$$f_c^{(p)}(x, u, u') = \sqrt{2\alpha} \, |u - u^\delta| \ .$$

By assumption, u is a minimizer of the convex functional $\mathcal{F}_c^{(p)}$. Consequently, the function u should satisfy the formal first-order optimality condition for $\mathcal{F}_c^{(p)}$ at the point x, that is,

$$0 \in \partial\big(f_c^{(p)}(x, u, u')\big) = \sqrt{2\alpha} \, \mathrm{sgn}(u - u^\delta) \, ,$$

which implies that $u(x) = u^\delta(x)$.

This formal argument shows that it can never happen that $\sqrt{2\alpha} \, |u'(x)|^p < |u(x) - u^\delta(x)|$. Recalling the definition of $f_c^{(p)}$ in (5.17), we obtain that $f_c^{(p)}(x, u, u') = f^{(p)}(x, u, u')$, and thus u is a minimizer of the *original non-convexified* functional $\mathcal{F}^{(p)}$.

The next result summarizes this argument. Moreover, a rigorous proof is cited.

Lemma 5.22. *Let u be a minimizer of $\mathcal{F}_c^{(p)}$. Then*

$$\sqrt{2\alpha} \, |u'(x)|^p \geq |u(x) - u^\delta(x)|$$

for almost every $x \in \Omega$. In particular, if $p > 1$, then u minimizes the functional $\mathcal{F}_c^{(p)}$, and if $p = 1$, the function u minimizes the functional

$$\tilde{\mathcal{F}}^{(1)}(u) := \int_\Omega \frac{(u - u^\delta)^2}{2 \, |u'|} + \alpha \mathcal{R}_1(u) \ .$$

Here we define $\dfrac{\big(u(x) - u^\delta(x)\big)^2}{2 \, |u'(x)|} := 0$, *if $u(x) = u^\delta(x)$ and $|u'(x)| = 0$.*

Proof. See [187, Lemma 4.15]. □

Recall that for $u \in BV(\Omega)$, $\Omega \subset \mathbb{R}$, the left and right limit $u^{(l)}(x)$ and $u^{(r)}(x)$ exist for every $x \in \Omega$ (see Theorem 9.89).

The following result states that minimization of $\mathcal{F}_c^{(1)}$ creates no additional jumps in the minimizer. More precisely, all jumps occurring in the minimizer u of $\mathcal{F}_c^{(1)}$ are already present in u^δ. Moreover, all existing jumps may only shrink.

Lemma 5.23. *Let u be a minimizer of $\mathcal{F}_c^{(1)}$ and $x_0 \in \Omega$. If $u^{(l)}(x_0) < u^{(r)}(x_0)$, then*

$$\operatorname*{ess\,lim\,inf}_{x \to x_0^-} u^\delta(x) \le u^{(l)}(x_0) < u^{(r)}(x_0) \le \operatorname*{ess\,lim\,sup}_{x \to x_0^+} u^\delta(x) \ .$$

Similarly, if $u^{(l)}(x_0) > u^{(r)}(x_0)$, then

$$\operatorname*{ess\,lim\,sup}_{x \to x_0^-} u^\delta(x) \ge u^{(l)}(x_0) > u^{(r)}(x_0) \ge \operatorname*{ess\,lim\,inf}_{x \to x_0^+} u^\delta(x) \ .$$

In particular, if u^δ is continuous in x_0, then so is u.

Proof. Suppose that there exists $c > 0$ such that

$$\operatorname*{ess\,lim\,inf}_{x \to x_0^+} u^\delta(x) > u^{(l)}(x_0) + c$$

and

$$u^{(l)}(x_0) + c < u^{(r)}(x_0) \ .$$

Then there exists $r > 0$ such that

$$u^\delta(x) > u^{(l)}(x) + c/2, \qquad x \in (x_0 - r, x_0) \ .$$

Define now

$$\tilde{u}(x) := \begin{cases} u(x) + c/2, & \text{if } x \in (x_0 - r, x_0), \\ u(x), & \text{if } x \notin (x_0 - r, x_0) \ . \end{cases}$$

Then,

$$f_c^{(1)}\big(x, \tilde{u}(x), \tilde{u}'(x)\big) < f_c^{(1)}\big(x, u(x), u'(x)\big)$$

for almost every $x \in (x_0 - r, x_0)$. On the other hand,

$$D^s \tilde{u} \llcorner \Omega \setminus \{x_0 - r, x_0\} = D^s u \llcorner \Omega \setminus \{x_0 - r, x_0\} \ ,$$

and

$$\begin{aligned} |D^s \tilde{u}| \left(\{x_0 - r, x_0\}\right) &= \left| \tilde{u}^{(r)}(x_0 - r) - \tilde{u}^{(l)}(x_0 - r) \right| + \left| \tilde{u}^{(r)}(x_0) - \tilde{u}^{(l)}(x_0) \right| \\ &\le \left| u^{(r)}(x_0 - r) - u^{(l)}(x_0 - r) \right| + \left| u^{(r)}(x_0) - u^{(l)}(x_0) \right| \\ &= |D^s u| \left(\{x_0 - r, x_0\}\right) \ . \end{aligned}$$

Thus, $|D^s \tilde{u}| \left(\Omega\right) \le |D^s u| \left(\Omega\right)$ and consequently, $\mathcal{F}_c^{(1)}(\tilde{u}) < \mathcal{F}_c^{(1)}(u)$. This gives a contradiction to the minimality of $\mathcal{F}_c^{(1)}(u)$.

All other inequalities in the claim can be shown similarly. $\qquad\square$

We now consider the Cantor part $D^c u$ of the distributional derivative of the minimizer u of $\mathcal{F}_c^{(1)}$. *A priori* it cannot be excluded that a Cantor part occurs. The next result, however, states that $D^c u$ vanishes whenever the Cantor part $D^c u^\delta$ of the original function u^δ is zero. Moreover, in every point x where the Cantor part of u does not vanish, we have $u(x) = u^\delta(x)$.

Lemma 5.24. *Assume that $u^\delta \in BV(\Omega)$. Let u be a minimizer of $\mathcal{F}_c^{(1)}$. Then,*

$$u(x) = u^\delta(x), \qquad |D^c u|\text{-a.e. } x \in \Omega.$$

Moreover, $|D^c u|(E) = 0$ for every $E \subset \Omega$ with $\left|D^c u^\delta\right|(E) = 0$.

Proof. See [187, Lemma 4.17]. $\qquad\qquad\qquad\qquad\qquad\qquad\qquad\qquad\qquad$ $\square$

5.6 Examples

Let $\Omega = (-1, 1)$ and $u^\delta = \chi_{[-c,c]}$ be the characteristic function of the closed interval $[-c, c]$ for some $0 < c < 1$. In the following, the exact minimizers u of $\mathcal{F}_c^{(1)}$ are given for all possible values of $c > 0$ and $\alpha > 0$. A derivation of the results can be found in [187].

1. $c > 1/2$:
   (a) If $1 - c \geq \sqrt{2\alpha}$, then $u = u^\delta$.
   (b) If $1 - c < \sqrt{2\alpha}$, then (cf. Fig. 5.1)

$$u(x) = \begin{cases} \dfrac{\sqrt{2\alpha} - 1 + c}{\sqrt{2\alpha} - 1 + |x|}, & \text{if } |x| \geq c, \\ 1, & \text{if } |x| < c. \end{cases}$$

2. $c < 1/2$:
   (a) If $c \geq \sqrt{2\alpha}$, then $u = u^\delta$.
   (b) If $c < \sqrt{2\alpha}$, then (cf. Fig. 5.1)

$$u(x) = \begin{cases} 1 - \dfrac{\sqrt{2\alpha} - c}{\sqrt{2\alpha} - |x|}, & \text{if } |x| \leq c, \\ 0, & \text{if } |x| > c. \end{cases}$$

3. $c = 1/2$:
   (a) If $\alpha \leq 1/8$, then $u = u^\delta$.
   (b) If $\alpha > 1/8$, then for every $0 \leq \lambda \leq 1$ the function

$$u_\lambda(x) = \begin{cases} (1 - \lambda)\dfrac{\sqrt{2\alpha} - 1/2}{\sqrt{2\alpha} - 1 + |x|}, & \text{if } |x| \geq 1/2, \\ 1 - \lambda\dfrac{\sqrt{2\alpha} - 1/2}{\sqrt{2\alpha} - |x|}, & \text{if } |x| < 1/2, \end{cases}$$

   is a minimizer of $\mathcal{F}_c^{(1)}$. In particular, the solution is not unique (cf. Fig. 5.2).

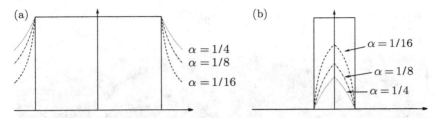

Fig. 5.1. Solution of NCBV regularization with **(a)** $u^\delta = \chi_{(-3/4,3/4)}$ and **(b)** $u^\delta = \chi_{(-1/4,1/4)}$ for different values of α.

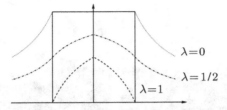

Fig. 5.2. Different solutions of NCBV regularization with $u^\delta = \chi_{(-1/2,1/2)}$ and $\alpha = 1/2$ for different values of λ.

We present some numerical result for the minimization of the discrete convexified NCBV functional

$$\mathcal{F}_h(\mathbf{u}) := h^2 \sum_{i,j} f_c\big(u_{ij} - u_{ij}^\delta, |v_{ij}|\big),$$

where $f_c(\xi, \mathbf{t})$ is the convexification of $f(\xi, \mathbf{t}) = \xi^2/(2\,|\mathbf{t}|) + \alpha\,|\mathbf{t}|$ with respect to $\mathbf{t}$, and $\mathbf{v}$ is a discrete gradient of $\mathbf{u}$.

Note that (2.32), which has been designed in Chapter 2 for removing sampling errors in noisy discrete images, can be considered a discretization of the NCBV functional. Taking into account that in the continuous setting the functional has to be convexified for guaranteeing existence of minimizers, we expect that the minimizer of the discrete convexified functional $\mathcal{F}_h$ approximates the minimizer of (2.32).

The result of filtering the "mountain" image with sampling errors (Fig. 5.3, left) is shown in Fig. 5.3, right. Additionally, we test the applicability of NCBV regularization to an image with sampling errors and Gaussian noise (see Fig. 5.4, left). The filtering result is shown in Fig. 5.4, right. In both cases, the distortion is removed feasibly well.

Figure 5.5 shows the result of filtering the ultrasound data by minimizing the NCBV functional with $\alpha = 2.5$ (middle) and $\alpha = 20$ (right).

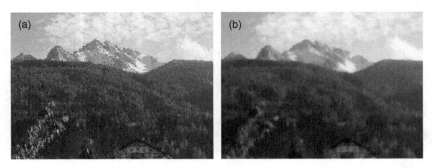

Fig. 5.3. NCBV Filter I. (**a**) Image with sampling point errors. (**b**) Result of NCBV filtering. The discretized NCBV functional was minimized by a steepest descent method.

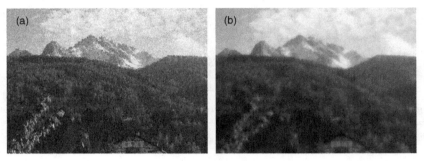

Fig. 5.4. NCBV Filter II. (**a**) Image with sampling point and intensity errors. (**b**) Result of NCBV filtering.

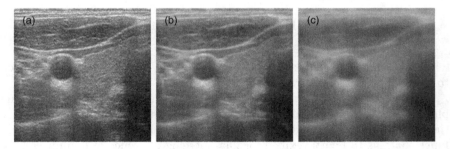

Fig. 5.5. NCBV Filter III. (**a**) Ultrasound image. (**b**) Result of NCBV filtering with $\alpha = 2.5$. (**c**) Result of NCBV filtering with $\alpha = 20$.

Further Literature on Direct Methods and Relaxation

Direct methods have been applied by several authors to the study of variational functionals. One of the main references is due to Morrey (see [279]), who mainly considered vector valued functions and introduced the notion of quasi-convexity for their treatment. Further results on lower semi-continuity of integral functionals in Sobolev spaces can be found, for instance, in [2, 74, 122, 123, 182, 220, 267, 268, 303].

Good references for the problem of relaxation on Sobolev spaces are [122, 123, 182, 365]. Recently, the focus has changed to the BV case. Here, we refer to [33, 42, 55, 167–169, 243, 254].

Finally, we want to mention the results of [130], where variational functionals depending on measures have been considered. The results here apply to the BV case, if the integrals only depend on the gradient ∇u.

The relation between non-convex regularization and level set segmentation algorithms [80, 82, 83] has been discussed in [172].

6

Semi-group Theory and Scale Spaces

Elegant methods for data analysis are evolutionary equations: Given data u^δ on $\Omega \subset \mathbb{R}^n$ to analyze, these methods consist in solving the evolution equation

$$
\begin{aligned}
\frac{\partial u}{\partial t} + A(u) \ni 0 \qquad &\text{in } \Omega \times (0, \infty)\,, \\
u(0) = u^\delta \qquad &\text{in } \Omega\,,
\end{aligned}
\tag{6.1}
$$

up to a certain $T > 0$ and considering $u(T)$ a filtered version of u^δ. The parameter T controls the amount of filtering and plays a similar role as the regularization parameter α used in Chapters 3–5.

The operator A in general will be a differential operator of second order satisfying appropriate boundary conditions and mapping a subset $\mathcal{D}$ of a Banach space U consisting of functions on Ω to the power set 2^U of all subsets of U.

In many applications, the operator A is set valued, and therefore (6.1) has to be considered an *inclusion equation.*

Some of the most prominent examples of diffusion filtering methods used in image processing are summarized in Table 6.1.

In this chapter, we establish the link between diffusion filtering, that is, solving (6.1), and variational regularization methods for denoising introduced in the previous chapters. This relation is derived via *semi-group theory.*

Definition 6.1. *Let $\mathcal{D} \subset U$. A family of mappings $S_t : \mathcal{D} \to \mathcal{D}$, $t \geq 0$, satisfying*

$$
S_{t+s} u = S_t S_s u\,, \qquad s, t \geq 0\,, \quad u \in \mathcal{D}\,,
$$

$$
\lim_{t \to 0^+} S_t u = S_0 u = u\,, \qquad u \in \mathcal{D}\,,
$$

is called strongly continuous semi-group *in $\mathcal{D}$.*

The family of mappings (S_t) is called contraction semi-group, *if it satisfies*

$$
\|S_t u - S_t \tilde{u}\| \leq \|u - \tilde{u}\|\,, \qquad t \geq 0\,, \quad u, \tilde{u} \in \mathcal{D}\,.
$$

O. Scherzer et al., *Variational Methods in Imaging,*
© Springer Science+Business Media, LLC 2009

Table 6.1. Summary of common diffusion filtering methods.

	$A(u)$
Heat flow	$-\Delta u$
Total variation flow (see, for instance, [22])	$-\nabla\cdot\left(\frac{1}{|\nabla u|}\nabla u\right)$
Perona–Malik [320]	$-\nabla\cdot\left(\frac{1}{1+|\nabla u|^2}\nabla u\right)$
Anisotropic diffusion [385]	$-\nabla\cdot(D\nabla u)$, (D matrix)
Mean curvature motion (MCM) [8]	$-\,|\nabla u|\,\nabla\cdot\left(\frac{1}{|\nabla u|}\nabla u\right)$
Affine invariant MCM (AIMCM) [8]	$-\,|\nabla u|\,\nabla\cdot\left(\frac{1}{|\nabla u|}\nabla u\right)^{1/3}$

Define for $t \geq 0$ the mapping $S_t : \mathcal{D} \subset U \to U$ setting $S_t u^\delta := u(t)$, where $u(t)$ is the solution of (6.1) at time t with initial data u^δ. Then we have the relations $S_{t+s}u^\delta = S_t S_s u^\delta$ and $S_0 u^\delta = u^\delta$ whenever the solution of (6.1) exists and is unique. If additionally $\lim_{t\to 0+} S_t u = u$ for every $u \in \mathcal{D}$, then the family of mappings (S_t) forms a continuous semi-group on $\mathcal{D}$.

In the following, we study the relation between the operator A and the semi-group S_t, $t \geq 0$, first in the case of a linear (but possibly unbounded) operator $A : \mathcal{D}(A) \subset U \to U$, and then in the general case of a non-linear set-valued operator $A : U \to 2^U$.

6.1 Linear Semi-group Theory

Let U be a Banach space, and let S_t, $t \geq 0$, be a semi-group consisting of bounded linear operators $S_t : U \to U$ in $\mathcal{D} = U$.

Under the semi-group condition $S_t S_s = S_{t+s}$, the continuity condition $S_t u \to u$ as $t \to 0$ can be shown to be equivalent to the weak continuity $S_t u \rightharpoonup u$ as $t \to 0$ for every $u \in U$ (see [401, Chap. IX.1, Thm.]). Thus, in the linear case, the concepts of strongly and weakly continuous semi-groups coincide.

For a linear semi-group, it can be shown (see [401, Chap. IX.1]) that the linear operators S_t satisfy the condition

$$\|S_t\|_{L(U,U)} \leq C \exp(-\beta t)\,, \qquad t \geq 0\,, \tag{6.2}$$

where $C > 0$ and $\beta \in \mathbb{R}$ are constants.

Remark 6.2. Note that S_t is a contraction semi-group, if and only if it satisfies (6.2) with $C = 1$ and $\beta = 0$, that is,

$$\|S_t\|_{L(U,U)} \leq 1\,, \qquad t \geq 0\,.$$

Definition 6.3. *Let (S_t) be a continuous semi-group on the Banach space U. The infinitesimal generator of (S_t) is the operator $A_S : \mathcal{D}(A_S) \to U$ defined by*

$$\mathcal{D}(A_S) = \left\{ u \in U : \lim_{t \to 0^+} \frac{S_t u - u}{t} \in U \text{ exists} \right\}, \tag{6.3}$$

and

$$A_S u = -\lim_{t \to 0^+} \frac{S_t u - u}{t}, \qquad u \in \mathcal{D}(A_S). \tag{6.4}$$

Denote $u(t) := S_t u^\delta$. Then (6.4) states that $-A_S u^\delta = \frac{\partial u}{\partial t}(0^+)$. The following result implies that, in fact, u solves the initial value problem (6.1).

Theorem 6.4. *Let (S_t) be a linear continuous semi-group with infinitesimal generator $A_S : \mathcal{D}(A_S) \to U$. The set $\mathcal{D}(A_S)$ is dense in U and $A_S : \mathcal{D}(A_S) \to U$ is closed.*

Let $u^\delta \in \mathcal{D}(A_S)$ and denote $u(t) := S_t u^\delta$. Then the function $u : [0, \infty) \to U$ is continuously differentiable and

$$\frac{\partial u}{\partial t}(t) = -A_S u(t) = -S_t A_S u^\delta, \qquad t \in [0, \infty).$$

Proof. See [38, Chap. 1, Prop. 3.1]. □

This theorem shows that every linear continuous semi-group indeed has an infinitesimal generator and thus can be constructed as solution of the differential equation (6.1). The more relevant question, however, is, under which conditions a given linear operator A on a subset of U generates a semi-group, in other words, under which conditions (6.1) has a solution. The main condition A has to satisfy turns out to be that the operator $(\text{Id} + \lambda A)$ is invertible for all $\lambda > 0$.

Theorem 6.5 (Hille–Yosida). *Let $A : \mathcal{D}(A) \subset U \to U$ be a linear operator with dense domain $\mathcal{D}(A)$.*

The operator A is the infinitesimal generator of a uniquely defined linear continuous semi-group (S_t) satisfying (6.2) with $C > 0$ and $\beta \in \mathbb{R}$, if and only if for all $n \in \mathbb{N}$ and $\lambda^{-1} > -\beta$ we have $(\text{Id} + \lambda A)^{-1} \in L(U, U)$ and

$$\left\| (\text{Id} + \lambda A)^{-n} \right\|_{L(U,U)} \leq \frac{C}{|1 + \lambda \beta|^n}.$$

In this case, $A = A_S$ and $\mathcal{D}(A) = \mathcal{D}(A_S)$ satisfy (6.4) and (6.3), respectively.

Proof. See [38, Chap. 1, Thm. 3.1]. □

In particular, it follows from Theorem 6.5 that we need not distinguish between the case where a semi-group (S_t) is defined by a generator A on the one hand, and the case where the operator A is defined by the semi-group (S_t) on the other hand.

Corollary 6.6. *The operator $A : \mathcal{D}(A) \subset U \to U$ with dense domain $\mathcal{D}(A)$ is the infinitesimal generator of a uniquely defined linear continuous contraction semi-group (S_t), if and only if $(\mathrm{Id} + \lambda A)^{-1} \in L(U,U)$, $\lambda > 0$, and*

$$\left\| (\mathrm{Id} + \lambda A)^{-1} \right\|_{L(U,U)} \leq 1, \qquad \lambda > 0 .$$

Proof. This is a direct consequence of Theorem 6.5 setting $C = 1$ and $\beta = 0$ (see Remark 6.2). □

Moreover, it is possible to construct the solution u of (6.1) by means of the following exponential type formula.

Theorem 6.7. *Let $A : \mathcal{D}(A) \subset U \to U$ be the infinitesimal generator of a linear continuous contraction semi-group (S_t). Then*

$$S_t u^\delta = \exp(-tA)\, u^\delta := \lim_{N \to \infty} \left(\mathrm{Id} + \frac{t}{N} A \right)^{-N} u^\delta , \qquad t \geq 0,\ u^\delta \in U . \quad (6.5)$$

Proof. See [319, Thm. 6.6]. □

Remark 6.8. Assume that U and V are Hilbert spaces and $A = L^* L$, where L^* denotes the adjoint of the densely defined linear operator $L : \mathcal{D}(L) \subset U \to V$ (see Theorem 8.26). Then it follows from Lemmas 10.15 and 10.16 that the function $u_{N,N} := \left(\mathrm{Id} + \frac{t}{N} A \right)^{-N} u^\delta$ can as well be obtained by iterative minimization with $u_{0,N} = u^\delta$ and

$$u_{k,N} := \arg\min \left(\frac{1}{2} \left\| u - u_{k-1,N} \right\|_U^2 + \frac{\alpha}{2} \left\| Lu \right\|_V^2 \right), \qquad k = 1, \dots, N ,$$

where $\alpha = \frac{t}{N}$. Each step of the variational method is a special instance of Tikhonov regularization with data $u_{k-1,N}$. This shows the fundamental relation between iterative regularization and evolution equations. ◇

Example 6.9. Assume that $\Omega \subset \mathbb{R}^n$, $n = 2, 3$, is bounded with C^1-boundary. Moreover, let $U = L_\diamond^2(\Omega)$, associated with the topology induced by the L^2 norm,

$$\mathcal{D}(-\Delta) := \left\{ u \in W^{2,2}(\Omega) \cap L_\diamond^2(\Omega) : \frac{\partial u}{\partial \mathbf{n}} = 0 \text{ on } \partial\Omega \right\} ,$$

and

$$A := -\Delta : \mathcal{D}(-\Delta) \subset U \to U , \qquad u \mapsto -\Delta u ,$$

the negative Laplacian. Here the condition $\frac{\partial u}{\partial \mathbf{n}} = 0$ is understood distributionally in the sense that

$$\int_\Omega \phi \, \nabla u = - \int_\Omega u \, \nabla \cdot (\phi) , \qquad \phi \in C^\infty(\mathbb{R}^n; \mathbb{R}^n) .$$

Now let $u \in L^2(\Omega)$. From Theorem 9.37, it follows that there exists a sequence $(u_k) \subset C_0^\infty(\Omega)$ with $\| u_k - u \|_2 \to 0$. Define $\tilde{u}_k := u_k - \mathcal{L}^n(\Omega)^{-1} \int_\Omega u_k$.

Then $\tilde{u}_k \in L^2_\diamond(\Omega) \cap C^\infty(\Omega)$, and $\frac{\partial \tilde{u}_k}{\partial \mathbf{n}} = 0$ on $\partial\Omega$, which implies that $(\tilde{u}_k) \subset \mathcal{D}(-\Delta)$. Moreover $\|\tilde{u}_k - u\|_2 \to 0$. This shows that A is densely defined in $L^2_\diamond(\Omega)$.

Moreover, from Green's formula (9.13), it follows that

$$\int_\Omega (-\Delta u) = -\int_{\partial\Omega} \frac{\partial u}{\partial \mathbf{n}} \, \mathrm{d}\mathcal{H}^{n-1} = 0, \qquad u \in \mathcal{D}(-\Delta) \,.$$

Therefore, $-\Delta u \in L^2_\diamond(\Omega)$ for $u \in \mathcal{D}(-\Delta)$.

Let $\lambda > 0$ and $y \in L^2_\diamond(\Omega)$. We denote by $u_\lambda \in L^2_\diamond(\Omega) \cap W^{2,2}(\Omega)$ the solution of

$$(\mathrm{Id} - \lambda\Delta) u = y \quad \text{in } \Omega \,,$$

$$\frac{\partial u}{\partial \mathbf{n}} = 0 \quad \text{in } \partial\Omega \,,$$

the existence and uniqueness of which follows from [195, Ex. 7.4.8]. Then from Green's formula (9.13), it follows that

$$\|u_\lambda\|_2^2 \le \int_\Omega u_\lambda^2 + \lambda \int_\Omega |\nabla u_\lambda|^2 \le \int_\Omega u_\lambda^2 - \lambda \int_\Omega u_\lambda \Delta u_\lambda = \int_\Omega u_\lambda \, y \le \|u_\lambda\|_2 \, \|y\|_2 \,.$$

This shows that $\|u_\lambda\|_2 \le \|y\|_2$ and therefore

$$\left\| (\mathrm{Id} - \lambda\Delta)^{-1} \right\| \le 1 \,.$$

From Corollary 6.6, it follows that $-\Delta$ generates a contraction semi-group on $L^2_\diamond(\Omega)$. Moreover, for $u^\delta \in \mathcal{D}(-\Delta)$ the solution defined by the exponential formula in Theorem 6.7 is continuously differentiable and satisfies (6.1). $\diamond$

Remark 6.10. We consider the variational method consisting in minimization of the functional

$$\mathcal{T}_{\alpha,u^\delta} : W^{1,2}_\diamond(\Omega) \to \mathbb{R} \,, \qquad u \mapsto \frac{1}{2} \int_\Omega (u - u^\delta)^2 + \frac{\alpha}{2} \int_\Omega |\nabla u|^2 \,,$$

for denoising data u^δ. We denote the minimizer of the functional by u_α.

Let $A = -\Delta$ as in Example 6.9. Then we have

$$u_\alpha = (\mathrm{Id} + \alpha A)^{-1} u^\delta \,.$$

Iterative minimization $u^{(k+1)} = \arg\min \mathcal{T}_{\alpha,u^{(k)}}$ with $u^{(0)} = u^\delta$ approximates a semi-group solution of

$$\frac{\partial u}{\partial t} = \Delta u \quad \text{in } \Omega \times (0,\infty) \,,$$

$$\frac{\partial u}{\partial \mathbf{n}} = 0 \quad \text{in } \partial\Omega \times (0,\infty) \,,$$

$$u(0) = u^\delta \,.$$

According to Example 6.9, a solution of this differential equation exists for

$$u^\delta \in \left\{ u \in W^{2,2}(\Omega) \cap L^2_\diamond(\Omega) : \frac{\partial u}{\partial \mathbf{n}} = 0 \text{ on } \partial\Omega \right\} = \mathcal{D}(-\Delta) \, .$$

In this case, it follows from (6.3) that $\left\| u(\alpha) - u^\delta \right\|_2 = O(\alpha)$.

The same result can be obtained from the convergence rates results for Tikhonov regularization in Chapter 3, in particular from the estimate (3.43). Let $F = \mathrm{i}$ the embedding from $U := W^{1,2}_\diamond(\Omega)$ into $V := L^2_\diamond(\Omega)$. The operator i is linear, and consequently it follows from Remark 3.37 that the convergence rates result Proposition 3.41 can be applied if $u^\delta \in \mathrm{Ran}(\mathrm{i}^*)$, which in turn is equivalent to $u^\delta \in \mathcal{D}(-\Delta)$. From (3.43), it then follows that

$$\left\| u_\alpha - u^\delta \right\|_2 = O(\alpha) \quad \text{and} \quad \int_\Omega \left| \nabla u_\alpha - \nabla u^\delta \right|^2 = O(\alpha) \, .$$

This example reveals a relation between the convergence rates results for Tikhonov regularization (see, for instance, Theorem 3.42) and the conditions for solutions of the associated evolutionary partial differential equations. In fact in this case, both variational regularization and diffusion equation satisfy the same L^2 estimate. $\diamond$

6.2 Non-linear Semi-groups in Hilbert Spaces

Many of the results for linear semi-groups can be translated to non-linear semi-groups, as long as the underlying space is a Hilbert space. Because in the non-linear case the defining operators are in general set-valued, it is, however, necessary to clarify some notation.

We first introduce some notation concerning set-valued mappings $A : U \to 2^U$. We denote by

$$\mathcal{D}(A) = \left\{ u : Au \neq \emptyset \right\}$$

the *domain* of A, by

$$\mathrm{Ran}(A) = \bigcup_{u \in \mathcal{D}(A)} Au$$

the *range* of A, and by

$$\mathcal{G}(A) = \left\{ (u,v) : u \in U, \, v \in Au \right\}$$

the *graph* of A. The *inverse* $A^{-1} : U \to 2^U$ of A is given by

$$A^{-1}v := \left\{ u : v \in Au \right\} \, .$$

Moreover, we define the *minimal section* $A^0 : U \to 2^U$ of A by

$$A^0 u = \left\{ v \in Au : \|v\| = \inf_{\tilde{v} \in Au} \|\tilde{v}\| \right\} \, . \tag{6.6}$$

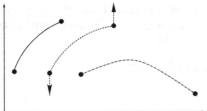
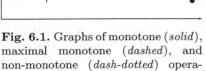
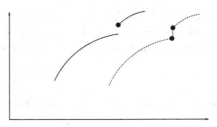

Fig. 6.1. Graphs of monotone (*solid*), maximal monotone (*dashed*), and non-monotone (*dash-dotted*) operators on $\mathbb{R}$.

Fig. 6.2. Graph of a monotone but not maximal monotone operator (*solid*), and graph of a maximal monotone operator (*dashed*).

In the linear case, two conditions have been essential for guaranteeing the existence of a (contraction) semi-group generated by some given operator $A : \mathcal{D}(A) \subset U \to U$; the first was the invertibility of $(\mathrm{Id} + \lambda A)$ for all $\lambda > 0$, and the second that $\left\| (\mathrm{Id} + \lambda A)^{-1} \right\|_{L(U,U)} \leq 1$, $\lambda > 0$. The first condition directly carries over to the non-linear case, the basic statement of the second one has to be formulated in a different way.

Definition 6.11 (Monotone operators). *Let* $A : U \to 2^U$. *The operator* A *is* monotone, *if*

$$\langle v - \tilde{v}, u - \tilde{u} \rangle \geq 0, \qquad u, \tilde{u} \in \mathcal{D}(A), \ v \in Au, \ \tilde{v} \in A\tilde{u}.$$

The operator A *is* maximal monotone, *if every monotone extension of* A *equals* A, *that is, whenever* $B : U \to 2^U$ *is a monotone operator with* $Au \subset Bu$, $u \in U$, *then* $A = B$.

Figures 6.1 and 6.2 show graphs of monotone and maximal monotone operators on $\mathbb{R}$.

Theorem 6.12 (Minty). *The operator* A *is maximal monotone, if and only if*

$$\mathrm{Ran}(\mathrm{Id} + \lambda A) = U, \qquad \lambda > 0, \tag{6.7}$$

and

$$\|u - \tilde{u}\| \leq \|u + \lambda v - (\tilde{u} + \lambda\tilde{v})\|, \qquad u, \tilde{u} \in \mathcal{D}(A), \ v \in Au, \ \tilde{v} \in A\tilde{u}, \ \lambda > 0. \tag{6.8}$$

Proof. See [38, Chap. II, Prop. 3.1, Thm. 3.1]. □

In particular, if A is a linear operator, then (6.7) implies that $(\mathrm{Id} + \lambda A)$ is surjective for all $\lambda > 0$, whereas (6.8) implies that $(\mathrm{Id} + \lambda A)$ is injective, and $\left\| (\mathrm{Id} + \lambda A)^{-1} \right\|_{L(U,U)} \leq 1$. This shows that, in the linear case, the maximal monotonicity of A is equivalent to the conditions required in Corollary 6.6.

Remark 6.13. The most important example of a maximal monotone operator on a Hilbert space U is the subdifferential of a convex, lower semi-continuous, and proper functional $\mathcal{R} : U \to \mathbb{R} \cup \{\infty\}$. In this case

$$\overline{\mathcal{D}(\partial \mathcal{R})} = \overline{\mathcal{D}(\mathcal{R})}$$

(see, for example, [38, Chap. II, Thm. 2.1]). $\Diamond$

Now we state the main results concerning semi-groups on Hilbert spaces. They are direct generalizations of the Hille–Yosida Theorem 6.5 and Theorem 6.7 to non-linear contraction semi-groups on Hilbert spaces. For the following results, recall the notion of the infinitesimal generator of a semi-group introduced in Definition 6.3.

Theorem 6.14. *Let $C \subset U$ be a non-empty, closed, and convex set, and (S_t) a (non-linear) semi-group of contractions on C. Then there exists a unique maximal monotone operator $A_S : U \to 2^U$, such that its minimal section A_S^0 is the infinitesimal generator of (S_t) in the sense of Definition 6.3.*

Conversely, if $A : U \to 2^U$ is maximal monotone, then there exists a unique semi-group S on $\overline{\mathcal{D}(A)}$ with infinitesimal generator A^0.

Proof. See [38, Chap. IV, Thm. 1.2]. $\square$

Theorem 6.15. *Let $A : U \to 2^U$ be maximal monotone, and let (S_t) be the semi-group generated by A^0. Then*

$$S_t u^\delta = \exp(-tA) = \lim_{N \to \infty} \left(\mathrm{Id} + \frac{t}{N} A \right)^{-N} u^\delta, \qquad t \geq 0, \ u^\delta \in \overline{\mathcal{D}(A)}.$$

Proof. See [38, Chap. IV, Thm. 1.4, Rem.]. $\square$

Finally, one can show that the semi-group generated by a maximal monotone operator A indeed satisfies the evolution equation (6.1).

Theorem 6.16. *Let $A : U \to 2^U$ be maximal monotone, and let (S_t) be the semi-group generated by A^0. Let $u^\delta \in \mathcal{D}(A)$, and define $u(t) := S_t u^\delta$. Then $u \in C\big([0, \infty); U\big) \cap W^{1,1}_{\mathrm{loc}}\big((0, \infty); U\big)$,*

$$\frac{\partial u}{\partial t}(t) \in -A\big(u(t)\big), \qquad a.e. \ t \in (0, \infty),$$

and $u(0) = u^\delta$.

Proof. See [60, Thm. 3.1]. $\square$

The main application we are interested in is the case where A is the subdifferential of a convex and lower semi-continuous function $\mathcal{R} : U \to \mathbb{R} \cup \{\infty\}$. In this case, Theorem 6.16 can be extended to initial values u^δ that are contained in the closure of the domain of A.

Theorem 6.17. *Let* $\mathcal{R} : U \to \mathbb{R} \cup \{\infty\}$ *be lower semi-continuous, convex, and proper, and let* (S_t) *be the semi-group generated by* $\partial^0 \mathcal{R} := (\partial \mathcal{R})^0$. *Assume that* $u^\delta \in \overline{\mathcal{D}(\mathcal{R})}$ *and denote* $u(t) := S_t u^\delta$.

Then $u \in C\big([0,\infty); U\big) \cap W^{1,2}_{\mathrm{loc}}\big((0,\infty); U\big)$, $u(0) = u^\delta$, $u(t) \in \mathcal{D}(\mathcal{R})$ *for* $t > 0$, *and*

$$\frac{\partial u}{\partial t}(t^+) = -\partial^0 \mathcal{R}\big(u(t)\big), \qquad t > 0 .$$

Proof. See [38, Chap. IV, Thm. 2.1, Thm. 2.2]. ☐

Remark 6.18. Let the assumptions of Theorem 6.17 be satisfied. We assume that $u^\delta \in \overline{\mathcal{D}(\mathcal{R})}$ and denote $u(t) := S_t u^\delta$. For every $v_0 \in \mathcal{D}(\mathcal{R})$, the following inequality holds (see [38, Chap. IV, Thm. 2.3]):

$$\left\| \frac{\partial u}{\partial t}(t^+) \right\| = \left\| \partial^0 \mathcal{R}\big(u(t)\big) \right\| \le \left\| \partial^0 \mathcal{R}(v_0) \right\| + \frac{1}{t} \left\| v_0 - u^\delta \right\| , \qquad t > 0 . \quad (6.9)$$

If additionally $\mathcal{R}$ attains a minimizer in U, then $u(t)$ converges to some minimizer of $\mathcal{R}$ as $t \to \infty$ (see [38, Chap. IV, Thm. 2.4, Rem.]). ◇

Example 6.19 (Total variation flow on $L^2(\Omega)$). Let $\Omega \subset \mathbb{R}^n$ be open, $U = L^2(\Omega)$, and $\mathcal{R} = \mathcal{R}_1 : U \to \mathbb{R} \cup \{\infty\}$ the total variation semi-norm. Then $\mathcal{R}$ is a lower semi-continuous, convex, and proper functional, which implies that the results of Theorem 6.17 can be applied to the *total variation flow* equation

$$\frac{\partial u}{\partial t}(t) \in -\partial \mathcal{R}\big(u(t)\big) =: \nabla \cdot \left(\frac{\nabla u(t)}{|\nabla u(t)|} \right) \quad (6.10)$$

with initial condition $u(0) = u^\delta \in L^2(\Omega)$. In particular, it follows that (6.10) has a unique solution $u \in C\big([0,\infty); L^2(\Omega)\big) \cap W^{1,2}_{\mathrm{loc}}\big((0,\infty), L^2(\Omega)\big)$. Moreover, $u(t) \in BV(\Omega) \cap L^2(\Omega)$ for all $t > 0$. Finally, it follows from Remark 6.18 that $u(t)$ converges to a function that is constant on each connected component of Ω as $t \to \infty$. In case $\Omega = \mathbb{R}^n$, it follows that $u(t) \to 0$ as $t \to \infty$. ◇

6.3 Non-linear Semi-groups in Banach Spaces

In the case of non-linear semi-groups in Banach spaces, the situation is notably more difficult. In general, it is possible that a given contraction semi-group has no infinitesimal generator in the sense of Definition 6.3. Conversely, it is as well possible that different operators generate the same semi-group by means of the exponential formula (6.5). Finally, it may happen that (6.5) yields a function that does not satisfy the evolution equation (6.1).

Due to the above problems, we revert the order of presentation compared with the previous sections. Moreover, we generalize the exponential formula, which can be seen as limit of an equidistant time discretization, by also allowing non-equidistant time steps. We start with considering existence and uniqueness of a limit of the time discrete schemes and afterwards discuss the question whether this limit solves the flow equation (6.1). Therefore, we first have to find a meaningful notion for the time continuous limit of a time discrete sequence. This is achieved by introducing ε-discrete and mild solutions:

Let $\varepsilon > 0$ and $[a, b] \subset [0, \infty)$. An ε-*discretization* of $[a, b]$ is a vector with entries $a \leq t_0 < t_1 < \ldots < t_N \leq b$ satisfying

$$t_i - t_{i-1} \leq \varepsilon, \quad i = 1, \ldots, N, \qquad t_0 - a \leq \varepsilon, \quad b - t_N \leq \varepsilon.$$

Definition 6.20. *Let* $t_0 < t_1 < \ldots < t_N$ *be an* ε-*discretization of the interval* $[a, b]$. *An* ε-*discrete solution of* $\frac{\partial u}{\partial t} + A(u) \ni 0$ *on* $[a, b]$ *according to the given* ε-*discretization is a piecewise constant function* $v : [t_0, t_N] \to U$ *satisfying*

$$\frac{v_i - v_{i-1}}{t_i - t_{i-1}} + A(v_i) \ni 0, \qquad i = 1, \ldots, N, \qquad (6.11)$$

where $v_0 = v(t_0)$ *and*

$$v(t) = v_i, \quad t \in (t_{i-1}, t_i], \qquad i = 1, \ldots, N.$$

Definition 6.21. *A* mild solution *of* $\frac{\partial u}{\partial t} + A(u) \ni 0$ *on* $[a, b]$ *is a function* $u \in C([a, b]; U)$ *such that for every* $\varepsilon > 0$, *there exists an* ε-*discrete solution* v *of* $\frac{\partial u}{\partial t} + A(u) \ni 0$ *satisfying*

$$\|u(t) - v(t)\| \leq \varepsilon, \qquad t_0 \leq t \leq t_N.$$

If $I \subset [0, \infty)$ *is an arbitrary not necessarily bounded interval, then a solution of* $\frac{\partial u}{\partial t} + A(u) \ni 0$ *on* I *is a function* $u \in C(I; U)$ *such that the restriction of* u *to every compact sub-interval* $[a, b] \subset I$ *is a mild solution of* $\frac{\partial u}{\partial t} + A(u) \ni 0$ *on* $[a, b]$.

Thus, a mild solution of $\frac{\partial u}{\partial t} + A(u) \ni 0$ is the pointwise limit of a sequence of piecewise constant time discrete approximations with varying step size.

Now the first question is, whether a mild solution is well-defined in the sense that it exists and is unique. Again, sufficient conditions can be found by generalizing the conditions needed for the Hilbert space case to general Banach spaces.

Definition 6.22. *An operator* $A : U \to 2^U$ *is* accretive *if*

$$\|u - \tilde{u}\| \leq \|u - \tilde{u} + \lambda(v - \tilde{v})\|, \qquad u, \tilde{u} \in U, \ v \in A(u), \ \tilde{v} \in A(\tilde{u}),$$

or, equivalently, if

$$\langle f, v - \tilde{v} \rangle_{U^*, U} \geq 0, \qquad u, \tilde{u} \in U, \ v \in A(u), \ \tilde{v} \in A(\tilde{u}), \ f \in \mathcal{J}(u - \tilde{u}),$$

where $\mathcal{J} : U \to 2^{U^*}$ *denotes the normalized duality mapping on* U.

The accretive operator A *is* m-accretive *if* $\mathrm{Ran}(\mathrm{Id} + \lambda A) = U$ *for all* $\lambda > 0$.

The equivalence of the two definitions of accretive operators above follows from [38, Chap. II, Prop. 3.1]. Moreover, it is shown in [38, Chap. II, Prop. 3.3] that the accretive operator A is m-accretive, if there exists some $\lambda > 0$ such that $\mathrm{Ran}(\mathrm{Id} + \lambda A) = U$.

If U is a Hilbert space, then the notions of m-accretivity and maximal monotonicity coincide (cf. Theorem 6.12). If U is an arbitrary Banach space, one can define A to be a maximal accretive operator by requiring that every accretive extension B of A equals A. Then it is possible to show that every m-accretive operator is maximal accretive (see [38, Chap. II, Thm. 3.1]), but the converse does not necessarily hold.

The defining equation (6.11) for an ε-discrete solution of $\frac{\partial u}{\partial t} + A(u) \ni 0$ can be rewritten as

$$\big(\mathrm{Id} + (t_i - t_{i-1})A\big)v_i \ni v_{i-1} \,. \tag{6.12}$$

Now the range condition $\mathrm{Ran}(\mathrm{Id} + \lambda A) = U$ implies that (6.12) has a solution v_i for every $v_{i-1} \in U$ and $t_i > t_{i-1}$. Consequently, if A is m-accretive, then (6.1) has ε-discrete solutions for every partition of $[0, T]$. The next result states that the accretivity of A implies that at most one limiting function of the different ε-discrete solutions may exist.

Theorem 6.23 (Uniqueness of mild solutions). *Assume that $A : U \to 2^U$ is accretive and $u^\delta \in \mathcal{D}(A)$. Then the evolution equation (6.13) has at most one mild solution u satisfying $u(0) = u^\delta$. Moreover, every sequence v_ε of ε-discrete solutions of $\frac{\partial u}{\partial t} + A(u) \ni 0$ on $[0, T]$ satisfying $v_\varepsilon(t_0^\varepsilon) \to u^\delta$ uniformly converges to u on $[0, T]$.*

Proof. See [319, Chap. 1, Thm. 3.1]. $\qquad\qquad\qquad\qquad\qquad\qquad\qquad\square$

The last result in particular shows that the choice of the discretization does not matter as long as a limiting function exists. The Crandall–Liggett Theorem 6.25 below states the existence of a limiting function for the equidistant discretization used in the exponential formula. These two results combined allow us to restrict ourselves to considering the exponential formula. For the Crandall–Liggett Theorem to hold, we use a condition on the operator A which is slightly weaker than m-accretivity.

Definition 6.24. *An accretive operator A satisfies the* range condition, *if*

$$\overline{\mathcal{D}(A)} \subset \mathrm{Ran}(\mathrm{Id} + \lambda A) \,, \qquad \lambda > 0 \,.$$

Theorem 6.25 (Crandall–Liggett). *Let A be accretive and satisfy the range condition. Define*

$$J_\lambda^N u^\delta := (\mathrm{Id} + \lambda A)^{-N} u^\delta \,, \qquad u^\delta \in \overline{\mathcal{D}(A)}, \ \lambda > 0, \ N \in \mathbb{N} \,.$$

Then, $J_{t/N}^N u^\delta$ converges to

$$\exp\left(-tA\right)u^\delta := \lim_{N\to\infty} J_{t/N}^N u^\delta = \lim_{N\to\infty}\left(\mathrm{Id}+\frac{t}{N}A\right)^{-N}u^\delta, \qquad u^\delta \in \overline{\mathcal{D}(A)}$$

uniformly with respect to t on every compact interval in $[0,\infty)$. *Moreover,* $S_t := \exp(-tA)$ *defines a semi-group of contractions on* $\overline{\mathcal{D}(A)}$.

Proof. See [119, Thm. I]. □

Note that the Crandall–Liggett Theorem does not state that the semigroup $\exp(-tA)$ is generated by A in the sense of Definition 6.3. Moreover, it may happen that $u(t) := \exp(-tA)u^\delta$ does not solve the evolution equation $\frac{\partial u}{\partial t} \in -A(u)$.

Before citing two results that imply that $\exp(-tA)u^\delta$ solves $\frac{\partial u}{\partial t} \in -A(u)$, we clarify the notion of a (strong) solution in the non-linear Banach space case.

Definition 6.26. *A function* $u : [0,\infty) \to U$ *is a* strong solution *of the evolution equation*

$$\frac{\partial u}{\partial t}(t) + A(u) \ni 0, \quad t \in (0,\infty),$$
$$u(0) = u^\delta, \tag{6.13}$$

if $u \in C\big([0,T];U\big)\cap W_{\mathrm{loc}}^{1,1}\big((0,T);U\big)$, $u(0) = u^\delta$, *and* $\frac{\partial u}{\partial t}+A(u) \ni 0$ *for almost every* $t \in (0,\infty)$.

The next result provides a relation between strong and mild solutions. In particular, it shows that most of the results of the Hilbert space case can be generalized to reflexive Banach spaces.

Theorem 6.27. *Every strong solution of* (6.1) *is a mild solution.*

Let U *be a reflexive Banach space,* A *an* m-*accretive operator on* U, *and* $u^\delta \in \mathcal{D}(A)$. *Then the mild solution of* (6.1), *the existence and uniqueness of which follows from Theorems 6.25 and 6.23, is a strong solution.*

Proof. See [357, Chap. IV, Prop. 8.2] for the first part of the theorem, and [319, Thm. 3.6, 5] for the second part. □

Finally, we provide a result stating that $\exp(-tA)u^\delta$ is a strong solution of (6.1), if it is sufficiently regular.

Theorem 6.28. *Let* A *be accretive and satisfy the range condition, and assume that* $\mathcal{D}(A)$ *is convex and* $\mathcal{G}(A) \subset U \times U$ *is closed. If* $u^\delta \in \mathcal{D}(A)$, *then* $u(t) = \exp(-tA)u^\delta$ *is a strong solution of* (6.1) *if and only if* $u(t)$ *is differentiable almost everywhere.*

Proof. See [119, Thm. II]. □

6.4 Axiomatic Approach to Scale Spaces

Strongly related to semi-group theory and evolutionary equations is the concept of scale spaces. Associated with a given image u^δ there is a family $u(t)$, $t \geq 0$, of images that are considered simplified versions of u^δ at scale t.

In the literature, the approach to scale spaces is not consistent. We follow the axiomatic approach given in [8, 194], where several axioms are introduced that imply that the scale space is governed by an evolution equation.

There is a theoretical and practical difference between the approach to scale spaces in [194] and the semi-group theory reviewed in the previous sections. Before, we have solved an evolution equation on a Banach space U with functional analytic methods. In particular, the operator governing the evolution was a mapping $A : U \to 2^U$. In this section, however, we assume that the evolution takes place in some space U of functions on $\Omega \subset \mathbb{R}^n$ and is governed by a purely local equation

$$\frac{\partial u}{\partial t}(\mathbf{x}, t) = F\big(t, \mathbf{x}, u, \nabla u, \nabla^2 u\big) \quad \text{in } \Omega \times (0, \infty) \,,$$

$$u(\mathbf{x}, 0) = u^\delta(\mathbf{x}) \qquad\qquad \text{in } \Omega \,.$$

As a consequence, these equations cannot be considered in the framework of the previous sections. Still, the existence of solutions can be shown using the theory of *viscosity solutions*. We will not consider this concept in this book, but refer to [41, 118, 194] for some fundamental references.

The following definitions and theorems are taken from [194].

Definition 6.29. *Let U be a space of functions on $\Omega \subset \mathbb{R}^n$. A* scale space *on U is a family of mappings $T_t : U \to U$, $t \geq 0$.*

The scale space (T_t) is pyramidal, *if there exists a family of operators $T_{t+h,t} : U \to U$, $t, h \geq 0$, such that*

$$T_{t+h,t}\, T_t = T_{t+h} \,, \qquad T_0 = \mathrm{Id} \,.$$

In a pyramidal scale space, it is possible to compute the function $u(t) := T_t u^\delta$ from the function $u(s)$, $0 < s < t$, without any knowledge of $u(s')$ for $0 \leq s' < s$.

Because we aim for simplifying operators T_t, we additionally require that a scale space does not add any new features to the data as t increases. This is achieved by the following definition.

Definition 6.30. *A pyramidal scale space (T_t) satisfies a* local comparison principle *if the following two conditions hold:*

- *For every u, $v \in U$ and $\mathbf{x} \in \Omega$ such that $u(\mathbf{y}) \leq v(\mathbf{y})$ in a neighborhood of $\mathbf{x}$, we have for all $t \geq 0$*

$$T_{t+h,t} u(\mathbf{x}) \leq T_{t+h,t} v(\mathbf{x}) + o(h) \,, \quad \text{as } h \to 0^+ \,.$$

- *If u, $v \in U$ satisfy $u(\mathbf{x}) \leq v(\mathbf{x})$ for all $\mathbf{x} \in \Omega$, then*

$$T_{t+h,t}u(\mathbf{x}) \leq T_{t+h,t}v(\mathbf{x}), \qquad t,\ h \geq 0,\ \mathbf{x} \in \Omega.$$

A function $u \in U$ is called *quadratic around* $\mathbf{x} \in \Omega$, if there exists $r > 0$ such that

$$u(\mathbf{y}) = c + \mathbf{p}^T(\mathbf{y}-\mathbf{x}) + \frac{1}{2}(\mathbf{y}-\mathbf{x})^T A\,(\mathbf{y}-\mathbf{x}), \qquad \mathbf{y} \in B_r(\mathbf{x}),$$

for some $c \in \mathbb{R}$, $\mathbf{p} \in \mathbb{R}^n$, and $A \in S^{n \times n}$, the set of symmetric $n \times n$ matrices. In this case $c = u(\mathbf{x})$, $\mathbf{p} = \nabla u(\mathbf{x})$, and $A = \nabla^2 u(\mathbf{x})$.

Definition 6.31. *A pyramidal scale space is regular, if there exists a function $F : \mathbb{R} \times \Omega \times \mathbb{R} \times \mathbb{R}^n \times S^{n \times n} \to \mathbb{R}$, continuous with respect to its last component, such that*

$$\lim_{h \to 0^+} \frac{T_{t+h,t}u(\mathbf{x}) - u(\mathbf{x})}{h} = F\big(t,\mathbf{x},u(\mathbf{x}),\nabla u(\mathbf{x}),\nabla^2 u(\mathbf{x})\big), \qquad t \geq 0, \quad (6.14)$$

for all quadratic functions u around $\mathbf{x} \in \Omega$.

Definition 6.32. *A pyramidal, regular scale space that satisfies a local comparison principle is called* causal.

The following theorem from [194] states that every causal scale space is governed by an evolution equation.

Theorem 6.33. *Let (T_t) be a causal scale space. Then (6.14) holds for all $u \in C^2(\Omega)$, $\mathbf{x} \in \Omega$, and $t \geq 0$. Moreover, the function F is non-decreasing with respect to its last component in the sense that*

$$F(t,\mathbf{x},c,\mathbf{p},A) \leq F(t,\mathbf{x},c,\mathbf{p},B), \quad A,B \in S^{n \times n}, \quad B-A \text{ positive semi-definite}.$$

Proof. See [194, Lemma 21.8, Thm. 21.9]. $\qquad\qquad\qquad\qquad\qquad\qquad\square$

Aside from the general properties of scale spaces, geometrical invariance properties are postulated in [8, 194]. There the following transformations are used:

For given $u \in U$, we consider *translation* operators $\tau_{\mathbf{z}}$,

$$(\tau_{\mathbf{z}}u)(\mathbf{x}) = u(\mathbf{x}-\mathbf{z}), \quad \mathbf{x},\mathbf{z} \in \mathbb{R}^n,$$

and *linear scaling* operators σ_c, ρ_A,

$$(\sigma_c u)(\mathbf{x}) = u(c\,\mathbf{x}), \quad c \in \mathbb{R}, \mathbf{x} \in \mathbb{R}^n,$$
$$(\rho_A u)(\mathbf{x}) = u(A\,\mathbf{x}), \quad A \in \mathbb{R}^{n \times n}.$$

In particular, it follows from these definitions that $\sigma_c = \rho_{c\,\mathrm{Id}}$.

Basic invariants of scale spaces are defined as follows:

Definition 6.34. *Let (T_t) be a causal scale space on a space U of functions on $\mathbb{R}^n$.*

- (T_t) is translation invariant, *if*

$$T_{t+h,t} \circ \tau_{\mathbf{z}} = \tau_{\mathbf{z}} \circ T_{t+h,t}, \quad \mathbf{z} \in \mathbb{R}^n.$$

- (T_t) is Euclidean invariant, *if for every orthogonal matrix O*

$$T_{t+h,t} \circ \rho_O = \rho_O \circ T_{t+h,t}.$$

- (T_t) is scale invariant, *if there exists a rescaling function $\theta : (0, \infty) \times [0, \infty) \to [0, \infty)$ satisfying the following conditions:*
  1. *The function θ is differentiable with respect to both variables, and $\frac{\partial \theta}{\partial c}(t, 1)$ is continuous and positive for all $t > 0$.*
  2. *The following equation holds:*

$$T_{t+h,t} \circ \sigma_c = \sigma_c \circ T_{\theta(c,t+h),\theta(c,t)}, \quad c > 0, \quad t, h \geq 0.$$

- *A scale invariant scale space (T_t) is* affine invariant, *if there exists $\hat{\theta} : \mathrm{GL}^n \times [0, \infty) \to [0, \infty)$, defined on the set of invertible matrices GL^n such that $\theta(c, \cdot) := \hat{\theta}(c\,\mathrm{Id}, \cdot)$, $c > 0$, satisfies the conditions of a rescaling function for a scale invariant scale space, and*

$$T_{t+h,t} \circ \rho_A = \rho_A \circ T_{\hat{\theta}(A,t+h),\hat{\theta}(A,t)}, \quad A \in \mathrm{GL}^n, \quad t, h \geq 0.$$

- (T_t) is invariant by gray level translations, *if*

$$T_{t+h,t}(0) = 0 \quad and \quad T_{t+h,t}(u + C) = T_{t+h,t}(u) + C, \quad C \in \mathbb{R}.$$

- (T_t) is contrast invariant, *if for every non-decreasing continuous function $g : \mathbb{R} \to \mathbb{R}$ and $u \in U$*

$$g\big((T_{t+h,t}u)(\mathbf{x})\big) = \big(T_{t+h,t}(g \circ u)\big)(\mathbf{x}), \quad t, h \geq 0, \mathbf{x} \in \mathbb{R}^n.$$

Example 6.35. In this example, we assume that $U \subset C(\mathbb{R}^n)$.

Let Δu denote the Laplacian of u with respect the space variable $\mathbf{x}$. The scale space (T_t) defined by $T_t u^\delta = u(t)$ where u is the solution of the heat equation on $\mathbb{R}^n$

$$\boxed{\frac{\partial u}{\partial t}(t) = \Delta u(t), \qquad u(0) = u^\delta,} \tag{6.15}$$

is translation, Euclidean, and gray level translation invariant. Up to a rescaling of time, the heat flow is the only *linear* causal scale space that satisfies these three properties (see [194, Sect. 21.5]).

Let $G : \mathbb{R} \times [0, \infty) \to \mathbb{R}$ be continuous and non-decreasing with respect to its first argument. Then the scale space (T_t) on $C(\mathbb{R}^2)$ generated by

$$\frac{\partial u}{\partial t}(t) = |\nabla u(t)| \, G\left(\nabla \cdot \left(\frac{\nabla u(t)}{|\nabla u(t)|}\right), t\right), \qquad u(0) = u^\delta, \qquad (6.16)$$

is gray level translation, translation, Euclidean, and contrast invariant. For $G(c, t) = c$, this equation is called the *mean curvature motion* (MCM) equation (also called *mean curvature flow equation*):

$$\frac{\partial u}{\partial t} \in |\nabla u| \, \nabla \cdot \left(\frac{\nabla u}{|\nabla u|}\right). \qquad (6.17)$$

Moreover, the scale space generated by the *affine invariant mean curvature motion* (AIMCM)

$$\frac{\partial u}{\partial t}(t) = |\nabla u(t)| \left(\nabla \cdot \left(\frac{\nabla u(t)}{|\nabla u(t)|}\right)\right)^{1/3}, \qquad u(0) = u^\delta,$$

is affine, gray level translation, translation, Euclidean, and contrast invariant.

It can be shown (see [194, Sect. 22.1]) that every translation, Euclidean, and contrast invariant causal scale space is, up to rescaling of time, of the form (6.16). Moreover, the affine invariant mean curvature motion is the only translation, affine, and contrast invariant scale space.   ◇

We summarize the results in Table 6.2.

Table 6.2. Invariance properties.

	Translation	Euclidean	Gray level translation	Contrast	Affine
Heat flow	✓	✓	✓		
MCM	✓	✓	✓	✓	
AIMCM	✓	✓	✓	✓	✓

6.5 Evolution by Non-convex Energy Functionals

The results of Sections 6.1–6.3 provide a strong connection between the solution of evolution equations and iterative minimization of convex variational functionals. A similar connection is not known to exist in the case of the scale spaces generated by mean curvature motion and its variants. In the following, we indicate how to formally link these scale spaces and iterative minimization of *non-convex* variational functionals.

We consider iterative minimization of the NCBV functional on $U = L^2(\Omega)$. Denoting as usual by $\mathcal{R}_1(u)$ the total variation semi-norm of u, we define for given data u^δ the iteration $J^0_{t/N} u^\delta := u^\delta$ and

$$J^k_{t/N} u^\delta := \arg\min\left(\int_\Omega \frac{\left(u - J^{k-1}_{t/N} u^\delta\right)^2}{2\,|\nabla u|} + \frac{t}{N}\,\mathcal{R}_1(u)\right), \qquad k \in \mathbb{N}\,. \quad (6.18)$$

Taking the limit $\lim_{N\to\infty} J^N_{t/N} u^\delta$, we formally obtain a semi-group $\exp(-tA)u^\delta$ for some operator $A : U \to 2^U$ as in Theorem 6.25.

We now proceed by deriving a generator of this semi-group. Note that the following computations are by no means mathematically rigorous. The generator A of $\exp(-tA)u^\delta$ can be obtained by writing J^1_λ in the form $(\mathrm{Id} + \lambda A_\lambda)^{-1}$ and considering the limit $\lambda \to 0^+$ (cf. Theorem 6.25). Note that we allow the operator A_λ to depend on λ, too. Denoting $u_\lambda := J^1_\lambda u^\delta$, we therefore have to find A_λ satisfying $(u^\delta - u_\lambda)/\lambda = A_\lambda u_\lambda$. The optimality condition for a minimizer u_λ of (6.18) (with $k = 1$ and $t/N = \lambda$) formally reads as (cf. Example 10.41)

$$0 \in \frac{u_\lambda - u^\delta}{|\nabla u_\lambda|} - \nabla\cdot\left(\left(\lambda - \frac{1}{2}\frac{(u_\lambda - u^\delta)^2}{|\nabla u_\lambda|^2}\right)\frac{\nabla u_\lambda}{|\nabla u_\lambda|}\right)\,.$$

Dividing by λ and multiplying by $|\nabla u_\lambda|$ shows that

$$\frac{u^\delta - u_\lambda}{\lambda} \in -|\nabla u_\lambda|\,\nabla\cdot\left(\left(1 - \frac{1}{2}\frac{(u_\lambda - u^\delta)^2}{\lambda^2}\frac{\lambda}{|\nabla u_\lambda|^2}\right)\frac{\nabla u_\lambda}{|\nabla u_\lambda|}\right)\,.$$

Consequently, we have

$$A_\lambda u_\lambda \in -|\nabla u_\lambda|\,\nabla\cdot\left(\left(1 - \lambda\frac{(A_\lambda u_\lambda)^2}{2\,|\nabla u_\lambda|^2}\right)\frac{\nabla u_\lambda}{|\nabla u_\lambda|}\right)\,.$$

Provided the term $A_\lambda u_\lambda/|\nabla u_\lambda|$ stays bounded, we obtain by passing to the limit $\lambda \to 0$ that

$$Au \in -|\nabla u|\,\nabla\cdot\left(\frac{\nabla u}{|\nabla u|}\right),$$

which is exactly the operator defining mean curvature motion (see (6.17)).

In a similar manner, the relation between AIMCM (6.35) and iterative minimization of the functionals

$$J^{k,\mathrm{AI}}_{t/N} u^\delta := \arg\min\left(\frac{1}{4}\int_\Omega \frac{\left(u - J^{k-1,\mathrm{AI}}_{t/N} u^\delta\right)^4}{|\nabla u|^3} + \frac{t}{N}\,\mathcal{R}_1(u)\right), \qquad k \in \mathbb{N},$$

with $J^{0,\mathrm{AI}}_{t/N} u^\delta := u^\delta$ can be established.

In [146], we have developed a preliminary analysis providing existence of the associated flow equations. Moreover, we have shown for rotationally symmetric data u^δ that the exponential formula generates in fact a classical solution of the MCM flow.

6.6 Enhancing

A common method for *enhancing* is to solve evolution equations based on partial differential equations *backward* in time. Given data u^δ to enhance, we determine $u(0)$ by solving

$$
\begin{aligned}
\frac{\partial u}{\partial t} + A(u) \ni 0 \quad &\text{in } \Omega \times (0, T), \\
u(T) = u^\delta \quad &\text{in } \Omega.
\end{aligned}
\tag{6.19}
$$

As in the examples above, A is typically a differential operator of second order; in most cases it is the subdifferential of an energy functional of first order, such as $\frac{1}{2} \int_\Omega |\nabla u|^2$ or $\mathcal{R}_1$. The function $u(0)$ is considered the enhanced data of u^δ, the parameter $T > 0$ controls the amount of enhancing. If, for example, A is an elliptic differential operator of second order, then (6.19) is extremely ill-posed. Thus, in practice, enhancing is used only for small parameters T.

Example 6.36. The following kinds of evolution equations are commonly used in practice.

- Solving (6.19) with $A(u) = -\Delta u$ is referred to as *backward linear diffusion*. Figure 6.3 shows the effect of enhancing a blurry image by backward linear diffusion.
- For $A(u) = \partial \mathcal{R}_1(u)$, we refer to the solution of (6.19) as *backward total variation flow*. $\diamond$

Remark 6.37 (Variational enhancing). Let $\mathcal{R}$ be a convex functional. In Chapter 4, we have studied convex denoising methods consisting in minimization of the functional

$$
\mathcal{T}_{\alpha, u^\delta}(u) := \frac{1}{2} \left\| u - u^\delta \right\|_2^2 + \alpha \mathcal{R}(u).
$$

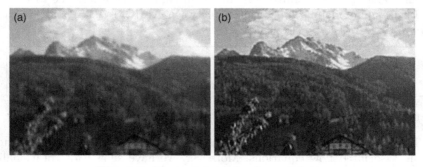

Fig. 6.3. Blurry data and enhanced data.

From the convexity of $\mathcal{R}$, it follows that u_α^δ is a minimizer of $\mathcal{T}_{\alpha,v^\delta}$ if and only if

$$u_\alpha^\delta \in u^\delta - \alpha\,\partial\mathcal{R}(u_\alpha^\delta) \,. \tag{6.20}$$

A *variational enhancing* procedure that stimulates certain features in the data u^δ is given by

$$u_e = u^\delta + \alpha\xi(u^\delta) \qquad \text{with} \qquad \xi(u^\delta) \in \partial\mathcal{R}(u^\delta) \,. \tag{6.21}$$

Note the difference between enhancing (6.21) and filtering (6.20): filtering is defined by an implicit Euler step, whereas enhancing is implemented by an explicit Euler step backward in time. We also mention that, in contrast with PDE enhancing, variational enhancing is defined by a single explicit Euler step. $\qquad\diamond$

Remark 6.38. Using the concept of enhancing, we can shed further light on the source condition (3.23) used in Chapter 3 for proving convergence rates results for variational regularization methods. Recall that, in the case of the regularization functional

$$\mathcal{T}_{\alpha,v}(u) = \frac{1}{2}\,\|F(u) - v\|_V^2 + \alpha\mathcal{R}(u)$$

with Gâteaux differentiable $F : U \to V$, this source condition reads as

$$F'(u^\dagger)^{\#}\omega^* \in \partial\mathcal{R}(u^\dagger)\,,$$

where $u^\dagger$ is an $\mathcal{R}$-minimizing solution of $F(u) = v$, and $\omega^* \in V^*$ (cf. Proposition 3.35). Exemplarily let

$$\mathcal{R}(u) = \frac{1}{2}\,\|u\|_2^2 + \beta\mathcal{R}_1(u)\,, \qquad \beta > 0\,.$$

In this case, we have

$$F'(u^\dagger)^{\#}\omega^* \in u^\dagger + \beta\,\partial\mathcal{R}_1(u^\dagger)\,.$$

In other words, the enhancing of $u^\dagger$ must be in the range of $F'(u^\dagger)^{\#}\omega^*$. $\qquad\diamond$

7

Inverse Scale Spaces

Consider again the problem of solving the operator equation

$$F(u) = v^\delta, \tag{7.1}$$

where $F : \mathcal{D}(F) \subset U \to V$ with Banach spaces U and V, and $v^\delta \in V$ are some given noisy data. In the case of denoising, where $F = \mathrm{Id} : U \to U$ and $v^\delta = u^\delta$, the scale space methods introduced in Chapter 6 can be applied and lead to regularized functions $u(t)$, which are solutions of the flow equation

$$\frac{\partial u}{\partial t}(t) + \partial \mathcal{R}\big(u(t)\big) \ni 0, \qquad u(0) = u^\delta.$$

Moreover, the Crandall–Liggett Theorem 6.25 implies that $u(t)$ can be approximated by a sequence (u_N) computed via the iteration $u_0 := u^\delta$ and

$$\boxed{\begin{aligned} u_k &:= \arg\min_{u \in U} \mathcal{T}_{t/N, u_{k-1}}(u) = \arg\min_{u \in U} \left(\frac{1}{2} \|u - u_{k-1}\|_U^2 + \frac{t}{N}\mathcal{R}(u) \right), \\ k &= 1, \dots, N. \end{aligned}}$$

If $F \neq \mathrm{Id}$, this ansatz cannot work, because it requires an initial condition that is the exact solution of equation (7.1). It is, however, possible to invert the flow direction. Starting from an initial guess u_0, one defines a flow equation, the solution of which converges to a solution of (7.1) as $t \to \infty$. Similarly to the semi-group methods of Chapter 6, the flow can be approximated by iterative minimization of a regularization functional. The difference is that, instead of the similarity term $\big\|F(u) - v^\delta\big\|_V^p$, the regularization term $\mathcal{R}$ is updated in each step.

For notational purposes, we add a superscript to the regularization functional in (3.7), and denote

$$\mathcal{T}_{\alpha, \tilde{v}}^{(\tilde{u})}(u) := \frac{1}{p} \|F(u) - \tilde{v}\|_V^p + \alpha \mathcal{R}(u - \tilde{u}), \qquad u \in \mathcal{D}(F) \subset U.$$

We first review the iterated Tikhonov–Morozov method and inverse scale space methods as introduced in [192], where $\mathcal{R}$ is a norm on U to some power $s \geq 1$. Later we consider Bregman distance regularization with respect to the total variation semi-norm $\mathcal{R}_1$ and the associated inverse scale space method (see also [307]).

7.1 Iterative Tikhonov Regularization

In the beginning, for motivation purposes, let $F : U \to V$ be a Gâteaux differentiable operator between two Hilbert spaces U and V. The *iterative Tikhonov–Morozov method* is defined by

$$
\boxed{
\begin{aligned}
u_0 &\in U, \qquad u_k = \arg\min \, \mathcal{T}^{(u_{k-1})}_{\alpha_k, v^\delta}, \qquad k \in \mathbb{N}, \\
\mathcal{T}^{(\tilde{u})}_{\alpha, v^\delta}(u) &= \frac{1}{2} \left\| F(u) - v^\delta \right\|_V^2 + \frac{\alpha}{2} \left\| u - \tilde{u} \right\|_U^2 .
\end{aligned}
}
$$

In applications, a typical choice for the initial function u_0 is a constant function.

The minimizers u_k of $\mathcal{T}^{(u_{k-1})}_{\alpha_k, v^\delta}$ satisfy the first-order optimality condition (cf. Example 10.35)

$$
F'(u_k)^* \big(F(u_k) - v^\delta \big) + \alpha_k (u_k - u_{k-1}) = 0, \qquad k \in \mathbb{N} .
$$

We now indicate that this optimality condition formally defines a flow on U.

By a *partition* of the interval $[0, \infty)$, we denote a sequence of positive numbers $\boldsymbol{\tau} = (\tau_k)$ such that

$$
|\boldsymbol{\tau}|_\infty := \sup_k \tau_k < \infty
$$

and the associated sequence $(t_k^\tau)_{k \in \mathbb{N}_0}$ defined by $\tau_k = t_k^\tau - t_{k-1}^\tau$ satisfies

$$
0 = t_0^\tau < t_1^\tau < \cdots < t_k^\tau < \cdots , \qquad \lim_k t_k^\tau = \infty .
$$

Now let (t_k), be an increasing sequence of discrete time instances with $t_k - t_{k-1}$ small. Setting $\alpha_k = 1/(t_k - t_{k-1})$, it follows that $(1/\alpha_k)$ is a partition of $[0, \infty)$. Consequently, $\alpha_k(u_k - u_{k-1})$ is an approximation of $\frac{\partial u}{\partial t}(t_k)$, and thus u_k can be considered as approximation at time t_k of the solution u of the *asymptotic Tikhonov–Morozov flow equation*

$$
\boxed{
\frac{\partial u}{\partial t}(t) + F'\big(u(t)\big)^* \big(F\big(u(t)\big) - v^\delta \big) = 0 , \qquad u(0) = u_0 .
}
\tag{7.2}
$$

If the functional $\mathcal{S}(u) := \frac{1}{2} \left\| F(u) - v^\delta \right\|_V^2$ is convex, proper, and lower semi-continuous on U, then (7.2) reads as

$$\frac{\partial u}{\partial t}(t) + \partial \mathcal{S}\big(u(t)\big) = 0, \qquad u(0) = u_0.$$

Thus it follows from Theorem 6.17 that (7.2) attains a unique solution for every $u_0 \in \overline{\mathcal{D}(\mathcal{S})} = U$. The stated properties of $\mathcal{S}$ are satisfied, if F is a bounded linear operator.

In the following example, we explicitly calculate the Tikhonov–Morozov flow equation if $F := i$, the embedding operator from $W_\diamond^{1,2}(\Omega)$ into $L_\diamond^2(\Omega)$ (cf. Example 3.8).

Example 7.1. Let $u^\delta \in V = L_\diamond^2(\Omega)$, and consider $U = W_\diamond^{1,2}(\Omega)$ associated with the norm $|u|_{1,2} = \sqrt{\int_\Omega |\nabla u|^2}$. For the embedding $F := i$ from $W_\diamond^{1,2}(\Omega)$ into $L_\diamond^2(\Omega)$, the iterative Tikhonov–Morozov method is given by

$$u_k = \underset{u \in W_\diamond^{1,2}(\Omega)}{\arg\min} \, \mathcal{T}_{\alpha_k, u^\delta}^{(u_{k-1})}(u), \qquad k \in \mathbb{N},$$

$$\mathcal{T}_{\alpha_k, u^\delta}^{(u_{k-1})}(u) = \frac{1}{2} \left\| u - u^\delta \right\|_2^2 + \frac{\alpha_k}{2} \left| u - u_{k-1} \right|_{1,2}^2.$$

Let $\mathcal{S}(u) = \frac{1}{2} \left\| u - u^\delta \right\|_2^2$. Then $\partial \mathcal{S}(u) = i^*(u - u^\delta)$, and the according flow equation reads as

$$\frac{\partial u}{\partial t}(t) = -\partial \mathcal{S}\big(u(t)\big) = -i^*\big(u(t) - u^\delta\big), \qquad u(0) = u_0.$$

From Theorem 6.17, it follows that this evolution equation has a unique solution for every $u^\delta \in L_\diamond^2(\Omega)$ and $u_0 \in W_\diamond^{1,2}(\Omega)$. Now note that, for sufficiently regular Ω, the adjoint of the embedding $i : W_\diamond^{1,2}(\Omega) \to L_\diamond^2(\Omega)$ can be obtained by inverting the Laplacian respecting Neumann boundary conditions (cf. Example 3.8). Accordingly, the asymptotic Tikhonov–Morozov method consists in solving the differential equation of third order

$$
\begin{aligned}
u(t) - u^\delta &= \Delta \frac{\partial u}{\partial t}(t) & &\text{in } \Omega \times (0, \infty), \\
\frac{\partial u}{\partial \mathbf{n}}(t) &= 0 & &\text{in } \partial\Omega \times (0, \infty), \\
u(0) &= u_0 & &\text{in } \Omega.
\end{aligned}
\tag{7.3}
$$

We now derive energy estimates for the solution $u : (0, \infty) \to W_\diamond^{1,2}(\Omega)$ of (7.3). In order to apply the estimate (6.9), we first clarify some notational differences. In (6.9), the function u^δ is used as initial data for the flow, whereas in the case of Tikhonov–Morozov flow it is a source term. Here, the initial function is denoted by $u_0 \in \overline{\mathcal{D}(\mathcal{S})} = W_\diamond^{1,2}(\Omega)$. We take an arbitrary $v_0 \in W_\diamond^{1,2}(\Omega)$. Then it follows from (6.9) that

$$\left| \frac{\partial u}{\partial t}(t^+) \right|_{1,2} \le \left| i^*(v_0 - u^\delta) \right|_{1,2} + \frac{1}{t} |v_0 - u_0|_{1,2}.$$

The operator $i : W_\diamond^{1,2}(\Omega) \to L_\diamond^2(\Omega)$ is injective, bounded, and linear and therefore $\overline{\mathrm{Ran}(i^*)} = W_\diamond^{1,2}(\Omega)$ (see, e.g., [340, Thm. 4.12]). Consequently, v_0 can be chosen arbitrarily close to u^δ, which shows that

$$\lim_{t\to\infty} \left| i^* \big(u(t) - u^\delta \big) \right|_{1,2} = \lim_{t\to\infty} \left| \frac{\partial u}{\partial t}(t^+) \right|_{1,2} = 0 \,.$$

$\diamondsuit$

We have shown in the previous example that the solution of (7.3) satisfies the *inverse fidelity* property

$$\boxed{\lim_{t\to\infty} u(t) = u^\delta \,, \qquad \lim_{t\to 0^+} u(t) = u_0 \,.}$$

Standard partial differential equations for diffusion filtering like the heat flow (6.15) or total variation flow (compare Table 6.1) satisfy

$$\boxed{\lim_{t\to 0^+} u(t) = u^\delta \,, \quad \lim_{t\to\infty} u(t) = \text{constant} \,.}$$

This is an important property of scale space methods (such as diffusion filtering methods), and as the approximation properties are obtained at the reverse timescale, we call (7.3) *inverse scale space* method.

Let Ω be bocL, $s > 1$, and $\mathcal{W}^{1,s}$ be either one of the spaces $W_\diamond^{1,s}(\Omega)$ or $W_0^{1,s}(\Omega)$, associated with the norm $|u|_{1,s} = \big(\int_\Omega |\nabla u|^s \big)^{1/s}$. Let moreover $\mathcal{J}_{1,s} := \mathcal{J}_{W^{1,s}_\diamond}$ or $\mathcal{J}_{1,s} := \mathcal{J}_{W^{1,s}_0}$ be the corresponding duality mapping (see Example 10.27).

We consider the Tikhonov–Morozov method in two settings:

- $\mathcal{W}^{1,s}$: The Tikhonov–Morozov method consists in choosing $u_0 \in \mathcal{W}^{1,s}$ and iteratively calculating

$$\boxed{u_k := \operatorname*{arg\,min}_{u\in\mathcal{W}^{1,s}} \left(\frac{1}{2} \left\| F(u) - v^\delta \right\|_2^2 + \frac{\alpha_k}{s} |u - u_{k-1}|_{1,s}^s \right), \qquad k \in \mathbb{N} \,.}$$

Using Asplund's Theorem 10.25, it follows that u_k has to satisfy

$$\frac{1}{\alpha_k} F'(u_k)^\# \big(F(u_k) - v^\delta \big) = -\mathcal{J}_{1,s}(u - u_{k-1}) \,.$$

Let (t_k) be a discretization of $(0, \infty)$ satisfying

$$\frac{1}{\alpha_k} = (t_k - t_{k-1})^{s-1} \,. \tag{7.4}$$

Then we find that the function u_k approximates the solution at t_k of

$$\mathcal{J}_{1,s}\left(\frac{\partial u}{\partial t}(t)\right) + F'\big(u(t)\big)^{\#}\big(F\big(u(t)\big) - v^\delta\big) = 0 \qquad \text{in } \Omega \times (0,\infty)\,,$$

$$u(0) = u_0 \quad \text{in } \Omega\,.$$

(7.5)

- $BV(\Omega)$: On the space of functions of bounded variation, the Tikhonov–Morozov method consists in calculating

$$u_k := \underset{u \in BV(\Omega)}{\arg\min}\left(\frac{1}{2}\left\|F(u) - v^\delta\right\|_2^2 + \alpha_k \mathcal{R}_1(u - u_{k-1})\right), \qquad k \in \mathbb{N}\,.$$

For $1 < s$, $s \neq 2$, the existence theory for (7.5) is not covered by standard semi-group theory. In some special cases of operators F, recent results from [12] are applicable and guarantee existence of a solution of the flow equation: Let $\mathcal{S} : \mathcal{W}^{1,s} \to \mathbb{R} \cup \{\infty\}$, defined by $u \mapsto \left\|F(u) - v^\delta\right\|_2^2$, be convex and proper. Moreover, we assume that the subdifferential $\partial \mathcal{S}$ is weak-weak*-closed in the sense that, if (u_k) weakly converges to u in $\mathcal{W}^{1,s}$, $\xi_k \in \partial \mathcal{S}(u_k)$ weakly* converges to ξ, and $\big(\mathcal{S}(u_k)\big)$ is uniformly bounded, it follows that $\xi \in \partial \mathcal{S}(u)$. Then [12, Thm. 2.3.3] guarantees the existence of an absolutely continuous function $u : [0,\infty) \to \mathcal{W}^{1,s}$ that solves (7.5). For instance, [12, Thm. 2.3.3] applies if F is linear, in which case $\mathcal{S}$ is convex. For general F, however, the solution theory is open.

For $s = 1$, the relation (7.4) degenerates in the sense that α_k does not depend on the choice of the sequence (t_k). This indicates that there is **no** asymptotic evolution equation corresponding to the Tikhonov–Morozov method on a space of functions with finite total variation. A scale space related to $s = 1$ can, however, be based on the Bregman distance.

7.2 Iterative Regularization with Bregman Distances

In this section, we consider iterative *Bregman distance regularization*, a variant of the inverse scale space method on the space of functions of bounded variation. We make the general assumptions that $p > 1$, Ω is bocL, and that $u^\delta \in L^p(\Omega)$. Recall that p_* denotes the conjugate of p (see Definition 8.22). As usual, we identify $\big(L^p(\Omega)\big)^*$ with $L^{p_*}(\Omega)$ and regard $\partial \mathcal{R}_1(u)$ as subset of $L^{p_*}(\Omega)$.

For $u^* \in L^{p_*}(\Omega)$ we consider

$$\mathcal{T}_{\alpha,u^\delta}^{(u^*)}(u) := \frac{1}{\alpha p}\left\|u - u^\delta\right\|_p^p - \int_\Omega u^* u + \mathcal{R}_1(u), \qquad u \in L^p(\Omega)\,.$$

Let $u_0 \in BV(\Omega)$ and $u_0^* \in \partial \mathcal{R}_1(u_0)$. *Iterative Bregman distance regularization* is defined by iterative calculation of

$$u_k := \arg\min_{u \in L^p(\Omega)} \mathcal{T}_{\alpha,u^\delta}^{(u_{k-1}^*)}(u) \,,$$

$$u_k^* := u_{k-1}^* + \frac{1}{\alpha} \mathcal{J}_p(u^\delta - u_k) \,,$$
$$k \in \mathbb{N} \,. \tag{7.6}$$

Lemma 7.2. *Iterative Bregman regularization is well-defined, that is, u_k, as defined in (7.6), exists and is unique, and satisfies*

$$u_k = \arg\min_{u \in L^p(\Omega)} \Big(\frac{1}{\alpha p} \big\| u - u^\delta \big\|_p^p + D_{u_{k-1}^*}(u, u_{k-1}) \Big) \,, \tag{7.7}$$

where $D_{u_{k-1}^*}(u, u_{k-1})$ is the Bregman distance of the total variation $\mathcal{R}_1$ at u_{k-1}. Moreover, the function u_k^*, as defined in (7.6), satisfies $u_k^* \in \partial\mathcal{R}_1(u_k)$.

Proof. We apply Theorem 3.22 with $U = V = L^p(\Omega)$, the identity operator $F = \mathrm{Id} : L^p(\Omega) \to L^p(\Omega)$, the weak $L^p(\Omega)$ topology $\tau_U = \tau_V$, and the regularizing semi-norm $\mathcal{R}_1$. For $u_k \in L^p(\Omega)$, the theorem provides existence of a minimizer of $\mathcal{T}_{\alpha,u^\delta}^{(u_{k-1}^*)}$. Because $p > 1$, the functional $u \mapsto \big\| u - u^\delta \big\|_p^p$ is strictly convex. Consequently, $\mathcal{T}_{\alpha,u^\delta}^{(u_{k-1}^*)}$ is strictly convex, and thus the minimizer is unique.

By definition

$$D_{u_{k-1}^*}(u, u_{k-1}) = \mathcal{R}_1(u) - \mathcal{R}_1(u_{k-1}) - \int_\Omega u_{k-1}^*(u - u_{k-1}) \,.$$

Thus $\mathcal{T}_{\alpha,u^\delta}^{(u_{k-1}^*)}(u)$ and the functional defined in (7.7) only differ by a constant independent of the argument u, which proves that minimization of $\mathcal{T}_{\alpha,u^\delta}^{(u_{k-1}^*)}$ yields the result (7.7).

It remains to show that $u_k^* \in \partial\mathcal{R}_1(u_{k-1})$. Denote

$$\mathcal{S}(u) := \frac{1}{\alpha p} \big\| u - u^\delta \big\|_p^p - \int_\Omega u_{k-1}^* u \,. \tag{7.8}$$

Then $\mathcal{T}_{\alpha,u^\delta}^{(u_{k-1}^*)} = \mathcal{S} + \mathcal{R}_1$. From the Kuhn–Tucker condition in Theorems 10.22 and 10.21, it follows that there exists $\tilde{u}^* \in \partial\mathcal{R}_1(u_k)$ with $-\tilde{u}^* \in \partial\mathcal{S}(u_k)$. Again, it follows from Asplund's Theorem 10.25 that

$$\partial\mathcal{S}(u_k) = \frac{1}{\alpha} \mathcal{J}_p(u_k - u^\delta) - u_{k-1}^* = -u_k^* \,.$$

This shows that $u_k^* = \tilde{u}^* \in \partial\mathcal{R}_1(u_k)$. □

For $p = 2$, iterative Bregman distance regularization consists in choosing $u_0 \in L^2(\Omega) \cap BV(\Omega)$ and iteratively calculating

$$u_k := \arg\min \Big(\frac{1}{2} \big\| u - (u^\delta - u_{k-1}) - (u_{k-1} + \alpha u_{k-1}^*) \big\|_2^2 + \alpha\mathcal{R}_1(u) \Big) \,, \quad k \in \mathbb{N} \,.$$

The difference $u^\delta - u_{k-1}$ is referred to as the *texture* part of the k-th iteration. The term $\hat{u}_{k-1} := u_{k-1} + \alpha u^*_{k-1}$ can be interpreted as an enhancing step (compare Sect. 6.6). We write

$$e_{k-1} := \underbrace{u^\delta - u_{k-1}}_{\text{texture}} + \underbrace{u_{k-1} + \alpha u^*_{k-1}}_{\text{enhanced smoothed data}} ,$$

and see that iterative Bregman distance regularization is total variation minimization with data e_{k-1}, which is enhanced data with added texture.

The single steps of iterative Bregman distance regularization are illustrated in Fig. 7.1.

We have demonstrated that regularization with Bregman distance can be considered a particular instance of *enhancing techniques*, which consist in filtering and enhancing the filtered part and back-substitution of the texture.

In (7.6), iterative Bregman distance regularization is written in a form that simultaneously computes the iterates (u_k) and dual functions (u^*_k). In the sequel, we derive the dual functional of $\mathcal{T}^{(u)}_{\alpha,u^\delta}$ and show that the dual functions (u^*_k) can be expressed without knowledge of the primal functions.

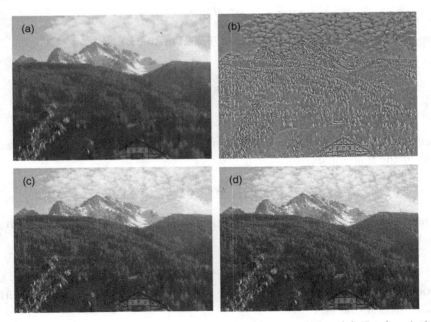

Fig. 7.1. The single steps of Bregman distance regularization. (**a**) Total variation denoising, u_{k-1}; (**b**) texture: $u^\delta - u_{k-1}$; (**c**) enhanced (filtered) data $\hat{u}_{k-1}$; (**d**) enhanced data + texture $e_{k-1} = u^\delta - u_{k-1} + \hat{u}_{k-1}$.

Dual Evolution

For simplicity of notation, we denote the Fenchel transform of $\mathcal{T}_{\alpha,u^\delta}^{(u_{k-1}^*)}$ by $\mathcal{T}_{\alpha,u_{k-1}^*}^*$ instead of $\big(\mathcal{T}_{\alpha,u^\delta}^{(u_{k-1}^*)}\big)^*$. It follows from Theorem 10.10 and Theorem 4.19 that

$$
\begin{aligned}
\mathcal{T}_{\alpha,u_{k-1}^*}^*(u^*) &:= \mathcal{S}^*(-u^*) + \mathcal{R}_1^*(u^*) \\
&= \frac{\alpha^{p_*-1}}{p_*}\left\|u^* - u_{k-1}^*\right\|_{p_*}^{p_*} - \int_\Omega (u^* - u_{k-1}^*)\,u^\delta + \mathcal{R}_1^*(u^*) \\
&= \begin{cases} \dfrac{\alpha^{p_*-1}}{p_*}\left\|u^* - u_{k-1}^*\right\|_{p_*}^{p_*} - \displaystyle\int_\Omega (u^* - u_{k-1}^*)\,u^\delta & \text{if } \|u^*\|_* \le 1, \\[2mm] \infty & \text{else}. \end{cases}
\end{aligned}
\tag{7.9}
$$

Using this dual functional $\mathcal{T}_{\alpha,u_{k-1}^*}^*$, we can reexpress the Bregman iteration (7.6).

Theorem 7.3. *The functions u_k and u_k^* defined in (7.6) satisfy*

$$
\begin{aligned}
u_k^* &= \operatorname*{arg\,min}_{u^* \in L^{p_*}(\Omega)} \mathcal{T}_{\alpha,u_{k-1}^*}^*(u^*), \\
u_k &= u^\delta - \alpha^{p_*} \mathcal{J}_{p_*}(u_k^* - u_{k-1}^*).
\end{aligned}
\tag{7.10}
$$

Proof. This is a direct consequence of Theorem 10.21.   □

In the following we denote by

$$
\overline{\mathcal{B}_{p_*}^*(0)} := \left\{ u^* \in L^{p_*}(\Omega) : \|u^*\|_* \le 1 \right\}
$$

the unit ball with respect to $\|\cdot\|_*$.

Remark 7.4. If $p = 2$, then minimization of $\mathcal{T}_{\alpha,u_{k-1}^*}^*$ is equivalent to minimization of the functional

$$
u^* \mapsto \frac{1}{2}\left\|u^* - \left(u_{k-1}^* + u^\delta/\alpha\right)\right\|_2^2 + \frac{1}{\alpha}\mathcal{R}_1^*(u^*).
$$

Now denote by $P_{\overline{\mathcal{B}_2^*(0)}}(u^*)$ the projection of u^* on $\overline{\mathcal{B}_2^*(0)}$, that is (see [403, 46.4]),

$$
P_{\overline{\mathcal{B}_2^*(0)}}(u^*) := \operatorname*{arg\,min}_{v^* \in \overline{\mathcal{B}_2^*(0)}} \|v^* - u^*\|_2, \qquad u^* \in L^2(\Omega).
$$

From Theorem 4.19, it follows that $u_k^* = P_{\overline{\mathcal{B}_2^*(0)}}(u_{k-1}^* + u^\delta/\alpha)$. Together with (7.10) we see that

$$
u_{k+1} = (u^\delta + \alpha u_k^*) - \alpha P_{\overline{\mathcal{B}_2^*(0)}}\left(u_k^* + u^\delta/\alpha\right).
$$

The dual formulation (7.10) is an equation for u_k^* that is independent of u_k. In contrast, in (7.6) the iterates u_k and u_k^* have to be considered coupled.

Because the Bregman distance is non-negative (Lemma 3.17), it follows from Lemma 7.2 that

$$\frac{1}{\alpha\,p}\left\|u_{k+1} - u^\delta\right\|_p^p \leq \mathcal{T}_{\alpha,u^\delta}^{(u_k^*)}(u_{k+1}) - \mathcal{R}_1(u_k) + \int_\Omega u_k^*\, u_k$$

$$\leq \mathcal{T}_{\alpha,u^\delta}^{(u_k^*)}(u_k) - \mathcal{R}_1(u_k) + \int_\Omega u_k^*\, u_k = \frac{1}{\alpha\,p}\left\|u_k - u^\delta\right\|_p^p . \qquad (7.11)$$

Therefore, the residuals are monotonously decreasing.

We now show the *discrete inverse fidelity property* of the iteration (7.6). There we use the following lemma:

Lemma 7.5. *Assume that (u_k^*) is a bounded sequence in $L^{p_*}(\Omega)$ such that $\|u_k^* - u^*\|_* \to 0$. Then $u_k^* \rightharpoonup u^*$ in $L^{p_*}(\Omega)$.*

Proof. We use the first convergence criterion (see Theorem 8.47), that is, $u_k^* \rightharpoonup u^*$ in $L^{p_*}(\Omega)$ if and only if (u_k^*) is a bounded sequence in $L^{p_*}(\Omega)$ and

$$\int_\Omega (u_k^* - u^*)\, u \to 0, \qquad u \in C_0^\infty(\Omega) .$$

From the definition of $\|\cdot\|_*$ in Definition 4.5, it follows that

$$\|u_k^* - u^*\|_* \geq \sup\left\{\int_\Omega (u_k^* - u^*)\, u : u \in C_0^\infty(\Omega),\ \mathcal{R}_1(u) = 1\right\} .$$

In particular, the assumption $\|u_k^* - u^*\|_* \to 0$ implies that $\int_\Omega (u_k^* - u^*)u \to 0$ for every $u \in C_0^\infty(\Omega)$, or in other words, that (u_k^*) weakly converges to u^*. $\quad\square$

Theorem 7.6 (Discrete inverse fidelity). *The sequence (u_k) defined by (7.6) satisfies*

$$\lim_k \left\|u_k - u^\delta\right\|_p = 0 .$$

Proof. From (7.10) and the definition of $\mathcal{J}_p$, it follows that

$$\left\|u_k - u^\delta\right\|_p^p = \alpha^{pp_*}\left\|\mathcal{J}_{p_*}(u_k^* - u_{k-1}^*)\right\|_p^p = \alpha^{pp_*}\left\|u_k^* - u_{k-1}^*\right\|_{p_*}^{p_*} . \qquad (7.12)$$

From (7.11), it follows that the sequence $\left(\left\|u_k - u^\delta\right\|_p^p\right)$ is monotonously decreasing. Together with (7.12), this shows that

$$\left\|u_k - u^\delta\right\|_p^p \leq \frac{1}{k}\sum_{i=1}^k \left\|u_i - u^\delta\right\|_p^p = \frac{\alpha^{pp_*}}{k}\sum_{i=1}^k \left\|u_i^* - u_{i-1}^*\right\|_{p_*}^{p_*} . \qquad (7.13)$$

Moreover, it follows from (7.9) that

$$\frac{\alpha^{p_*-1}}{p_*} \left\| u_k^* - u_{k-1}^* \right\|_{p_*}^{p_*} - \int_\Omega (u_k^* - u_{k-1}^*)\, u^\delta = T_{\alpha, u_{k-1}^*}^* (u_k^*) \leq T_{\alpha, u_{k-1}^*}^* (u_{k-1}^*) = 0 \,.$$
(7.14)

Combining (7.13) and (7.14), and using the fact that $pp_* = p + p_*$, it follows that

$$\left\| u_k - u^\delta \right\|_p^p \leq \frac{p_* \alpha^{p+1}}{k} \sum_{i=1}^k \int_\Omega (u_k^* - u_{k-1}^*) u^\delta = p_* \alpha^{p+1} \int_\Omega \frac{u_k^* - u_0^*}{k}\, u^\delta \,. \quad (7.15)$$

Because $\|u_k^*\|_* \leq 1$ for all k and thus $\|u_k^*/k\|_* \to 0$, it follows from Lemma 7.5 that u_k^*/k weakly converges to 0, which in turn implies that

$$\int_\Omega \frac{u_k^* - u_0^*}{k}\, u^\delta \leq \int_\Omega \frac{u_k^*}{k}\, u^\delta + \frac{1}{k} \left\| u_0^* \right\|_{p_*} \left\| u^\delta \right\|_p \to 0 \,.$$

Thus the assertion follows from (7.15). □

Continuous Inverse Scale Space Flow

In the following, we derive the gradient flow equation associated with the iteration (7.6). We make the general assumptions that $p > 1$, Ω is bocL, and that $u^\delta \in L^p(\Omega)$. A detailed analysis of the continuous inverse scale space flow is omitted but can be found in [61].

For a given partition $\tau = (\tau_1, \tau_2, \ldots)$ and initial values $u_0 \in BV(\Omega) \cap L^p(\Omega)$ and $u_0^* \in \partial \mathcal{R}_1(u_0)$, we define

$$U_\tau^0 = u_0, \qquad\qquad\qquad U_\tau^{*,0} = u_0^*,$$
$$U_\tau^k = \arg\min_{u \in L^p(\Omega)} T_{1/\tau_k, u^\delta}^{(U_\tau^{*,k-1})}(u), \quad U_\tau^{*,k} = \arg\min_{u^* \in L^{p_*}(\Omega)} T_{1/\tau_k, U_\tau^{*,k-1}}^*(u^*) \,. \tag{7.16}$$

The sequences (U_τ^k) and $(U_\tau^{*,k})$ are extended to piecewise constant functions $\overline{U}_\tau : [0, \infty) \to L^p(\Omega)$ and $\overline{U}_\tau^* : [0, \infty) \to L^{p_*}(\Omega)$ as follows:

$$\overline{U}_\tau(t) = U_\tau^k, \quad \overline{U}_\tau^*(t) = U_\tau^{*,k}, \qquad t \in \left(t_{k-1}^\tau, t_k^\tau \right] \,.$$

It has been shown in [61] by applying the results of [12] that for $k \to \infty$, a limiting function exists, satisfies smoothness properties, and can be considered a solution of (7.16).

Theorem 7.7. *Assume that (τ_l) is a sequence of partitions of $[0, \infty)$ such that $\lim_l |\tau_l|_\infty = 0$. Then there exists $u^* \in C\big((0, \infty); \mathcal{B}_{p_*}^*(0) \big)$, which is uniformly continuous, differentiable almost everywhere in $[0, \infty)$, such that*

$$\overline{U}_{\tau_l}^*(t) \to u^*(t) \text{ in } L^{p_*}(\Omega), \qquad t \in [0, \infty) \,.$$

Moreover, the function u^* satisfies the growth property

$$\left\|u^*(t)\right\|_{p_*}^{p_*} \le \left\|u_0^*\right\|_{p_*}^{p_*} + t \left\|u_0 - u^\delta\right\|_p^p, \qquad t \ge 0,$$

and

$$\mathcal{J}_{p_*}\left(\frac{\partial u^*}{\partial t}(t)\right) \in -\partial^0 \phi\big(u^*(t)\big) \qquad \text{a.e. in } [0, \infty),$$

$$u^*(0) = u_0^*,$$

(7.17)

where

$$\phi(u^*) := \chi_{\overline{B_{p_*}^*(0)}}(u^*) - \int_\Omega u^\delta u^*,$$

and $\partial^0 \phi$ denotes the minimal section of $\partial\phi$ (see (6.6)). In particular, for $p = 2$, it follows that $\overline{U}_{\tau_l}^* \to u^*$ with respect to the L^2 norm for every $t \in [0, \infty)$ and uniformly on $[0, T]$ for every $T > 0$.

The above result shows that the solution u^* of the flow equation (7.17) is approximated by iterative minimization $u_{k+1}^* = \arg\min \mathcal{T}_{\alpha, u_k^*}^*(u)$ and piecewise constant extension.

Theorem 7.7 shows the existence of a solution of the dual flow. The existence of a solution of the flow for the primal variable is guaranteed by the following proposition where in addition several other results from [61] are summarized.

Proposition 7.8 (Properties of the Bregman distance flow).

1. There exists a solution (u, u^*) of

$$\boxed{\begin{aligned} \frac{\partial u^*}{\partial t}(t) &= \mathcal{J}_p\big(u^\delta - u(t)\big), & u^*(t) &\in \partial\mathcal{R}_1\big(u(t)\big), \\ u^*(0) &= u_0^*, & u(0) &= u_0, \end{aligned}}$$

(7.18)

which satisfies

$$u^* \in C\big([0, \infty); L^{p_*}(\Omega)\big), \qquad u \in L^\infty\big([0, \infty); L^p(\Omega)\big).$$

Moreover, $u(t) \in BV(\Omega)$ for all $t \in [0, \infty)$.

2. For $p = 2$, the solution (u, u^*) of (7.18) is unique.

3. Let (τ_l) be a sequence of partitions of $[0, \infty)$ such that $|\tau_l|_\infty \to 0$. Then

$$\lim_l \left\|\overline{U}_{\tau_l}(t) - u(t)\right\|_p = 0 \qquad \text{a.e. in } [0, \infty).$$

4. The function u satisfies the inverse fidelity property

$$\lim_{t \to \infty} \left\|u(t) - u^\delta\right\|_p = 0.$$

If, in addition, $u^\delta \in BV(\Omega)$, then

$$\left\|u(t) - u^\delta\right\|_p^p \le \mathcal{R}_1(u^\delta)/t, \qquad \text{a.e. in } [0, \infty).$$

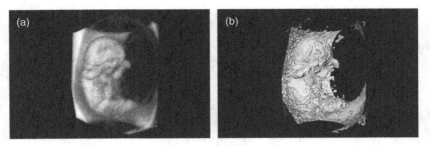

Fig. 7.2. (a) Volumetric view and (b) level set of original data.

Note that so far for the general case $p \neq 2$, no uniqueness result has been given.

The following example shows an application of Bregman flows for surface smoothing. For the evolution of the ultrasound image, it can be observed that the level set surfaces are smoothed and pick up more and more edges over time. The example shows 3D ultrasound data of a fetus with a resolution of $93 \times 186 \times 158$. A volumetric view as well as the view of one level set are displayed in Fig. 7.2. Figure 7.3 shows numerical approximations of $u(t)$, $t = 2, 4, \ldots, 12$.

Remark 7.9. We have presented two inverse scale space methods for solving $F(u) = v^\delta$, the Tikhonov–Morozov flow, and the Bregman distance flow. Exemplarily, let $s > 1$ and $\mathcal{W}^{1,s}$ be either $W_0^{1,s}(\Omega)$ with $\Omega = \mathbb{R}^n$ or $W_\diamond^{1,s}(\Omega)$ with Ω bocL, both associated with the norm $|\cdot|_{1,s}$. We consider a Gâteaux differentiable operator $F : \mathcal{W}^{1,s} \to L^2(\Omega)$.

- The Tikhonov–Morozov flow, as stated in (7.5), is

$$F'\big(u(t)\big)^{\#}\big(F\big(u(t)\big) - v^\delta\big) + \mathcal{J}_{1,s}\left(\frac{\partial u}{\partial t}(t)\right) = 0 \qquad \text{in } \Omega \times (0, \infty),$$

$$u(0) = u_0 \quad \text{in } \Omega.$$

- The L^2-*Bregman distance flow* on $\mathcal{W}^{1,s}$ is derived from iterative minimization of the functional

$$\mathcal{T}_{\alpha, u_k^*}(u) := \frac{1}{2\alpha}\left\|F(u) - v^\delta\right\|_2^2 + \frac{1}{s}\int_\Omega |\nabla u|^s - \int_\Omega u_k^* u,$$

where (note that for $s > 1$ the subdifferential is single valued)

$$u_k^* = \partial\left(\frac{1}{s}\int_\Omega |\nabla u|^s\right)(u_k) = \mathcal{J}_{1,s}(u_k).$$

The associated flow equation is

$$F'\big(u(t)\big)^{\#}\big(F\big(u(t)\big) - v^\delta\big) + \frac{\partial \mathcal{J}_{1,s}\big(u(t)\big)}{\partial t} = 0 \qquad \text{in } \Omega \times (0, \infty),$$

$$u(0) = u_0 \quad \text{in } \Omega.$$

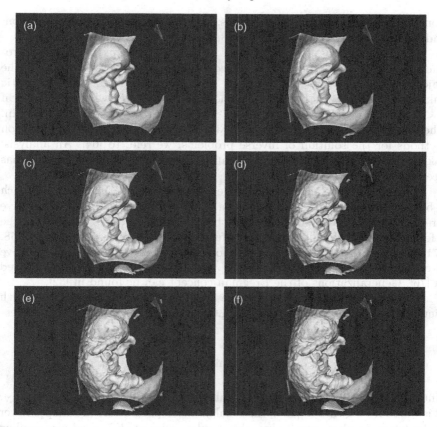

Fig. 7.3. Denoised surfaces: Numerical approximations at time (**a**) $t = 2$, (**b**) $t = 4$, (**c**) $t = 6$, (**d**) $t = 8$, (**e**) $t = 10$, (**f**) $t = 12$.

Therefore, the difference between Tikhonov–Morozov flows and Bregman distance flows is that the duality operator and time differentiation are interchanged. In general, interchanging the order of time differentiation and duality mapping gives different equations.

$\diamondsuit$

7.3 Recent Topics on Evolutionary Equations for Inverse Problems

Evolutionary equations for image analysis play a significant role in modern image processing. In the following, we give a few references to evolutionary equations used for image analysis and for the solution of inverse problems.

A standard reference for image analysis is [385]. There, references on this field up to 1998 can be found. Evolutionary morphological differential equations for image processing applications, such as the mean curvature motion, and axiomatics have been studied in [8, 9, 194].

Level set methods for the solution of inverse problems have been introduced in [341]. This approach is based on a gradient descent flow for the object to be recovered. The resulting flow is analogous to the asymptotic Tikhonov–Morozov method (7.2) in the case $F = G \circ P$, where $P(\phi) = 0$ if $\phi < 0$ and 1 else. The set where $P(\phi) \geq 1$ characterizes the evolving domain. The idea of this approach goes back to [311]. For the topic of level set evolution methods for the solution of inverse problems, we refer to [64]. An analysis, taking into account that the classification operator P is discontinuous, has been developed in [175].

Inverse scale space methods have been introduced in [192]. This approach is based on the Tikhonov–Morozov idea, while asymptotical limits of iterative Bregman distance regularization have been proposed in [62]. Aside from the references stated already in the text, further relevant references are [65, 258, 271, 356, 393]. In the discrete setting, one of the first references on iterative Bregman distance regularization is [75]. Related methods have been surveyed in [76]. Generalizations of the Bregman concept can be found in [32].

In [366], it is suggested to use the ROF functional in combination with hierarchical decompositions (cf. Sect. 4.6) by considering the iterative process

$$
v_0 := u^\delta \,, \qquad u_0 = 0 \,,
$$
$$
v_k := v_{k-1} - u_k \,, \quad u_k = \arg\min \mathcal{T}^{2,1}_{2^{k-1}\alpha, v_{k-1}}(u) \,, \quad k \in \mathbb{N} \,.
$$

Thus the method provides a hierarchical decomposition of $u^\delta = \sum_{k=1}^N u_k + v_N$. It is worth noting that in [366], the regularization parameters are adapted over scale. Recently, these results have been extended (see [367]) and also applied to multiplicative noise models.

Mathematical Foundations

Mathematical notations

8

Functional Analysis

In the following, we give an overview on results of topology and functional analysis frequently used in this book. We assume that the reader is familiar with the basic notions of linear algebra and calculus.

8.1 General Topology

We recall some basic results of topology collected from [149, 234].

Definition 8.1. *Let X be a set. A* topology *τ on X is a collection of subsets of X, called* open sets, *such that:*

1. *The empty set and the whole space are open, that is, $\emptyset \in \tau$ and $X \in \tau$.*
2. *If U_1, $U_2 \in \tau$, then $U_1 \cap U_2 \in \tau$, that is, the intersection of two open sets is open.*
3. *If $\{U_i\}_{i \in I}$ is a family of sets $U_i \in \tau$, then $\bigcup_i U_i \in \tau$, that is, the union of arbitrarily many open sets is open.*

A set X together with a topology is called topological space.

A set $K \subset X$ is called *closed*, if its complement is open, that is, $X \setminus K \in \tau$. It is easy to see that the union of two closed sets and the intersection of arbitrarily many closed sets are closed.

Let (X, τ) be a topological space, let $x \in X$ and $A \subset X$. The set A is called a *neighborhood* of x, if there exists an open set $U \subset X$ such that $x \in U \subset A$. In particular, an open set U is a neighborhood of x if and only if $x \in U$.

Let (X, τ) be a topological space, and $A \subset X$. The *interior* $\mathring{A}$ of A is the largest open set contained in A. The *closure* $\bar{A}$ of A is the smallest closed set containing A. We have

$$\mathring{A} = \bigcup_{U \subset A \text{ open}} U, \qquad \bar{A} = \bigcap_{K \supset A \text{ closed}} K.$$

O. Scherzer et al., *Variational Methods in Imaging*,
© Springer Science+Business Media, LLC 2009

The *boundary* ∂A of A is defined as $\bar{A} \setminus \overset{\circ}{A}$.

Let $A \subset K \subset X$. Then A is called *dense* in K, if for every open set U satisfying $K \cap U \neq \emptyset$ also the intersection $A \cap U$ is non-empty. In particular, A is dense in its closure $\bar{A}$. A topological space X is called *separable* if there exists a countable set that is dense in X.

A *metric* on a set X is a function $d : X \times X \to \mathbb{R}_{\geq 0}$ satisfying

- $d(x,y) = 0$, if and only if $x = y$,
- $d(x,y) = d(y,x)$ for all $x,\, y \in X$,
- $d(x,z) \leq d(x,y) + d(y,z)$ for all $x,\, y,\, z \in X$.

The set X together with a metric is called *metric space*.

A metric induces a topology on X in the following manner: A set $U \subset X$ is open, if and only if for every $x \in U$ there exists $\varepsilon > 0$ such that $\{y \in X : d(x,y) < \varepsilon\} \subset U$. Unless noted otherwise, we always consider a metric space as a topological space equipped with the topology induced by the metric.

A topological space (X, τ) is called *metrizable*, if there exists a metric that induces the topology on X. In general, this metric is not unique.

In a metric space X, we can define the *distance* of a point $x \in X$ to a set $A \subset X$ by

$$\operatorname{dist}(x, A) := \inf\{d(x,y) : y \in A\}.$$

Moreover, we define the *diameter* of $A \subset X$ by

$$\operatorname{diam}(A) := \sup\{d(x,y) : x,y \in A\}.$$

A *sequence* in a set X is a mapping $\phi : \mathbb{N} \to X$, where $\mathbb{N}$ denotes the set of natural numbers. In this book, we will always write $x_k := \phi(k)$ for the elements in the sequence and denote the sequence as a whole by (x_k).

A sequence (x_k) in a topological space X converges to an element $x \in X$, denoted $x_k \to x$ or $x = \lim_k x_k$, if for every open set U containing x there exists an index k_0 such that $x_k \in U$ for all $k \geq k_0$. In the case X is a metric space, the sequence converges to x, if and only if the sequence of real numbers $d(x_k, x)$ converges to zero.

A *subsequence* of a sequence (x_k) is itself a sequence $(x_{k'})$ such that there exists a strictly increasing mapping $N : \mathbb{N} \to \mathbb{N}$ with $x_{k'} = x_{N(k)}$. We have the following quite useful lemma that characterizes the convergence of a sequence in a topological space by the convergence of subsequences.

Lemma 8.2. *Let (x_k) be a sequence in a topological space X. Then (x_k) converges to $x \in X$ if and only if every subsequence $(x_{k'})$ of (x_k) itself has a subsequence $(x_{k''})$ converging to x.*

Proof. First note that the convergence of (x_k) implies the convergence of every subsequence; thus one implication is trivial.

Now assume that (x_k) does not converge to x. From the definition of convergence, it follows that there exist an open set U containing x and a subsequence $(x_{k'})$ of (x_k) such that $x_{k'} \notin U$ for all k'. Now, if $(x_{k''})$ is any subsequence of $(x_{k'})$, then also $x_{k''} \notin U$ for all k'', which shows that $(x_{k''})$ cannot converge to x. This shows the assertion. $\square$

An element $x \in X$ is called *cluster point* of the sequence (x_k), if for every open set U containing x and $k_0 \in \mathbb{N}$ there exists $k \geq k_0$ such that $x_k \in U$. If (x_k) has a subsequence $(x_{k'})$ converging to x, then x is a cluster point of (x_k). The converse holds, if for instance X is a metrizable space.

A set $K \subset X$ is called *sequentially closed*, if K coincides with the set of all cluster points of sequences in K. Every closed set is sequentially closed. If X is a metrizable space, then sequential closedness and closedness are equivalent.

A set $K \subset X$ is *compact*, if every family $\{U_j : j \in J\}$ of open sets U_j satisfying $K \subset \bigcup_j U_j$ has a finite subfamily $U_1, \ldots, U_k$, such that $K \subset \bigcup_{j=1}^k U_j$. A set K is *pre-compact*, if its closure $\bar{K}$ is compact.

A set $K \subset X$ is called *sequentially compact*, if every sequence $(x_k) \subset K$ has a subsequence $(x_{k'})$ converging to some $x \in K$. It is called *sequentially pre-compact*, if every sequence $(x_k) \subset K$ has a subsequence $(x_{k'})$ converging to some $x \in X$ – but the limit need not be in K.

Let $A \subset E \subset X$. We say that A is *compactly contained* in E, in short $A \subset\subset E$, if the closure of A is compact and contained in E.

Lemma 8.3. *Let X be a metrizable space and $K \subset X$. Then K is compact, if and only if K is sequentially compact.*

Proof. See [234, Thm. 5.5]. $\square$

Note, however, that for general topological spaces, neither implication needs to hold (cf. [361, Ex. 43]).

Let X and Y be topological spaces. A mapping $\mathcal{F} : X \to Y$ is called *continuous*, if for every open set $U \subset Y$ its pre-image $\mathcal{F}^{-1}(U) \subset X$ is open. It is called *sequentially continuous*, if for every sequence (x_k) in X converging to $x \in X$, the sequence $(\mathcal{F}(x_k))$ converges to $\mathcal{F}(x) \in Y$.

Every continuous mapping is sequentially continuous. If X and Y are metrizable spaces, then the converse also holds, that is, continuity is equivalent to sequential continuity.

Let X and Y be topological spaces, and $\mathcal{F} : X \to Y$. The mapping $\mathcal{F}$ is an *isomorphism* if it is continuous, bijective, and its inverse $\mathcal{F}^{-1} : Y \to X$ is continuous. The spaces X and Y are called *isomorph*, if there exists an isomorphism $\mathcal{F} : X \to Y$.

Let τ_1 and τ_2 be two topologies on X. We say that τ_1 is *weaker* than τ_2, if τ_1 is contained in τ_2. In other words, every open set with respect to τ_1 is open with respect to τ_2. The topology τ_1 is weaker than τ_2, if and only if the *identity mapping* $\mathrm{Id} : (X, \tau_2) \to (X, \tau_1)$, $x \mapsto x$, is continuous.

A sequence (x_k) in a metric space is called *Cauchy sequence*, if for every $\varepsilon > 0$ there exists $k_0 \in \mathbb{N}$ such that $d(x_k, x_l) < \varepsilon$ for all $k, l \geq k_0$. A metric space X is *complete*, if every Cauchy sequence (x_k) in X converges to some element $x \in X$.

Definition 8.4. *Let X be a topological space and $Y = \mathbb{R}$ or $Y = \mathbb{R} \cup \{\infty\}$. We define the* level sets *of $\mathcal{F} : X \to Y$ by*

$$\mathrm{level}_t(\mathcal{F}) := \{x \in X : \mathcal{F}(x) \leq t\}, \qquad t \in Y,$$

and the according level lines *by $\partial \,\mathrm{level}_t(\mathcal{F})$.*

The functional $\mathcal{F}$ is lower semi-continuous, *if the level sets $\mathrm{level}_t(\mathcal{F})$ are closed for every $t \in Y$.*

The functional $\mathcal{F}$ is sequentially lower semi-continuous, *if $\liminf_k \mathcal{F}(x_k) \geq \mathcal{F}(x)$ whenever $(x_k) \to x$.*

Note that lower semi-continuity implies sequential lower semi-continuity.

Definition 8.5. *Let X and Y be topological spaces. An operator $F : G \subset X \to Y$ is* closed, *if its graph*

$$\mathcal{G}(F) := \big\{(x, F(x)) : x \in G\big\} \subset X \times Y$$

is closed in $X \times Y$. It is sequentially closed, *if $\mathcal{G}(F)$ is sequentially closed in $X \times Y$.*

An operator $F : G \subset X \to Y$ is sequentially closed, if and only if for every sequence (x_k) converging to $x \in X$ such that $\big(F(x_k)\big)$ converges to $y \in Y$, we have that $x \in G$ and $F(x) = y$.

8.2 Locally Convex Spaces

Assume that X is a *linear space* (also called *vector space*) over the real numbers $\mathbb{R}$.

Definition 8.6. *A* semi-norm *on X is a function $p : X \to \mathbb{R}_{\geq 0}$ such that*

- *the triangle inequality $p(x + y) \leq p(x) + p(y)$ holds for all $x, y \in X$, and*
- *p is positively homogeneous, that is, $p(\lambda x) = |\lambda| \, p(x)$ for all $x \in X$ and $\lambda \in \mathbb{R}$.*

If p additionally satisfies

- *$p(x) = 0$, if and only if $x = 0$,*

then p is called a norm *on X. In this case, the norm of $x \in X$ is denoted by $\|x\|_X := p(x)$. If the particular norm can be identified from the context, we simply write $\|x\|$ instead. A linear space X together with a norm $\|\cdot\|_X$ is called a* normed linear space.

A subspace *of a linear space is an arbitrary, not necessarily closed, algebraic subspace.*

Let $(p_j)_{j \in J}$, be a *(not necessarily countable) family of semi-norms on X. The family of semi-norms is called* separating *if*

$$x = 0, \quad \text{if and only if} \quad p_j(x) = 0 \text{ for all } j \in J.$$

A linear space X together with a separating family of semi-norms is called a locally convex space.

In particular, a normed linear space is a locally convex space where the family of semi-norms consists of a single element.

On a locally convex space equipped with the family of semi-norms $(p_j)_{j \in J}$, the following (strong) topology is considered: $U \subset X$ is open, if for every $x \in U$ there exist $\varepsilon > 0$ and a finite non-empty set $J' \subset J$ of indices such that

$$\bigcap_{j \in J'} \{y \in X : p_j(y - x) < \varepsilon\} \subset U.$$

A sequence (x_k) converges to $x \in X$, if and only if $p_j(x_k - x) \to 0$ for all $j \in J$.

Let X be a locally convex space and $B \subset X$. The set B is *bounded*, if for every open neighborhood U of 0 there exists $\alpha_U > 0$ such that $\alpha_U B \subset U$.

In a normed linear space X, the set

$$B_r(x) := \{y \in X : \|y - x\| < r\}$$

is called the (open) *ball* of radius r centered at x. A set $B \subset X$ is bounded, if and only if there exists $r > 0$ such that B is contained in the ball $B_r(0)$.

Example 8.7. Let $1 \leq p < \infty$ and $n \in \mathbb{N}$. The *p-norm* of a vector $\mathbf{v} = (v_1, \ldots, v_n) \in \mathbb{R}^n$ is defined as

$$|\mathbf{v}|_p := \left(\sum_k |v_k|^p \right)^{1/p}.$$

The norm $|\cdot|_2$ is called *Euclidean norm*. If no confusion is possible, we omit the subscript and simple write $|\mathbf{v}|$ instead of $|\mathbf{v}|_2$.

Moreover, we define the *maximum norm*

$$|\mathbf{v}|_\infty := \sup_k |v_k|.$$

$\diamondsuit$

Remark 8.8. A normed linear space is a metric space with metric $d(x, y) := \|x - y\|_X$. In particular, a set $U \subset X$ is open, if for every $x \in U$ there exists $\varepsilon > 0$ such that $B_\varepsilon(x) \subset U$. Moreover, a sequence (x_k) converges to x with respect to the topology of the normed space X if and only if the sequence of real numbers $(\|x_k - x\|_X)$ converges to zero. A complete, normed linear space is called a *Banach space*.

Let X be a linear space, and let $\|\cdot\|_1$ and $\|\cdot\|_2$ be two norms on X. The norms are called *equivalent*, if there exist $c_2 \geq c_1 > 0$ such that

$$c_1 \|x\|_1 \leq \|x\|_2 \leq c_2 \|x\|_1, \qquad x \in X .$$

In this (and only this) case, they induce the same topology on X.

Lemma 8.9. *Let X be a normed linear space. There exists a Banach space $\bar{X}$, called the* completion *of X, satisfying $X \subset \bar{X}$, $\|x\|_X = \|x\|_{\bar{X}}$ for every $x \in X$, and X is dense in $\bar{X}$ with respect to the topology induced by $\|\cdot\|_{\bar{X}}$. The space $\bar{X}$ is unique up to isomorphisms.*

Proof. See [401, Sect. I.10, Thm.].   □

Definition 8.10. *An* inner product *(also called* scalar product*) on a linear space X is a function $\langle \cdot, \cdot \rangle_X : X \times X \to \mathbb{R}$ such that for all x, y, $z \in X$ and $\lambda \in \mathbb{R}$, the following conditions are satisfied:*

- $\langle x, y \rangle_X = \langle y, x \rangle_X$ *(symmetry)*,
- $\langle x, y + \lambda z \rangle_X = \langle x, y \rangle_X + \lambda \langle x, z \rangle_X$ *(linearity in the second argument)*,
- $\langle x, x \rangle_X \geq 0$ *for all $x \in X$, and $\langle x, x \rangle_X = 0$ if and only if $x = 0$ (positive definiteness)*.

In the case that the particular inner product can be identified from the context, we simply write $\langle x, y \rangle$ instead of $\langle x, y \rangle_X$.

Two elements x, $y \in X$ are called orthogonal *(to each other), if $\langle x, y \rangle = 0$. The inner product defines a norm on X by*

$$\|x\|_X := \langle x, x \rangle_X^{1/2} .$$

A linear space X together with an inner product is called a pre-Hilbert space. *If X is complete (that is, X is a Banach space), it is called a* Hilbert space.

Remark 8.11. In the case $X = \mathbb{R}^n$, $n \in \mathbb{N}$, the (standard) scalar product is defined by

$$\mathbf{x} \cdot \mathbf{y} := \langle \mathbf{x}, \mathbf{y} \rangle := \sum_k x_k y_k , \qquad \mathbf{x}, \mathbf{y} \in \mathbb{R}^n .$$

◇

Lemma 8.12. *Let X be a Banach space and $G \subset X$ a closed linear subspace. Then G, endowed with the restriction of the norm on X to G, is a Banach space. If X is a Hilbert space and $G \subset X$ a closed linear subspace, then G associated with the restriction of the inner product on X to $G \times G$ is a Hilbert space.*

Proof. It is clear that G is a normed linear space (pre-Hilbert space). Thus, it remains to show that G is complete. From standard results of topology (see [149, Thm. 4.3.6]), it follows that a subset of a complete space is complete, if it is closed. Because G is closed by assumption, the assertion follows.   □

8.3 Bounded Linear Operators and Functionals

Assume that X and Y are linear spaces. An *operator* $L : X \to Y$ is *linear*, if

$$L(x + y) = Lx + Ly, \quad L(\lambda x) = \lambda Lx, \quad x, y \in X, \lambda \in \mathbb{R}.$$

If $Y = \mathbb{R}$, then we refer to L as *linear functional*. The *kernel* of a linear operator $L : X \to Y$ is defined as

$$\ker(L) = \{ x \in X : Lx = 0 \}.$$

The *range* is defined as

$$\text{Ran}(L) = \{ y \in Y : \text{ there exists } x \in X \text{ with } Lx = y \}.$$

Lemma 8.13. *Assume that X and Y are locally convex spaces, $G \subset X$ is a linear subspace, and $L : G \to Y$ is a linear operator. The operator L is continuous, if and only if L is bounded, that is, for every semi-norm q on Y, there exist a semi-norm p on X and $C \geq 0$ such that*

$$q(Lx) \leq Cp(x), \quad x \in G.$$

If X and Y are normed linear spaces, the operator is continuous, if and only if there exists $C \geq 0$ such that

$$\|Lx\|_Y \leq C \|x\|_X, \quad x \in G.$$

A *bounded linear mapping* $i : X \to Y$ is called an embedding, *if i is injective.*

Proof. See [401, Sect. I.6, Thm. 1]. $\qquad\qquad\qquad\qquad\qquad\qquad\qquad\qquad$ $\square$

By $L(X, Y)$, we denote the space of bounded linear operators from X to Y. The space $L(X, Y)$ is a linear space with pointwise addition and scalar multiplication,

$$(L + \lambda \hat{L})(x) = Lx + \lambda \hat{L}x, \quad L, \hat{L} \in L(X, Y), \ x \in X, \ \lambda \in \mathbb{R}.$$

If X and Y are normed linear spaces, a norm on $L(X, Y)$ is defined by

$$\|L\|_{L(X,Y)} := \sup\{ \|Lx\|_Y : \|x\|_X \leq 1 \} = \sup \left\{ \frac{\|Lx\|_Y}{\|x\|_X} : x \neq 0 \right\}.$$

If Y is a Banach space, then so is $L(X, Y)$, independent of the completeness of the normed linear space X.

Definition 8.14. *Let X and Y be Banach spaces, and let $S_X := \{ x \in X : \|x\| = 1 \}$ denote the unit sphere in X. An operator $L \in L(X, Y)$ is compact, if the closure $\overline{L(S_X)}$ of the image of S_X under L is compact in Y.*

Another useful characterization of compact operators is as follows: A bounded linear operator L between Banach spaces X and Y is compact, if and only if every bounded sequence (u_k) in X has a subsequence $(u_{k'})$ such that $(Lu_{k'})$ converges in Y (compare with Lemma 8.3).

Definition 8.15. *Assume that X is a locally convex space. The* dual $X^* := L(X, \mathbb{R})$ *is the space of all bounded linear functionals $L : X \to \mathbb{R}$. If $L \in X^*$, we often write its evaluation at $x \in X$ as*

$$\langle L, x \rangle := \langle L, x \rangle_{X^*, X} := Lx .$$

Definition 8.16. *Let X be a locally convex space. The topology induced by the family of semi-norms*

$$p_B(L) := \sup\{|\langle L, x \rangle_{X^*, X}| : x \in B\}, \qquad B \subset X \text{ is bounded, } L \in X^*,$$

is called strong topology *on X^*.*

Lemma 8.17. *Let X be a normed linear space. The strong topology on X^* is induced by the norm*

$$\|L\|_{X^*} = \sup\left\{|\langle L, x \rangle_{X^*, X}| : \|x\|_X \leq 1\right\} .$$

Moreover, X^* with the norm $\|\cdot\|_{X^*}$ is a Banach space.

Proof. See [401, Sect. IV.7, Thm. 1].   □

If X is a locally convex space, then X^* is again locally convex when endowed with the family of semi-norms given in Definition 8.16. Therefore its dual $X^{**} := (X^*)^*$, the *bi-dual* of X, can be defined. Moreover, the relation

$$\langle i(x), L \rangle_{X^{**}, X^*} := \langle L, x \rangle_{X^*, X} , \qquad L \in X^*, x \in X , \tag{8.1}$$

defines an embedding $i : X \to X^{**}$ (see [401, Sect. IV.8, Cor.]).

If X is a normed linear space, then the operator $i : X \to X^{**}$ is a linear *isometry* (see [401, Sect. IV.8, Thm. 2]), that is, $\|i(x)\|_{X^{**}} = \|x\|_X$ for every $x \in X$. If in addition i is an isomorphism, then X is called *reflexive*. In this case, X^{**} can be identified with X via the isomorphism i.

Proposition 8.18. *Let X and Y be locally convex spaces, and $L \in L(X, Y)$. There exists a unique bounded linear operator $L^\# \in L(Y^*, X^*)$ such that*

$$\langle L^\# y^*, x \rangle_{X^*, X} = \langle y^*, Lx \rangle_{Y^*, Y} , \qquad y^* \in Y^*, \ x \in X .$$

The operator $L^\#$ is called the dual-adjoint *of L.*
If X and Y are normed linear spaces, then

$$\|L\|_{L(X,Y)} = \|L^\#\|_{L(Y^*, X^*)} .$$

Proof. See [401, Sect. VII.1, Thm. 2, Thm. 2']. $\qquad\square$

Remark 8.19. Let U be a linear subspace of a locally convex space X. Then the embedding $i : U \to X$, $i(x) = x$, is a bounded linear operator. Consequently, its dual adjoint $i^\# : X^* \to U^*$ is well-defined. Now let $x^* \in X^*$. Then $i^\#$ is defined by

$$\langle i^\# x^*, u \rangle_{U^*,U} = \langle x^*, i(u) \rangle_{X^*,X} = \langle x^*, u \rangle_{X^*,X} , \qquad u \in U .$$

Therefore $i^\# x^* = x^*|_U$ equals the restriction of x^* to U. $\qquad\diamond$

Theorem 8.20 (Hahn–Banach). *Assume that X is a locally convex space and $G \subset X$ is a linear subspace. For every bounded linear functional $L : G \to \mathbb{R}$ there exists an extension $\hat{L} \in X^*$, that is, a bounded linear functional $\hat{L} : X \to \mathbb{R}$ satisfying $\hat{L}x = Lx$ for all $x \in G$.*

If X is a normed linear space, then $\hat{L}$ can be chosen in such a way that

$$\|\hat{L}\|_{X^*} = \sup \{|Lx| : x \in G, \|x\|_X \le 1\} = \|L\|_{G^*} .$$

Proof. For the proof of the first part, we refer to [340, Thm. 3.6]; the second part follows from [340, Thm. 3.3] by choosing $p(x) = \|L\|_{G^*}$ there. $\qquad\square$

Lemma 8.21. *Let X, Y be normed linear spaces, let $L \in L(X,Y)$ and $x^* \in X^*$. Then $x^* \in \mathrm{Ran}(L^\#)$ if and only if there exists $C > 0$ such that*

$$\left|\langle x^*, x \rangle_{X^*,X}\right| \le C \|Lx\|_Y , \qquad x \in X . \tag{8.2}$$

Proof. Assume first that $x^* \in X^*$ satisfies (8.2). Then $\langle x^*, x \rangle_{X^*,X} = 0$ whenever $x \in \ker(L)$. Thus x^* defines a bounded linear functional ξ^* on $\mathrm{Ran}(L) \subset Y$ by

$$\langle \xi^*, Lx \rangle_{Y^*,Y} := \langle x^*, x \rangle_{X^*,X} , \qquad x \in X .$$

From the Hahn–Banach Theorem 8.20, it follows that ξ^* can be extended to a bounded linear functional $\tilde{\xi}^*$ on Y. The definition of the dual-adjoint in Proposition 8.18 shows that $x^* = L^\# \tilde{\xi}^*$, which proves that $x^* \in \mathrm{Ran}(L^\#)$.

Now let $x^* \in \mathrm{Ran}(L^\#)$. Then there exists $y^* \in Y^*$ with $x^* = L^\# y^*$. Consequently, for all $x \in X$ we have

$$\left|\langle x^*, x \rangle_{X^*,X}\right| = \left|\langle L^\# y^*, x \rangle_{X^*,X}\right| = \left|\langle y^*, Lx \rangle_{Y^*,Y}\right| \le \|y^*\|_{Y^*} \|Lx\|_Y .$$

Setting $C := \|y^*\|_{Y^*}$, this proves (8.2). $\qquad\square$

Definition 8.22. *The* conjugate p_* *of p, $1 \le p \le \infty$, is the solution of the equation*

$$1/p + 1/p_* = 1 .$$

We use the convention that $1_* = \infty$.

Example 8.23. The space $l^p(\mathbb{N})$, $1 \le p < \infty$, consists of all sequences $\mathbf{x} = (x_k) \subset \mathbb{R}$ satisfying

$$\|\mathbf{x}\|_p := \left(\sum_k |x_k|^p \right)^{1/p} < \infty .$$

For every $1 \le p < \infty$, the space $l^p(\mathbb{N})$ is a Banach space. It is reflexive, if $p > 1$. In this case, the dual can be identified with $l^{p_*}(\mathbb{N})$. This means that there exists an isometric isomorphism $\Im_p : \left(l^p(\mathbb{N}) \right)^* \to l^{p_*}(\mathbb{N})$ such that

$$L\mathbf{x} = \langle L, \mathbf{x} \rangle = \sum_k (\Im_p L)_k \, x_k , \qquad \mathbf{x} \in l^p(\mathbb{N}) .$$

The space $l^2(\mathbb{N})$ is a Hilbert space with the inner product

$$\langle \mathbf{x}, \mathbf{y} \rangle := \sum_k x_k y_k .$$

The dual of $l^1(\mathbb{N})$ can be identified via a linear isometry $\Im_1 : \left(l^1(\mathbb{N}) \right)^* \to l^\infty(\mathbb{N})$ with the space $l^\infty(\mathbb{N})$ of all bounded sequences satisfying

$$\|\mathbf{x}\|_\infty := \sup_k |x_k| < \infty .$$

Let

$$c_0(\mathbb{N}) := \left\{ \mathbf{x} \in l^\infty(\mathbb{N}) : x_k \to 0 \right\} .$$

The space $c_0(\mathbb{N})$ is a closed subspace of $l^\infty(\mathbb{N})$, and $\left(c_0(\mathbb{N}) \right)^*$ is isometrically isomorph to $l^1(\mathbb{N})$ (see [131, p. 15 & p. 43]), that is, the pre-dual of $l^1(\mathbb{N})$ is $c_0(\mathbb{N})$.

We have the following relation between l^p spaces:

$$l^{p_1}(\mathbb{N}) \subset l^{p_2}(\mathbb{N}), \qquad 1 \le p_1 \le p_2 \le \infty .$$

$\diamond$

Remark 8.24. In the following, we show that the dual of $l^\infty(\mathbb{N})$ is strictly larger than $l^1(\mathbb{N})$, which implies that $l^1(\mathbb{N})$ is not reflexive (see also [390, Satz III.1.11]).

Let

$$G := \left\{ \mathbf{x} \in l^\infty(\mathbb{N}) : \lim_k x_k \text{ exists} \right\} .$$

Then G is a linear subspace of $l^\infty(\mathbb{N})$. For $\mathbf{x} \in G$, define $L\mathbf{x} := \lim_k x_k$. Because $|\lim_k x_k| \le \|\mathbf{x}\|_\infty$, it follows that L is a bounded linear operator on G. From Theorem 8.20, it follows that there exists a bounded extension $\hat{L}$ of L to $l^\infty(\mathbb{N})$.

Assume that there exists $\mathbf{x}^* \in l^1(\mathbb{N})$ such that

$$\hat{L}\mathbf{x} = \sum_k x_k^* x_k , \qquad \mathbf{x} \in l^\infty(\mathbb{N}) .$$

If we choose $\mathbf{x} = \mathbf{e}_k$ the k-th unit vector in $l^\infty(\mathbb{N})$, then we see that

$$0 = \hat{L}\mathbf{e}_k = x_k^*, \qquad k \in \mathbb{N},$$

which implies that $x_k^* = 0$ for all k.

On the other hand, if $\mathbf{x}$ is a constant sequence $x_k = c$ for some $c \neq 0$, then by definition

$$c = \lim_k x_k = L\mathbf{x} = \sum_k c x_k^* = 0,$$

which gives a contradiction.

This shows that $\hat{L}$ cannot be represented by any element of $l^1(\mathbb{N})$. In particular, $l^1(\mathbb{N})$ is not reflexive. $\diamond$

8.4 Linear Operators in Hilbert Spaces

Throughout this section, let X and Y be Hilbert spaces.

Theorem 8.25 (Riesz representation). *For $x \in X$, define $\mathcal{J}_X x \in X^*$ by*

$$\langle \mathcal{J}_X x, y \rangle_{X^*, X} = \langle x, y \rangle_X, \qquad y \in X.$$

The mapping $\mathcal{J}_X : X \to X^*$ is an isometric isomorphism. In particular, every Hilbert space is reflexive.

Proof. See [401, Sect. III.6].   □

Theorem 8.26. *Let $G \subset X$ be a dense linear subspace and $L : G \to Y$ a linear operator. There exists a unique linear operator $L^* : \mathcal{D}(L^*) \subset Y \to X$ such that*

$$\langle L^* y, x \rangle_X = \langle y, Lx \rangle_Y, \qquad x \in G \text{ and } y \in \mathcal{D}(L^*),$$

where

$$\mathcal{D}(L^*) := \{ y \in Y : \text{ the functional } x \mapsto \langle y, Lx \rangle \text{ is continuous on } G \}.$$

The operator L^* is called the adjoint *of L.*

Proof. See [387, Chap. 4.4].   □

Theorem 8.27. *Assume that $L \in L(X, Y)$ is bounded. Then $\mathcal{D}(L^*) = Y$, $L^* \in L(Y, X)$, and $\|L\|_{L(X,Y)} = \|L^*\|_{L(Y,X)}$.*

Proof. See [387, Thm. 4.14].   □

Lemma 8.28. *Assume that $L : X \to Y$ is closed. Then $(L^*)^* = L$.*

Proof. See [401, Sect. VII.2, Cor.].

Theorem 8.29. *Let $G \subset X$ be a dense linear subspace and $L_1 : G \to Y$ be a linear operator. Moreover, let Z be a Hilbert space and $L_2 \in L(Y, Z)$ be bounded. Then $(L_2 L_1)^* = L_1^* L_2^*$.*

Proof. See [387, Thm. 4.19]. $\qquad\qquad\qquad\qquad\qquad\qquad\qquad\qquad\qquad\square$

Remark 8.30. If $L \in L(X, Y)$ is bounded, its adjoint L^* is related with the dual-adjoint $L^\#$ by the equality

$$L^* = \mathcal{J}_X^{-1} L^\# \mathcal{J}_Y .$$

$\qquad\qquad\qquad\qquad\qquad\qquad\qquad\qquad\qquad\qquad\qquad\qquad\qquad\qquad\qquad\diamond$

Lemma 8.31. *Let X, Y be Hilbert spaces, let $L \in L(X, Y)$ and $x \in X$. Then $x \in \text{Ran}(L^*)$ if and only if there exists $C > 0$ such that*

$$\left| \langle x, u \rangle_X \right| \le C \left\| Lu \right\|_Y , \qquad u \in X .$$

Proof. This is a direct consequence of Lemma 8.21. $\qquad\qquad\qquad\qquad\square$

Corollary 8.32. *Let X, Y, Z be Hilbert spaces, let $U \subset X$ be a linear subspace, let $L_1 \in L(X, Y)$ and $L_2 \in L(X, Z)$. Assume that there exists $C \ge 1$ such that*

$$C^{-1} \left\| L_1 u \right\|_Y \le \left\| L_2 u \right\|_Z \le C \left\| L_1 u \right\|_Y , \qquad u \in U .$$

Then $\text{Ran}(L_1^*) \cap U = \text{Ran}(L_2^*) \cap U$.

Proof. Without loss of generality, assume that U is closed, else we may replace U by its closure $\bar{U}$. Let $x \in \text{Ran}(L_1^*) \cap U$. From Lemma 8.31, it follows that there exists $\tilde{C} > 0$ such that

$$\left| \langle x, u \rangle_X \right| \le \tilde{C} \left\| L_1 u \right\|_Y , \qquad u \in X .$$

Consequently,

$$\left| \langle x, u \rangle_X \right| \le \tilde{C} \left\| L_1 u \right\|_Y \le \tilde{C} C \left\| L_2 u \right\|_Z , \qquad u \in U .$$

Again applying Lemma 8.31, this shows that $x \in i^* \text{Ran}(L_2^*)$, where $i^* : X \to U$ is the adjoint of the inclusion $i : U \to X$, $i(u) = u$. Now note that $i \circ i^*(u) = u$ for every $u \in U$. Thus, $x = i(x) \in i \circ i^* \big(\text{Ran}(L_2^*) \big) = \text{Ran}(L_2^*) \cap U$, which implies that $\text{Ran}(L_1^*) \cap U \subset \text{Ran}(L_2^*) \cap U$.

The converse inclusion follows analogously. $\qquad\qquad\qquad\qquad\qquad\square$

Definition 8.33. *An operator $L : G \subset X \to X$ is self-adjoint if $L^* = L$ (which in particular requires that $\mathcal{D}(L^*) = G$).*

Lemma 8.34. *An operator $L \in L(X, Y)$ is compact, if and only if the composition $L^* L$ is compact.*

Proof. See [387, Thm. 6.4]. □

Definition 8.35. *An* orthonormal system *on a Hilbert space* X *is a family* $(u_k) \subset X$ *such that* $\langle u_k, u_l \rangle = 0$ *for all* $k \neq l$ *(that is, all elements* u_k *are mutually orthogonal), and* $\|u_k\| = 1$ *for every* k.

The orthonormal system (u_k) *is called* complete *if no orthonormal system* (v_k) *contains* (u_k) *as proper subset. In this case,* (u_k) *is also called an* orthonormal basis *of* X.

Theorem 8.36. *A Hilbert space* X *has at least one orthonormal basis. If* X *is separable, it has an at most countable orthonormal basis.*

Proof. See [401, Sect. III.4, Thm. 1; Sect. III.5, Cor.]. □

Theorem 8.37. *Let* (u_k) *be an orthonormal basis of the Hilbert space* X. *Then*

$$\|x\|^2 = \sum_k |\langle x, u_k \rangle|^2 \,, \qquad x \in X \,.$$

In particular, for every $x \in X$ *there exist at most countably many* u_k *such that* $\langle x, u_k \rangle \neq 0$. *Moreover we have*

$$x = \sum_k \langle x, u_k \rangle u_k \,.$$

Proof. See [401, Sect. III.4, Thm. 2, Cor. 1]. □

Definition 8.38. *Let* $G \subset X$ *be a dense linear subspace and* $L : G \to Y$ *a linear operator. A* singular value decomposition *of* L, *in short SVD, is a (possibly finite) sequence of triples* (u_k, v_k, σ_k) *such that* (u_k) *and* (v_k) *are orthonormal systems on* X *and* Y, *respectively,* $\sigma_k > 0$ *for all* k, *and*

$$Lx = \sum_k \sigma_k \langle u_k, x \rangle_X v_k \,, \qquad x \in G \,. \tag{8.3}$$

The numbers σ_k *are called the* singular values *of* L.

If $X = Y$, *a sequence of pairs* (u_k, σ_k) *is called an* eigensystem *of* L, *if* (u_k) *is an orthonormal system,* $\sigma_k \neq 0$, *and equation (8.3) holds with* v_k *replaced by* u_k. *In this case, the numbers* σ_k *are the non-vanishing eigenvalues of* L, *that is,* $Lu_k = \sigma_k u_k$ *for all* k. *Note that, in contrast with singular values, the eigenvalues may be negative.*

Theorem 8.39. *Let* $L \in L(X, Y)$ *be compact. Then there exists a singular value decomposition* (u_k, v_k, σ_k) *of* L *such that either* (σ_k) *is finite or is countable and converges to zero.*

If in addition $X = Y$ *and* L *is self-adjoint, then* L *has an eigensystem* (u_k, σ_k). *Again, either* (σ_k) *is finite or converges to zero.*

Proof. See [387, Thm. 7.6, Thm. 7.2]. □

Note that the singular value decomposition may be empty, which is the case if and only if $L = 0$.

Theorem 8.40. *Let $L \in L(X, Y)$ be compact with singular value decomposition (u_k, v_k, σ_k). Then (v_k, u_k, σ_k) is a singular value decomposition of L^*. Moreover, L^*L and LL^* have the eigensystems (u_k, σ_k^2) and (v_k, σ_k^2), respectively.*

Proof. See [387, Thm. 7.6]. $\square$

Definition 8.41. *An operator $L \in L(X, X)$ is called* non-negative *if*

$$\langle Lx, x \rangle \geq 0, \qquad x \in X .$$

Lemma 8.42. *A self-adjoint and compact operator is non-negative, if and only if all eigenvalues are non-negative.*

Proof. See [340, Thm. 13.31]. $\square$

Theorem 8.43. *Let $E \in L(X, X)$ be compact, self-adjoint, and non-negative. Then there exists exactly one self-adjoint and non-negative operator $E^{1/2} \in L(X, X)$ having the property that $E^{1/2}E^{1/2} = E$. It is called the* square root *of E.*

If $E = L^*L$, with $L \in L(X, Y)$ compact, then $\mathrm{Ran}(E^{1/2}) = \mathrm{Ran}(L^*)$.

Proof. See [387, Thm. 7.4] and [152, Prop. 2.18]. $\square$

The singular value decomposition is also defined for matrices $M \in \mathbb{R}^{m \times n}$.

Definition 8.44. *Let $M \in \mathbb{R}^{m \times n}$, with $m, n \in \mathbb{N}$. A* singular value decomposition (SVD) *of M is a triple (U, V, Σ) of matrices such that $U \in \mathbb{R}^{m \times m}$ and $V \in \mathbb{R}^{n \times n}$ are orthogonal, that is, $U^T U = \mathrm{Id}$ and $V^T V = \mathrm{Id}$, $\Sigma \in \mathbb{R}^{m \times n}$ is a diagonal matrix with non-negative entries $\sigma_1 \geq \sigma_2 \geq \ldots \geq 0$, and*

$$M = U \Sigma V^T .$$

Lemma 8.45. *Every matrix $M \in \mathbb{R}^{m \times n}$ has an SVD (U, V, Σ). If $m = n$ and M is symmetric, that is, $M^T = M$, and positive semi-definite, that is, $\mathbf{x}^T M \mathbf{x} \geq 0$ for all $\mathbf{x} \in \mathbb{R}^n$, then there exists an SVD with $U = V$.*

Proof. See [217, Thms. 7.3.5, 4.1.5, 7.2.1]. $\square$

8.5 Weak and Weak* Topologies

Definition 8.46. *Let X be a locally convex space and X^* its dual. For every finite set $\{L_1, \ldots, L_l\} \subset X^*$, we define the* semi-norm

$$p_{L_1, \ldots, L_l}(x) := \sup_k |\langle L_k, x \rangle| , \qquad x \in X .$$

The topology on X induced by the family of semi-norms

$$\{p_{L_1,\ldots,L_l} : L_1,\ldots,L_l \in X^*, \ l \in \mathbb{N}\}$$

is called the weak topology *on X. It is the weakest topology on X with respect to which every $L \in X^*$ is continuous.*

Similarly, we define for a finite set $\{x_1,\ldots,x_l\} \subset X$ the semi-norm

$$p_{x_1,\ldots,x_l}(L) := \sup_k |\langle L, x_k\rangle|, \qquad L \in X^*.$$

The topology on X^* induced by the family of semi-norms

$$\{p_{x_1,\ldots,x_l} : x_1,\ldots,x_l \in X, \ l \in \mathbb{N}\}$$

is called the weak* topology *on X^*.*

We say that (x_k) converges weakly to x and symbolize it with $x_k \rightharpoonup x$, if (x_k) converges with respect to the weak topology. We say that (L_k) weakly converges to L, in signs $L_k \overset{*}{\rightharpoonup} L$, if L_k converges to L with respect to the weak* topology.*

If X is reflexive, then the weak and weak* topology coincide. This easily follows from the definition of the weak* topology on X^{**}, as it uses the same semi-norms as the weak topology on X.

Theorem 8.47 (First convergence criterion). *Assume that X is a normed linear space. A sequence (x_k) in X weakly converges to $x \in X$, if and only if*

$$\sup_k \|x_k\|_X < \infty, \quad \text{and} \quad \langle L, x_k\rangle \to \langle L, x\rangle, \quad L \in D^*,$$

where $D^* \subset X^*$ is dense with respect to the strong topology on X^*.

Similarly, if X is a Banach space, then a sequence (L_k) in X^* weak converges to $L \in X^*$, if and only if*

$$\sup_k \|L_k\|_{X^*} < \infty, \quad \text{and} \quad \langle L_k, x\rangle \to \langle L, x\rangle, \quad x \in D,$$

where $D \subset X$ is dense with respect to the strong topology on X.

Proof. See [401, Sect. V.1, Thm. 3, Thm. 10]. □

In Hilbert spaces, we have the following characterization of strong convergence by means of weak convergence:

Lemma 8.48. *Let X be a Hilbert space. A sequence (x_k) in X converges strongly to $x \in X$, if and only if it converges weakly to x and $(\|x_k\|)$ converges to $\|x\|$.*

Proof. See [401, Sect. V.1, Thm. 8].

Lemma 8.49. *Assume that X and Y are locally convex spaces. Then every $L \in L(X,Y)$ is continuous with respect to the weak topologies on X and Y, respectively.*

Proof. See [57, Chap. IV.3]. $\square$

For the next results, recall the definition of convex sets (see Definition 10.1 below).

Lemma 8.50. *Assume that $E \subset X$ is a convex subset of the locally convex space X. Then the closure of E with respect to the weak topology is equal to the closure of E with respect to the strong topology. In particular, every (strongly) closed convex subset of X is weakly closed.*

Proof. See [340, Thm. 3.12]. $\square$

Theorem 8.51 (Alaoglu–Bourbaki–Kakutani). *Assume that X is a locally convex space. Every bounded, closed, and convex set $K \subset X^*$ is weakly* compact. If, in addition, X is separable, then K is also weakly* sequentially compact.*

The closed unit ball in a Banach space X is weakly compact, if and only if X is reflexive. If additionally X is separable, then it is also weakly sequentially compact.

Proof. See [340, Thm. 3.15, 3.17] and [401, V.App.3, Thm. 2]. $\square$

As a consequence of Theorem 8.51, we obtain from the definition of weak sequential compactness that:

Corollary 8.52. *Assume that X is a reflexive Banach space. Then, every sequence (x_k) in X satisfying $\sup_k \|x_k\|_X < \infty$ has a subsequence $(x_{k'})$ weakly converging to some $x \in X$.*

Because by Theorem 8.25 every Hilbert space is reflexive, Corollary 8.52 in particular applies to this case.

Let G be a closed subspace of a Banach space X (for instance, the kernel of a bounded linear operator). A norm on the *factor space* X/G is defined as follows

$$\|x + G\|_{X/G} := \inf \left\{ \|y\|_X : y - x \in G \right\}.$$

Lemma 8.53. *Let X be a Banach space, and let $G \subset X$ be a closed linear subspace. Then G and X/G are Banach spaces. Denote by*

$$G^\perp := \{ L \in X^* : \langle L, x \rangle = 0, \quad x \in G \}.$$

The duals of G and X/G, respectively, are given by

$$G^* = X^*/G^\perp, \quad (X/G)^* = G^\perp,$$

respectively. If X is reflexive (a Hilbert space), then G and X/G are reflexive (Hilbert spaces).

Proof. See [340, Thm. 4.9]. $\square$

8.6 Spaces of Differentiable Functions

In the following, let $\Omega \subset \mathbb{R}^n$ be an open set.

A *multi-index* $\boldsymbol{\gamma} = (\gamma_1, \ldots, \gamma_n) \in \mathbb{N}_0^n$ is an n-tuple of non-negative integers. The *length* of $\boldsymbol{\gamma}$ is defined as $|\boldsymbol{\gamma}| := \sum_{i=1}^n \gamma_i$. For $\boldsymbol{\gamma} \in \mathbb{N}_0^n$, the derivative of $u : \Omega \to \mathbb{R}$ (whenever defined in an appropriate sense) is denoted by

$$\partial^{\boldsymbol{\gamma}} u(\mathbf{x}) := \frac{\partial^{|\boldsymbol{\gamma}|} u}{\partial x_1^{\gamma_1} \cdots \partial x_n^{\gamma_n}}(\mathbf{x}) .$$

The number $|\boldsymbol{\gamma}|$ is called the *order* of the derivative $\partial^{\boldsymbol{\gamma}} u$.

For $l \in \mathbb{N}_0$, we define

$$\overline{\mathcal{N}}(l) := |\{\boldsymbol{\gamma} \in \mathbb{N}_0^n : |\boldsymbol{\gamma}| \le l\}| , \qquad \mathcal{N}(l) := |\{\boldsymbol{\gamma} \in \mathbb{N}_0^n : |\boldsymbol{\gamma}| = l\}| , \qquad (8.4)$$

the number of multi-indices of length smaller than l and of length l, respectively.

We order the set of multi-indices in the following manner: $\boldsymbol{\gamma} < \boldsymbol{\sigma}$ if either $|\boldsymbol{\gamma}| < |\boldsymbol{\sigma}|$, or $|\boldsymbol{\gamma}| = |\boldsymbol{\sigma}|$ and there exists $1 \le k \le n$ such that $\gamma_i = \sigma_i$ for $1 \le i < k$, and $\gamma_k < \sigma_k$. This is a total ordering of $\mathbb{N}_0^n$.

We define the l-th order *gradient* of an l-times differentiable function $u : \Omega \to \mathbb{R}$ as the vector valued function

$$\nabla^l u := (\partial^{\boldsymbol{\gamma}} u)_{|\boldsymbol{\gamma}|=l} : \Omega \to \mathbb{R}^{\mathcal{N}(l)} ,$$

more precisely, the k-th component of $\nabla^l u$ is the k-th partial derivative of order l of u with respect to the ordering on $\mathbb{N}_0^n$ defined above.

Similarly, if $\mathbf{u} = (u_1, \ldots, u_m) : \Omega \to \mathbb{R}^m$ is vector valued, we define

$$\nabla^l \mathbf{u}(\mathbf{x}) := \big(\nabla^l u_1(\mathbf{x}), \ldots, \nabla^l u_m(\mathbf{x})\big) : \Omega \to \mathbb{R}^{\mathcal{N}(l) \times m}.$$

Let $l \in \mathbb{N}$ and $\mathbf{u} : \Omega \to \mathbb{R}^{\mathcal{N}(l)}$ be l-times differentiable. We define the l-th order *divergence*

$$\big(\nabla^l \cdot \mathbf{u}\big)(\mathbf{x}) := \sum_{|\boldsymbol{\gamma}|=l} \partial^{\boldsymbol{\gamma}} \mathbf{u}_{\boldsymbol{\gamma}}(\mathbf{x}) .$$

Now we define spaces of differentiable functions that are used in the book.

- By $C(\Omega; \mathbb{R}^m) = C^0(\Omega; \mathbb{R}^m)$, we denote the space of $\mathbb{R}^m$-valued continuous functions from Ω to $\mathbb{R}^m$. The space $C(\Omega; \mathbb{R}^m)$ becomes a locally convex space with the family of semi-norms

$$p_K(\mathbf{u}) := \max_{\mathbf{x} \in K} |\mathbf{u}(\mathbf{x})|, \qquad K \subset\subset \Omega .$$

- For $l \in \mathbb{N}$, we denote by $C^l(\Omega; \mathbb{R}^m)$ the space of all l-times continuously differentiable functions $\mathbf{u} : \Omega \to \mathbb{R}^m$. On $C^l(\Omega; \mathbb{R}^m)$, we define the semi-norms

$$p_{K,\boldsymbol{\gamma}}(\mathbf{u}) := \sup_{\mathbf{x} \in K} |\partial^{\boldsymbol{\gamma}} \mathbf{u}(\mathbf{x})| , \qquad K \subset\subset \Omega \text{ and } |\boldsymbol{\gamma}| \le l . \qquad (8.5)$$

- By $C_B^l(\Omega; \mathbb{R}^m)$, we denote the space of all $\mathbf{u} \in C^l(\Omega; \mathbb{R}^m)$ satisfying

$$\|\mathbf{u}\|_{C_B^l(\Omega; \mathbb{R}^m)} := \sup\{|\partial^\gamma \mathbf{u}(\mathbf{x})| : \mathbf{x} \in \Omega, \ |\gamma| \leq l\} < \infty \, .$$

The space $C_B^l(\Omega; \mathbb{R}^m)$ is a Banach space.

- By $C^l(\overline{\Omega}; \mathbb{R}^m)$, we denote the space of all $\mathbf{u} \in C_B^l(\Omega; \mathbb{R}^m)$ such that $\partial^\gamma(\mathbf{u})$ can be continuously extended to $\overline{\Omega}$ for all $|\gamma| \leq l$.

- By $C_0^l(\Omega; \mathbb{R}^m)$, we denote the space of all l-times continuously differentiable functions $\mathbf{u} : \Omega \to \mathbb{R}^m$ such that the support

$$\mathrm{supp}(\mathbf{u}) := \overline{\{\mathbf{x} \in \Omega : \mathbf{u}(\mathbf{x}) \neq 0\}}$$

of $\mathbf{u}$ is a compact subset of Ω. We define a topology on $C_0^l(\Omega; \mathbb{R}^m)$ as follows: Let $K \subset \Omega$,

$$C_K^l(\Omega; \mathbb{R}^m) := \{\mathbf{u} \in C_0^l(\Omega; \mathbb{R}^m) : \mathrm{supp}(\mathbf{u}) \subset K\} \, ,$$

and let $p_{K,\gamma}$ be as in (8.5). Then, $C_K^l(\Omega; \mathbb{R}^m)$ associated with the family of semi-norms

$$\{p_{K,\gamma} : |\gamma| \leq l\}$$

is a locally convex space. For $K \subset \Omega$ compact, denote $i_K : C_K^l(\Omega; \mathbb{R}^m) \to C_0^l(\Omega; \mathbb{R}^m)$ the inclusion $i_K \mathbf{u} = \mathbf{u}$. The topology on $C_0^l(\Omega; \mathbb{R}^m)$ is defined as the finest locally convex topology such that all operators i_K are continuous. A set $U \subset C_0^l(\Omega; \mathbb{R}^m)$ is open, if and only if $i_K^{-1}(U) \subset C_K^l(\Omega; \mathbb{R}^m)$ is open for all $K \subset \Omega$ compact. In particular, a sequence $(\mathbf{u}_k) \subset C_0^l(\Omega; \mathbb{R}^m)$ converges to $\mathbf{u}$, if and only if there exists $K \subset\subset \Omega$ such that $\mathrm{supp}(\mathbf{u}_k) \subset K$ for all k, $\mathrm{supp}(\mathbf{u}) \subset K$, and $p_{K,\gamma}(\mathbf{u}_k - \mathbf{u}) \to 0$ for all $|\gamma| \leq l$.

- By $C^\infty(\Omega; \mathbb{R}^m) := \bigcap_l C^l(\Omega; \mathbb{R}^m)$, we denote the space of all arbitrarily differentiable functions $\mathbf{u} : \Omega \to \mathbb{R}^m$. The topology on $C^\infty(\Omega; \mathbb{R}^m)$ is defined by the family of semi-norms $p_{K,\gamma}$, $K \subset \Omega$ compact and $\gamma \in \mathbb{N}^n$.

- By $C_0^\infty(\Omega; \mathbb{R}^m)$, we denote the space of all arbitrarily differentiable functions $\mathbf{u} : \Omega \to \mathbb{R}^m$ such that $\mathrm{supp}(\mathbf{u}) \subset K$ for some compact set $K \subset \Omega$. The topology on $C_0^\infty(\Omega; \mathbb{R}^m)$ is defined similarly as for $C_0^l(\Omega; \mathbb{R}^m)$.

- The space $C_0^\infty(\overline{\Omega}; \mathbb{R}^m)$ is defined as the space of all functions $\mathbf{u} \in C_0^\infty(\mathbb{R}^n; \mathbb{R}^m)$ satisfying $\mathbf{u} = 0$ on $\mathbb{R}^n \setminus \Omega$. This space is a closed subspace of $C_0^\infty(\mathbb{R}^n; \mathbb{R}^m)$.

- For $T > 0$, we denote by $C_{\mathrm{per},0}^\infty\big((0,T) \times \Omega; \mathbb{R}^m\big)$ the space of all restrictions $\mathbf{u}|_{(0,T) \times \Omega}$ to $(0,T) \times \Omega$ of functions $\mathbf{u} \in C^\infty(\mathbb{R} \times \Omega; \mathbb{R}^m)$ such that $\mathbf{u}(t + T, \mathbf{x}) = \mathbf{u}(t, \mathbf{x})$ for $t \in \mathbb{R}$ and $\mathbf{x} \in \mathbb{R}^n$, and there exists a compact subset $K \subset \Omega$, with $\mathbf{u}(t, \mathbf{x}) = 0$ for $t \in \mathbb{R}$ and $\mathbf{x} \notin K$.

When we write $C(\Omega)$, $C^l(\Omega)$,…, we always mean that the regarded functions are scalar valued. In the literature, the space $C_0^\infty(\Omega)$ is often also called *Schwartz space* and denoted by $\mathcal{D}(\Omega)$.

9

Weakly Differentiable Functions

In this chapter we review some important results from *measure theory*, *Sobolev spaces*, *Bochner spaces*, and the *space of functions of bounded variation*. Mostly, the results are quoted and not proved.

9.1 Measure and Integration Theory

There exist several approaches to measure and integration theory in the literature. We will mainly follow the approach taken in [157].

Measure Theory

The following definitions are taken from [157, Sect. 1.1].

Let X be a set and denote by

$$2^X := \{E : E \subset X\}$$

the *power set* of X consisting of all subsets of X. We say that a function $\mu : 2^X \to [0, \infty]$ is a *measure* on X, if

1. $\mu(\emptyset) = 0$,
2. μ is monotone, that is,

$$\mu(E) \leq \mu(F), \qquad E \subset F \subset X,$$

3. μ is countably subadditive, that is, for every at most countable collection (E_i) of subsets of X we have

$$\mu\left(\bigcup_i E_i\right) \leq \sum_i \mu(E_i).$$

A set $E \subset X$ with $\mu(E) = 0$ is called *negligible*.

We say that a set $E \subset X$ is μ-measurable, or simply *measurable*, if

$$\mu(F) = \mu(F \cap E) + \mu(F \setminus E), \quad F \subset X .$$

This definition in particular implies that every negligible set is measurable. If E is measurable, then so is its complement $X \setminus E$. Moreover, the countable union or intersection of measurable sets is again measurable.

For a μ-measurable subset E of X, we define the restriction $\mu \llcorner E$ of μ to E setting

$$\mu \llcorner E(F) := \mu(F \cap E), \quad F \subset X .$$

The measure μ is called *finite*, if $\mu(X) < \infty$. It is called *σ-finite*, if there exists an ascending sequence of measurable sets (X_k) such that $\mu(X_k) < \infty$ for all $k \in \mathbb{N}$, and $\bigcup_k X_k = X$.

A classical way of defining measures is by introducing σ-algebras (see below) on which measures are defined. In order to be able to measure arbitrary subsets of X, which need not be contained in the σ-algebra, one has to perform a completion step. Although our definition of measures requires no σ-algebras, we still need them for the definition of Radon measures.

Definition 9.1 (σ-algebra). *Let $X \neq \emptyset$ be a set and let $\mathcal{E} \subset 2^X$ be a collection of subsets of X. We say that $\mathcal{E}$ is a σ-algebra, if*

- $\emptyset \in \mathcal{E}$,
- *whenever $E \in \mathcal{E}$, then $X \setminus E \in \mathcal{E}$, that is, $\mathcal{E}$ is closed with respect to taking complements,*
- *whenever (E_i) is a countable collection of sets in $\mathcal{E}$, then $\bigcup_i E_i \in \mathcal{E}$, that is, $\mathcal{E}$ is closed with respect to forming countable unions.*

If X is a topological space, the Borel σ-algebra $\mathcal{B}(X)$ is defined as the smallest σ-algebra containing all open subsets of X. A set $E \subset X$ is a Borel set, if it is an element of the Borel σ-algebra of X.

Definition 9.2 (Regular measures). *Let X be a topological space and μ a measure on X.*

- *The measure μ is regular, if for every $E \subset X$ there exists a measurable set F such that $E \subset F$ and $\mu(E) = \mu(F)$.*
- *The measure μ is Borel, if every Borel set is measurable.*
- *The measure μ is Borel regular, if μ is Borel, and for every $E \subset X$ there exists a Borel set F such that $E \subset F$ and $\mu(E) = \mu(F)$.*
- *The measure μ is a positive Radon measure, if μ is Borel regular, and $\mu(K) < \infty$ for every compact set $K \subset X$.*

Note that in [157] simply the term Radon measure instead of positive Radon measure is used.

The most important example for a positive Radon measure is the *Lebesgue measure*, denoted $\mathcal{L}^n$, which is the unique positive Radon measure on $\mathbb{R}^n$ such that $\mathcal{L}^n(E + t) = \mathcal{L}^n(E)$ for all Borel sets $E \subset \mathbb{R}^n$ and $t \in \mathbb{R}^n$, and $\mathcal{L}^n([0,1]^n) = 1$.

Moreover, for $s \in \mathbb{R}_{\geq 0}$, we can define the s-dimensional *Hausdorff measure* $\mathcal{H}^s$, which is intended to measure the s-dimensional volume of subsets of $\mathbb{R}^n$. The measure $\mathcal{H}^s$ is defined in two steps. First we define for $\delta > 0$ and $E \subset \mathbb{R}^n$

$$\mathcal{H}^s_\delta(E) := \frac{\omega_s}{2^s} \inf \left\{ \sum_k \mathrm{diam}(E_k)^s : E \subset \bigcup_k E_k \text{ and } \mathrm{diam}(E_k) < \delta \text{ for all } k \right\},$$

where $\omega_s := \pi^{s/2} / \Gamma(1 + s/2)$ with $\Gamma(s) := \int_0^\infty e^{-x} x^{s-1}$ being the Γ-function (in particular, if $s \in \mathbb{N}$, then $\Gamma(s)$ is the volume of an s-dimensional unit ball). Then we set

$$\mathcal{H}^s(E) := \lim_{\delta \to 0} \mathcal{H}^s_\delta(E) = \sup_{\delta > 0} \mathcal{H}^s_\delta(E) . \tag{9.1}$$

The measures $\mathcal{H}^s$ have the following properties (see [157, Sect. 2.1]):

- For every $s \geq 0$ the measure $\mathcal{H}^s$ is a Borel regular positive measure.
- If $s = 0$, it is the counting measure, that is, $\mathcal{H}^0(E) = |E|$.
- The measure $\mathcal{H}^n$ coincides with the n-dimensional Lebesgue measure on $\mathbb{R}^n$.
- If $\mathcal{H}^s(E) > 0$, then $\mathcal{H}^t(E) = \infty$ for all $t < s$.
- If $\mathcal{H}^s(E) = 0$, then $\mathcal{H}^t(E) = 0$ for all $t > s$.
- For every $E \subset \mathbb{R}^n$, $t \in \mathbb{R}^n$ and $\lambda > 0$ we have

$$\mathcal{H}^s(\lambda E + t) = \lambda^s \mathcal{H}^s(E) .$$

Let μ be a measure on X and let Y be a topological space. A function $u : X \to Y$ is called μ-*measurable*, or simply *measurable*, if for every open set $U \subset Y$ its preimage $u^{-1}(U)$ is measurable. If X is a topological space, then $u : X \to Y$ is called *Borel function*, if for every open set $U \subset Y$ its preimage $u^{-1}(U)$ is a Borel set. In this case the function u is μ-measurable for every Borel measure μ.

Now assume that $u : X \to Y$ is measurable and $g : Y \to Z$ is continuous. Then also $g \circ u$ is measurable. In particular, if $Y = Z = [-\infty, +\infty]$, the functions $|u|^p$, $1 \leq p < \infty$,

$$u^+ := \max\{u, 0\} , \qquad u^- := -\min\{u, 0\}$$

are measurable.

Integration in $\mathbb{R}^n$

For the definition of the integral of a measurable function we follow [11]. In the following we assume that μ is a positive Radon measure on a Borel set $\Omega \subset \mathbb{R}^n$.

Let s be a simple function on Ω, that is,

$$s = \sum_{k=1}^{m} c_k \, \chi_{E_k} \, ,$$

where c_k are real numbers, $E_k \subset \Omega$ are measurable sets, and χ_E denotes the *characteristic function* of the set E, defined by $\chi_E(x) = 1$ if $x \in E$ and $\chi_E(x) = 0$ if $x \notin E$.

For a measurable set $E \subset \Omega$ and a simple function s we define

$$\int_E s \, d\mu := \sum_{k=1}^{m} c_k \, \mu(E_k \cap E) \, .$$

In the case $c_k = 0$ and $\mu(E \cap E_k) = \infty$, we use the convention that $0 \cdot \infty = 0$.

If $u : \Omega \to [0, \infty]$ is a measurable function and $E \subset \Omega$, then we define

$$\int_E u \, d\mu := \sup \int_E s \, d\mu \, , \tag{9.2}$$

where the supremum is taken over all simple functions s such that $0 \le s \le u$. The number $\int_E u \, d\mu$ in (9.2) is called the *integral* of u on E with respect to μ. In the case $\mu = \mathcal{L}^n$, the n-dimensional Lebesgue measure, we write

$$\int_E u := \int_E u \, d\mathcal{L}^n \, .$$

Now let $u : \Omega \to [-\infty, +\infty]$ be μ-measurable. The integral of u on $E \subset \Omega$ is defined by

$$\int_E u \, d\mu := \int_E u^+ \, d\mu - \int_E u^- \, d\mu \, ,$$

provided at least one of the integrals on the right hand side is finite. Note that in our terminology the integral can be infinite. If the integral exists, we call u μ-integrable. In the case $\mu = \mathcal{L}^n$ we simply say that u is integrable. If two μ-integrable functions u and v are identical μ-almost everywhere on Ω, that is,

$$\mu\big(\{\mathbf{x} \in \Omega : u(\mathbf{x}) \neq v(\mathbf{x})\}\big) = 0 \, ,$$

then

$$\int_E u \, d\mu = \int_E v \, d\mu \, , \qquad E \subset \Omega \text{ measurable} \, .$$

Therefore, u and v can be identified in the class of integrable functions. In particular, we will identify an integrable function u with the equivalence class of all functions that coincide with u μ-almost everywhere.

Spaces of Integrable Functions

Definition 9.3. *Let $\Omega \subset \mathbb{R}^n$ be μ-measurable. For $p \in [1, \infty)$, the space $L^p(\Omega; \mu)$ consists of all μ-measurable functions u which satisfy*

$$\int_\Omega |u|^p \, d\mu < \infty \, .$$

In the case $\mu = \mathcal{L}^n$ we simply write $L^p(\Omega)$ instead of $L^p(\Omega; \mathcal{L}^n)$. We define the norm

$$\|u\|_p := \left(\int_\Omega |u|^p \, d\mu \right)^{1/p} \, , \qquad u \in L^p(\Omega; \mu) \, .$$

A measurable function u satisfying $\|u\|_1 < \infty$ is called summable.

Let u be a μ-measurable function and $V \subset \Omega$. Then the *essential supremum* of u on V is defined as

$$\operatorname{ess\,sup}_V u := \inf \left\{ t \in \mathbb{R} : \mu(\{ \mathbf{x} \in V : u(\mathbf{x}) \geq t \}) = 0 \right\} \, .$$

Similarly, the *essential infimum* of u on V is defined as

$$\operatorname{ess\,inf}_V u := \sup \left\{ t \in \mathbb{R} : \mu(\{ \mathbf{x} \in V : u(\mathbf{x}) \leq t \}) = 0 \right\} \, .$$

Here we define

$$\inf \emptyset := +\infty, \qquad \sup \emptyset := -\infty \, .$$

In case $V = \Omega$, we write $\operatorname{ess\,sup} u := \operatorname{ess\,sup}_\Omega u$ and $\operatorname{ess\,inf} u := \operatorname{ess\,inf}_\Omega u$ instead.

Definition 9.4. *The space $L^\infty(\Omega; \mu)$ is the space of measurable functions u satisfying*

$$\|u\|_\infty := \operatorname{ess\,sup} |u| < \infty \, .$$

In the case of vector valued functions $\mathbf{u} : \Omega \to \mathbb{R}^m$, $m > 1$, the definitions of the L^p spaces are similar, but one has to pay attention to the fact that the actual L^p norm strongly depends on the norm chosen on $\mathbb{R}^m$.

We define the space $L^p(\Omega; \mu; \mathbb{R}^m)$ as the space of all measurable functions $\mathbf{u} : \Omega \to \mathbb{R}^m$ satisfying

$$\|\mathbf{u}\|_p := \left(\int_\Omega |\mathbf{u}|^p \, d\mu \right)^{1/p} = \left(\int_\Omega \left(\sum_{k=1}^m u_k^2 \right)^{p/2} d\mu \right)^{1/p} < \infty \, .$$

Similarly, we define $L^\infty(\Omega; \mu; \mathbb{R}^m)$ as the space of all measurable functions $\mathbf{u} : \Omega \to \mathbb{R}^m$ satisfying

$$\|\mathbf{u}\|_\infty := \operatorname{ess\,sup} |\mathbf{u}| < \infty \, .$$

A measurable function u is locally p-integrable, in short $u \in L^p_{\mathrm{loc}}(\Omega; \mu)$, if the restriction $u|_V$ to every measurable set V compactly contained in Ω is in $L^p(V; \mu \llcorner V)$. In other words, if $1 \leq p < \infty$, then $u \in L^p_{\mathrm{loc}}(\Omega; \mu)$, if and only if

$$\int_V |u|^p \, \mathrm{d}\mu < \infty, \qquad V \subset\subset \Omega.$$

Similarly, u is locally bounded, in short $u \in L^\infty_{\mathrm{loc}}(\Omega; \mu)$, if and only if

$$\operatorname{ess\,sup}_V |u| < \infty, \qquad V \subset\subset \Omega.$$

We call a function $u : \Omega \to [-\infty, \infty]$ *locally summable* if $u \in L^1_{\mathrm{loc}}(\Omega; \mu)$.

Definition 9.5. *A sequence (u_k) of measurable functions converges to a function u pointwise almost everywhere, if there exists a set E with $\mu(E) = 0$ such that $u_k(\mathbf{x}) \to u(\mathbf{x})$ for all $\mathbf{x} \in \Omega \setminus E$.*

Lemma 9.6. *Let $1 \leq p \leq \infty$. Assume that the sequence $(u_k) \subset L^p(\Omega; \mu; \mathbb{R}^m)$ converges to $u \in L^p(\Omega; \mu; \mathbb{R}^m)$ with respect to the L^p norm. Then there exists a subsequence $(u_{k'})$ converging to u pointwise almost everywhere.*

Proof. See [11, Sect. 1.2]. □

The following results treat the main convergence results for integrals (see [11, Thms. 1.19–1.21]).

Theorem 9.7 (Monotone convergence). *Let (u_k) be an increasing sequence of integrable functions $u_k : \Omega \to [-\infty, +\infty]$. Assume moreover that there exists $v \in L^1(\Omega; \mu)$ with $u_k \geq v$ for all k. Then*

$$\lim_k \int_\Omega u_k \, \mathrm{d}\mu = \int_\Omega \lim_k u_k \, \mathrm{d}\mu.$$

Theorem 9.8 (Fatou's lemma). *Let (u_k) be a sequence of integrable functions $u_k : \Omega \to [-\infty, +\infty]$. Assume that there exists $v \in L^1(\Omega; \mu)$ such that $u_k \geq v$ for all k. Then*

$$\int_\Omega \liminf_k u_k \, \mathrm{d}\mu \leq \liminf_k \int_\Omega u_k \, \mathrm{d}\mu.$$

Theorem 9.9 (Dominated convergence). *Let (u_k) be a sequence of integrable functions $u_k : \Omega \to [-\infty, +\infty]$. Assume that u_k converges to a function u pointwise almost everywhere, and that*

$$\int_\Omega \sup_k |u_k| \, \mathrm{d}\mu < \infty.$$

Then

$$\lim_k \int_\Omega u_k \, \mathrm{d}\mu = \int_\Omega u \, \mathrm{d}\mu.$$

Standard result from functional analysis (see e.g. [3] or [11, Sect. 1.2]) state that for all $1 \leq p \leq \infty$ the space $L^p(\Omega; \mu; \mathbb{R}^m)$ is a Banach space. If $1 < p < \infty$, then $L^p(\Omega; \mu; \mathbb{R}^m)$ is reflexive. Moreover, the space $L^2(\Omega; \mu; \mathbb{R}^m)$ is a Hilbert space.

For the next results recall that p_* is defined by the equation $1/p + 1/p_* = 1$ (see Definition 8.22).

Lemma 9.10 (Hölder's inequality). *Let $u \in L^p(\Omega; \mu)$ and $v \in L^{p_*}(\Omega; \mu)$. Then $uv \in L^1(\Omega; \mu)$, and*

$$\|uv\|_1 \leq \|u\|_p \|v\|_{p_*} . \tag{9.3}$$

In the special case $p = p_* = 2$, this inequality is widely known as the Cauchy–Schwarz *inequality.*

Lemma 9.11. *Let $1 < p < \infty$. Then the dual space of $L^p(\Omega; \mu)$ can be identified with $L^{p_*}(\Omega; \mu)$. That is, there exists an isometric isomorphism*

$$\Im_p : \left(L^p(\Omega; \mu)\right)^* \to L^{p_*}(\Omega; \mu) ,$$

such that

$$\langle L, u \rangle_{(L^p)^*, L^p} = \int_\Omega \Im_p L \, u \, \mathrm{d}\mu , \qquad L \in \left(L^p(\Omega; \mu)\right)^*, \ u \in L^p(\Omega; \mu) . \tag{9.4}$$

In particular, $\|L\|_{(L^p)^*} = \|\Im_p L\|_{p_*}$.

If μ is σ-finite, the dual space of $L^1(\Omega; \mu)$ can be identified with $L^\infty(\Omega; \mu)$, that is, there exists an isometric isomorphism $\Im_1 : \left(L^1(\Omega; \mu)\right)^* \to L^\infty(\Omega; \mu)$ such that (9.4) holds with $p = 1$, $p_* = \infty$.

In the case of spaces $L^p(\Omega; \mu; \mathbb{R}^m)$ of vector valued functions, the dual space again can be identified with $L^{p_*}(\Omega; \mu; \mathbb{R}^m)$. Here, the dual pairing of two functions $\mathbf{v} = \Im_p L$ and $\mathbf{u}$ is the integral of their inner product in $\mathbb{R}^m$,

$$\langle \mathbf{v}, \mathbf{u} \rangle = \int_\Omega \mathbf{u} \cdot \mathbf{v} \, \mathrm{d}\mu .$$

Note, though, that in general the dual of $L^\infty(\Omega; \mu)$ is strictly larger than $L^1(\Omega; \mu)$. As a consequence, the space $L^1(\Omega; \mu)$ is not reflexive.

Lemma 9.12. *If μ is a finite measure, and $1 \leq p \leq q \leq \infty$, then*

$$L^q(\Omega; \mu; \mathbb{R}^m) \subset L^p(\Omega; \mu; \mathbb{R}^m) .$$

In particular, this shows that every p-integrable function u on a finite measure space is summable.

Moreover, if μ is a positive Radon measure and $1 \leq p \leq q \leq \infty$, then we always have

$$L^q_{\mathrm{loc}}(\Omega; \mu; \mathbb{R}^m) \subset L^p_{\mathrm{loc}}(\Omega; \mu; \mathbb{R}^m) .$$

Definition 9.13. *Let $\Omega \subset \mathbb{R}^n$ and let μ be a finite measure on Ω. For $p \in [1, \infty)$, the space $L_\diamond^p(\Omega; \mu)$ is the subspace of all functions $u \in L^p(\Omega; \mu)$ with zero mean, that is, for every $u \in L_\diamond^p(\Omega; \mu)$*

$$\int_\Omega u \, \mathrm{d}\mu = 0 .$$

Remark 9.14. Define $L \in \big(L^p(\Omega; \mu)\big)^*$ setting $Lu = \int_\Omega u \, \mathrm{d}\mu$. Then $L_\diamond^p(\Omega; \mu) = \ker L$, which shows that $L_\diamond^p(\Omega; \mu)$ is a closed subspace of $L^p(\Omega; \mu)$. From Lemma 8.53 it follows that $L_\diamond^p(\Omega; \mu)$ is a Banach space, reflexive if $1 < p < \infty$, and a Hilbert space, if $p = 2$. $\diamond$

Theorem 9.15 (Fubini). *Let X and Y be sets, and μ, ν be σ-finite measures on X and Y, respectively. There exists a unique measure $\mu \times \nu$ on $X \times Y$, called product measure, such that $(\mu \times \nu)(E \times F) = \mu(E) \nu(F)$ whenever $E \subset X$ and $F \subset Y$ are measurable.*

If $f \in L^1(X \times Y; \mu \times \nu)$, then for μ-almost every $x \in X$ the function $f(x, \cdot)$ is ν-summable, and for ν-almost every $y \in Y$ the function $f(\cdot, y)$ is μ-summable. Moreover

$$\int_{X \times Y} f \, \mathrm{d}(\mu \times \nu) = \int_X \int_Y f(x, y) \, \mathrm{d}\nu(y) \, \mathrm{d}\mu(x) = \int_Y \int_X f(x, y) \, \mathrm{d}\mu(x) \, \mathrm{d}\nu(y) .$$

Proof. See [11, Thm. 1.74] and [157, Sect. 1.4, Thm. 1]. $\square$

The following result is an interesting consequence of Fubini's Theorem:

Corollary 9.16. *Assume that $u \in L^p(\Omega)$, $v \in L^{p_*}(\Omega)$, and $\int_\Omega u = 0$. Then*

$$\int_\Omega u \, v = \int_{-\infty}^{+\infty} \int_{\{v \geq t\}} u \, \mathrm{d}\mathbf{x} \, \mathrm{d}t .$$

Proof. Define $w \in L^1(\Omega \times \mathbb{R})$,

$$w(\mathbf{x}, t) := \begin{cases} u(\mathbf{x}), & \text{if } 0 \leq t \leq v(\mathbf{x}) , \\ -u(\mathbf{x}), & \text{if } v(\mathbf{x}) < t < 0 , \\ 0, & \text{else} . \end{cases}$$

For almost every $\mathbf{x} \in \Omega$ we have

$$\int_{-\infty}^{+\infty} w(\mathbf{x}, t) \, \mathrm{d}t = u(\mathbf{x}) v(\mathbf{x}) .$$

Consequently, it follows from Fubini's Theorem 9.15 that

$$\int_{\Omega \times \mathbb{R}} w \, \mathrm{d}\mathcal{L}^{n+1} = \int_\Omega \int_{\mathbb{R}} w(\mathbf{x}, t) \, \mathrm{d}t \, \mathrm{d}\mathbf{x} = \int_\Omega u \, v \, \mathrm{d}\mathbf{x} .$$

Now note that from the assumption $\int_\Omega u \, d\mathbf{x} = 0$ it follows that

$$\int_{\Omega \cap \{v < t\}} u \, d\mathbf{x} = - \int_{\Omega \cap \{v \geq t\}} u \, d\mathbf{x}, \qquad t \in \mathbb{R}.$$

Using Fubini's Theorem it follows that

$$\begin{aligned}
\int_{\Omega \times \mathbb{R}} w \, d\mathcal{L}^{n+1} &= \int_{-\infty}^{+\infty} \int_\Omega w(\mathbf{x}, t) \, d\mathbf{x} \, dt \\
&= \int_{-\infty}^{0} \int_\Omega w(\mathbf{x}, t) \, d\mathbf{x} \, dt + \int_{0}^{+\infty} \int_\Omega w(\mathbf{x}, t) \, d\mathbf{x} \, dt \\
&= - \int_{-\infty}^{0} \int_{\Omega \cap \{v < t\}} u \, d\mathbf{x} \, dt + \int_{0}^{+\infty} \int_{\Omega \cap \{v \geq t\}} u \, d\mathbf{x} \, dt \\
&= \int_{-\infty}^{0} \int_{\Omega \cap \{v \geq t\}} u \, d\mathbf{x} \, dt + \int_{0}^{+\infty} \int_{\Omega \cap \{v \geq t\}} u \, d\mathbf{x} \, dt \\
&= \int_{-\infty}^{+\infty} \int_{\Omega \cap \{v \geq t\}} u \, d\mathbf{x} \, dt,
\end{aligned}$$

which proves the assertion. □

Radon Measures

Recall that $C_0(\Omega; \mathbb{R}^m)$ denotes the space of all continuous $\mathbb{R}^m$-valued functions on Ω with compact support, and that $C_0(\Omega; \mathbb{R}^m)$ can be given the structure of a locally convex space.

Definition 9.17. *The dual space*

$$\mathcal{M}(\Omega; \mathbb{R}^m) := C_0(\Omega; \mathbb{R}^m)^*$$

is called the space of $\mathbb{R}^m$-valued Radon measures *on Ω.*

The next theorem shows the relation between Radon measures and the positive Radon measures defined above.

Theorem 9.18 (Riesz representation). *Let $\boldsymbol{\mu} \in \mathcal{M}(\Omega; \mathbb{R}^m)$. Then there exist a unique positive Radon measure $|\boldsymbol{\mu}|$ on Ω, called* total variation *of $\boldsymbol{\mu}$, and a unique function $\boldsymbol{\sigma} \in L^1_{\mathrm{loc}}(\Omega; \boldsymbol{\mu}; \mathbb{R}^m)$ satisfying $|\boldsymbol{\sigma}(\mathbf{x})| = 1$ for $|\boldsymbol{\mu}|$-almost every $\mathbf{x} \in \Omega$, such that*

$$\langle \boldsymbol{\mu}, \boldsymbol{\phi} \rangle = \int_\Omega \boldsymbol{\phi} \cdot \boldsymbol{\sigma} \, d|\boldsymbol{\mu}|, \qquad \boldsymbol{\phi} \in C_0(\Omega; \mathbb{R}^m).$$

If moreover $m = 1$ and $\langle \mu, \phi \rangle \geq 0$ for every non-negative function ϕ, then $\sigma(\mathbf{x}) = 1$ almost everywhere. Consequently, μ can be regarded as positive Radon measure.

Proof. See [157, Sect. 1.8, Thm. 1, Cor. 1].   □

Using the Riesz representation theorem it is possible to regard Radon measures as generalized measures and define integration with respect to a Radon measure by

$$\int_\Omega \mathbf{u} \, \mathrm{d}\boldsymbol{\mu} := \int_\Omega \mathbf{u} \cdot \boldsymbol{\sigma} \, \mathrm{d}\,|\boldsymbol{\mu}| \,,$$

if $\mathbf{u} \in L^1(\Omega; |\boldsymbol{\mu}| \,; \mathbb{R}^m)$, or

$$\int_\Omega u \, \mathrm{d}\boldsymbol{\mu} := \int_\Omega u \, \boldsymbol{\sigma} \, \mathrm{d}\,|\boldsymbol{\mu}| \in \mathbb{R}^m \,,$$

if $u \in L^1(\Omega; |\boldsymbol{\mu}|)$.

Theorem 9.19 (Radon–Nikodým). *Let $\boldsymbol{\mu} \in \mathcal{M}(\Omega; \mathbb{R}^m)$, and let ν be a σ-finite positive Radon measure on Ω. Then there exist a unique function $\mathrm{d}\boldsymbol{\mu}/\mathrm{d}\nu \in L^1(\Omega; \nu; \mathbb{R}^m)$ and a unique Radon measure $\boldsymbol{\mu}^s$, such that*

$$\boldsymbol{\mu} = \frac{\mathrm{d}\boldsymbol{\mu}}{\mathrm{d}\nu}\, \nu + \boldsymbol{\mu}^s \,,$$

and $|\boldsymbol{\mu}^s|$ and ν are mutually singular, *in short $|\boldsymbol{\mu}^s| \perp \nu$, that is, there exists a set $E \subset \Omega$ such that $|\boldsymbol{\mu}^s|\,(E) = 0$ and $\nu(\Omega \setminus E) = 0$.*

The function $\mathrm{d}\boldsymbol{\mu}/\mathrm{d}\nu$ is called Radon–Nikodým derivative *of $\boldsymbol{\mu}$ with respect to ν, and $\boldsymbol{\mu}^s$ the* singular part *of $\boldsymbol{\mu}$ with respect to ν. The decomposition $\boldsymbol{\mu} = (\mathrm{d}\boldsymbol{\mu}/\mathrm{d}\nu)\nu + \boldsymbol{\mu}^s$ is called* Lebesgue decomposition *of $\boldsymbol{\mu}$ with respect to ν.*

Here, the product $\mathrm{d}\boldsymbol{\mu}/\mathrm{d}\nu \, \nu \in \mathcal{M}(\Omega; \mathbb{R}^m)$ is defined by

$$\left\langle \frac{\mathrm{d}\boldsymbol{\mu}}{\mathrm{d}\nu} \nu, \boldsymbol{\phi} \right\rangle := \int_\Omega \frac{\mathrm{d}\boldsymbol{\mu}}{\mathrm{d}\nu} \cdot \boldsymbol{\phi} \, \mathrm{d}\nu \,, \qquad \boldsymbol{\phi} \in C_0(\Omega; \mathbb{R}^m) \,.$$

Proof. See [11, Thm. 1.28].   □

9.2 Distributions and Distributional Derivatives

Definition 9.20. *A bounded linear operator*

$$L : C_0^\infty(\Omega) \to \mathbb{R}$$

is called a distribution on Ω.

Here $C_0^\infty(\Omega)$ is the space of infinitely differentiable functions $\phi : \Omega \to \mathbb{R}$ with compact support in Ω.

Lemma 9.21. *The operator $L : C_0^\infty(\Omega) \to \mathbb{R}$ is bounded (and hence a distribution), if and only if for every compact set $K \subset \Omega$ there exist $C > 0$ and $k \in \mathbb{N}$ such that*

$$|L(\phi)| \le C \sum_{|\gamma| \le k} \sup_{\mathbf{x} \in K} |\partial^\gamma \phi(\mathbf{x})| \,, \qquad \phi \in C_K^\infty(\Omega) \,. \tag{9.5}$$

Proof. See [401, Chap. I.8, Cor.].   □

The smallest number $k \in \mathbb{N}$ such that (9.5) holds for every compact set $K \subset \Omega$ (but not necessarily with the same $C > 0$) is called the *order* of the distribution L. If there exists no such number k, the distribution L is said to be of *infinite order*.

In the following we give some examples of distributions:

Example 9.22.

1. A locally summable function $u \in L^1_{\mathrm{loc}}(\Omega)$ can be identified with the distribution of order zero

$$L_u \phi := \int_\Omega u\,\phi\,, \qquad \phi \in C_0^\infty(\Omega)\,.$$

2. A scalar valued Radon measure μ on Ω can be identified with the distribution of order zero

$$L_\mu \phi := \int_\Omega \phi\,\mathrm{d}\mu\,, \qquad \phi \in C_0^\infty(\Omega)\,.$$

3. The *Dirac δ-distribution* is defined by

$$\delta^{(\gamma)}(\phi) := (-1)^{|\gamma|}\partial^\gamma \phi(0)\,, \qquad \phi \in C_0^\infty(\Omega)\,.$$

This distribution is of order $|\gamma|$.
The *Dirac δ-distribution* centered at $\mathbf{x} \in \Omega$ is given by

$$\delta_{\mathbf{x}}^{(\gamma)}(\phi) := (-1)^{|\gamma|}\partial^\gamma \phi(\mathbf{x})\,, \qquad \phi \in C_0^\infty(\Omega)\,.$$

If $\gamma = 0$ we write δ, $\delta_{\mathbf{x}}$, instead.   ◇

If a distribution L can be represented as locally summable function u, then u is uniquely determined almost everywhere. Similarly, if L can be represented as Radon measure, then the corresponding Radon measure is unique.

If L is a distribution on Ω and γ a multi-index, then we define the *distributional derivative*

$$(\partial^\gamma L)(\phi) := (-1)^{|\gamma|}L(\partial^\gamma \phi)\,.$$

The distributional derivative $\partial^\gamma L$ is again a distribution on Ω.

Distributional derivatives are formally motivated by Green's formula (cf. Theorem 9.31 below): if u is an $|\gamma|$-times continuously differentiable function, then from Green's formula it follows that

$$\int_\Omega (\partial^\gamma u)\,\phi = (-1)^{|\gamma|}\int_\Omega u\,\partial^\gamma \phi\,, \qquad \phi \in C_0^\infty(\Omega)\,.$$

Thus in this situation the function $\partial^\gamma u$ can be identified with the distribution $\partial^\gamma L_u$. This shows that differentiation of distributions is a concept generalizing the differentiation of functions.

9.3 Geometrical Properties of Functions and Domains

Definition 9.23. *Let $\Omega \subset \mathbb{R}^n$ be open and $u : \Omega \to \mathbb{R}$. The function u is called* Lipschitz *with* Lipschitz constant $\text{Lip}(u)$, *if*

$$\text{Lip}(u) := \sup \left\{ \frac{|u(\mathbf{x}) - u(\mathbf{y})|}{|\mathbf{x} - \mathbf{y}|} : \mathbf{x} \neq \mathbf{y} \in \Omega \right\} < \infty .$$

In particular, if Ω is convex, then every differentiable function $u \in C_B^1(\Omega)$ is Lipschitz with $\text{Lip}(u) \leq \|u\|_{C_B^1(\Omega)}$. Conversely, Rademacher's Theorem (see [157, p. 81]) states that every Lipschitz function is differentiable almost everywhere on its domain.

We say that $\partial\Omega$ is Lipschitz *if for each $\mathbf{x} \in \partial\Omega$, there exist $r > 0$ and a Lipschitz mapping $\gamma : \mathbb{R}^{n-1} \to \mathbb{R}$ such that – if necessary upon rotating and relabelling the coordinate axes – we have*

$$\Omega \cap Q(\mathbf{x}, r) = \{\mathbf{y} : \gamma(y_1, \ldots, y_{n-1}) < y_n\} \cap Q(\mathbf{x}, r) ,$$

where $Q(\mathbf{x}, r) := \{\mathbf{y} : |y_i - x_i| < r, i = 1, \ldots, n\}$ is an open rectangle around $\mathbf{x}$. Compare the definition with Fig. 9.1.
The normal vector *to Ω is defined for $\mathcal{H}^{n-1}$-almost every $\mathbf{x} \in \partial\Omega$ by*

$$\mathbf{n}(\mathbf{x}) = \frac{\left(\nabla\gamma(\hat{\mathbf{x}}), -1\right)^T}{\sqrt{1 + |\nabla\gamma(\hat{\mathbf{x}})|^2}} , \tag{9.6}$$

where $\hat{\mathbf{x}} := (x_1, \ldots, x_{n-1})$. We say that $\partial\Omega$ is C^l, $l \in \mathbb{N} \cup \{\infty\}$, if for each $\mathbf{x} \in \partial\Omega$ the mapping $\gamma : \mathbb{R}^{n-1} \to \mathbb{R}$ is C^l. If $\partial\Omega$ is C^2, then the Gauss curvature K and the mean curvature H of $\partial\Omega$ at $\mathbf{x}$ are defined as

$$K := \det\left(\partial^i \partial^j \gamma(\hat{\mathbf{x}})\right)_{ij} , \qquad H := \frac{1}{n-1} \sum_i (\partial^i)^2 \gamma(\hat{\mathbf{x}}) . \tag{9.7}$$

Note that the definitions of normal vector and curvature are independent of the defining function γ.

Definition 9.24. *A set $\Omega \subset \mathbb{R}$ is* bocL *if it is a bounded, open, connected domain with Lipschitz boundary.*

Definition 9.25. *We say that a bounded domain $\Omega \subset \mathbb{R}^2$ is* starlike *with respect to the center c if there exists a one-to-one Lipschitz function $r : [0, 2\pi) \to \mathbb{R}_{>0}$ satisfying $r(0) = \lim_{t \to 2\pi^-} r(t)$ and*

$$\partial\Omega = \left\{ c + r(\phi)\big(\cos(\phi), \sin(\phi)\big)^T : \phi \in [0, 2\pi) \right\} .$$

Lemma 9.26. *If $\Omega \subset \mathbb{R}^2$ is starlike then $\partial\Omega$ is Lipschitz.*

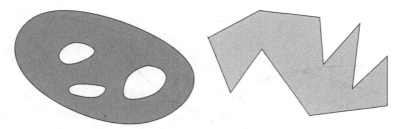

Fig. 9.1. A Lipschitz domain may have holes and a "rough" boundary.

Let $\Omega \subset \mathbb{R}^n$ be bounded with $\partial\Omega$ Lipschitz. Due to the compactness of $\partial\Omega$, there exists a finite family $\{Q(\mathbf{x}_k, r_k) : k = 1, \ldots, m\}$ of open rectangles and a corresponding family of Lipschitz functions $\{\gamma_k : k = 1, \ldots, m\}$ covering $\partial\Omega$ such that

$$\Omega \cap Q(\mathbf{x}_k, r_k) = \{\mathbf{y} : \gamma_k(y_1, \ldots, y_{n-1}) < y_n\} \cap Q(\mathbf{x}_k, r_k), \qquad k = 1, \ldots, m .$$

In particular there exists a constant M such that

$$\mathrm{Lip}(\gamma_k) \le M , \qquad k = 1, \ldots, m .$$

In the sequel we always associate with a Lipschitz domain a finite cover and a uniform Lipschitz constant M.

Assume that $\Omega \subset \mathbb{R}^n$ is bounded with $\partial\Omega$ Lipschitz. We select a minimal cover

$$\{Q(\mathbf{x}_k, r_k) : k = 1, \ldots, m\} .$$

- If $n = 2$, then the *normal vector* $\mathbf{n}$ to γ_k at $(s, \gamma_k(s))^T$ is given by (after possible relabelling of the coordinate axes, see Fig. 9.2)

$$\mathbf{n}(s) = \frac{(\gamma_k'(s), -1)^T}{\sqrt{1 + |\gamma_k'(s)|^2}} .$$

We assume that the domain Ω is above the graph of γ. The normal vector of Ω pointing outwards corresponds to the normal vector of the function γ.

- If $n = 3$, then the *normal vector* $\mathbf{n}$ to γ_k at $\left(s_1, s_2, \gamma_k(s_1, s_2)\right)^T$ is given by (after possibly relabelling of the coordinate axes)

$$\mathbf{n}(s_1, s_2) = - \begin{pmatrix} 1 \\ 0 \\ \frac{\partial \gamma_k}{\partial s_1} \end{pmatrix} \times \begin{pmatrix} 0 \\ 1 \\ \frac{\partial \gamma_k}{\partial s_2} \end{pmatrix}$$

where $\times$ denotes the *outer product*, which is defined for $\mathbf{a}, \mathbf{b} \in \mathbb{R}^3$ by

$$\mathbf{a} \times \mathbf{b} = \left(a_2 b_3 - b_2 a_3, -a_1 b_3 + b_1 a_3, a_1 b_2 - b_1 a_2\right)^T .$$

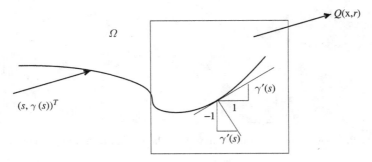

Fig. 9.2. The normal vector on a curve γ.

This in particular shows that

$$\mathbf{n}(s_1, s_2) = \left(\frac{\partial \gamma_k}{\partial s_1}(s_1, s_2), \frac{\partial \gamma_k}{\partial s_2}(s_1, s_2), -1 \right)^T .$$

Geometrical Properties of Functions

Recall that the t-level sets of a function $\phi : \mathbb{R}^n \to \mathbb{R}$ are defined as $\mathrm{level}_t(\phi) = \{\mathbf{x} \in \mathbb{R}^n : \phi(\mathbf{x}) \leq t\}$. In the following we relate the properties of ϕ to geometrical properties of the level sets of ϕ and the according level lines $\partial \, \mathrm{level}_t(\phi)$. In particular we derive a relation between ϕ and the *curvature* of $\partial \, \mathrm{level}_t(\phi)$.

Definition 9.27. *Let $\Omega \subset \mathbb{R}^n$ be open bounded and Lipschitz. A level set function for Ω is a Lipschitz function $\phi : \mathbb{R}^n \to \mathbb{R}$ such that*

$$\Omega = \mathrm{level}_0(\phi), \qquad \partial \Omega = \big\{ \mathbf{x} \in \mathbb{R}^n : \phi(\mathbf{x}) = 0 \big\},$$

and $|\nabla \phi| > 0$ almost everywhere in a neighborhood of $\partial \Omega$. Moreover, we require that ϕ is differentiable $\mathcal{H}^{n-1}$-almost everywhere on $\partial \Omega$.

Example 9.28. A typical level set function ϕ is the *signed distance function* defined by

$$\phi(\mathbf{x}) := \begin{cases} -\,\mathrm{dist}(\mathbf{x}, \partial \Omega), & \text{if } \mathbf{x} \in \Omega, \\ +\,\mathrm{dist}(\mathbf{x}, \partial \Omega), & \text{if } \mathbf{x} \in \mathbb{R}^n \setminus \Omega. \end{cases}$$

$\diamondsuit$

Lemma 9.29. *Let $\Omega \subset \mathbb{R}^n$ be bocL with level set function ϕ. Then the normal vector $\mathbf{n}$ on $\partial \Omega$ satisfies*

$$\mathbf{n} = \frac{\nabla \phi}{|\nabla \phi|} \qquad \mathcal{H}^{n-1}\text{-a.e. on } \partial \Omega .$$

Proof. Let $\gamma(\hat{\mathbf{x}})$ be a local parametrization of $\partial\Omega$ at $\mathbf{x} = (\hat{\mathbf{x}}, x_n)^T$. Without loss of generality we assume that

$$\Omega \cap Q(\mathbf{x}, r) = \{\mathbf{y} = (\hat{\mathbf{y}}, y_n) : \gamma(\hat{\mathbf{y}}) < y_n\} \ .$$

Since ϕ is a level set function for Ω, it follows that $\phi(\mathbf{y}) > 0$ for $\gamma(\hat{\mathbf{y}}) > y_n$, and $\phi(\mathbf{y}) < 0$ for $\gamma(\hat{\mathbf{y}}) < y_n$. In particular $\partial^n\phi(\mathbf{x}) < 0$. From the implicit function theorem (see [228, Thm. 10.1]) it follows that

$$\nabla\gamma(\hat{\mathbf{x}}) = -\frac{\nabla_{\hat{\mathbf{x}}}\phi\big(\hat{\mathbf{x}}, \gamma(\hat{\mathbf{x}})\big)}{\partial^n\phi\big(\hat{\mathbf{x}}, \gamma(\hat{\mathbf{x}})\big)} \ . \tag{9.8}$$

For the sake of simplicity, we omit the arguments of ϕ and γ for the rest of the proof. Inserting (9.8) in the definition for $\mathbf{n}$ (see (9.6)) we find, using the fact that $\partial^n\phi < 0$, that

$$\mathbf{n}(\mathbf{x}) = \frac{(\nabla\gamma, -1)^T}{\sqrt{1 + |\nabla\gamma|^2}} = -\frac{\big(\nabla_{\hat{\mathbf{x}}}\phi/\partial^n\phi, 1\big)^T}{\sqrt{1 + (\nabla_{\hat{\mathbf{x}}}\phi/\partial^n\phi)^2}}$$

$$= -\frac{\partial^n\phi}{|\partial^n\phi|}\frac{\big(\nabla_{\hat{\mathbf{x}}}\phi, \partial^n\phi\big)^T}{\sqrt{(\partial^n\phi)^2 + (\nabla_{\hat{\mathbf{x}}}\phi)^2}} = \frac{\nabla\phi}{|\nabla\phi|} \ .$$

$\square$

Lemma 9.30. *Let $\partial\Omega$ be C^2 and ϕ a level set function for Ω. If $\phi \in C^2(\mathbb{R}^n)$, then the curvature H of $\partial\Omega$ is*

$$H = \frac{1}{n-1}\,\nabla\cdot\left(\frac{\nabla\phi}{|\nabla\phi|}\right) \ .$$

Proof. For every $\mathbf{x} \in \mathbb{R}^n$ we write $\mathbf{x} = (\hat{\mathbf{x}}, x_n)^T$. Let $\gamma(\hat{\mathbf{x}})$ be a local parametrization of $\partial\Omega$ at $\mathbf{x}$. Without loss of generality we assume that

$$\Omega \cap Q(\mathbf{x}, r) = \{\mathbf{y} = (\hat{\mathbf{y}}, y_n) : \gamma(\hat{\mathbf{y}}) < y_n\} \text{ and } \nabla\gamma(\hat{\mathbf{x}}) = 0 \ .$$

From the implicit function theorem (see [228, Thm. 10.1]) it follows that

$$\nabla\gamma(\hat{\mathbf{x}}) = -\frac{\nabla_{\hat{\mathbf{x}}}\phi(\hat{\mathbf{x}}, \gamma(\hat{\mathbf{x}}))}{\partial^n\phi(\hat{\mathbf{x}}, \gamma(\hat{\mathbf{x}}))} \ . \tag{9.9}$$

For the sake of simplicity, we again omit the arguments of ϕ and γ for the rest of the proof. Using the definition of H, see (9.7), we derive with (9.9) that

$$H = \frac{1}{n-1}\sum_{i=1}^{n-1}(\partial^i)^2\gamma = \frac{1}{n-1}\sum_{i=1}^{n-1}\partial^i\left(-\frac{\partial^i\phi}{\partial^n\phi}\right)$$

$$= -\frac{1}{n-1}\sum_{i=1}^{n-1}\frac{(\partial^i)^2\phi\,\partial^n\phi - \partial^i\phi\,\partial^i\partial^n\phi}{(\partial^n\phi)^2} \tag{9.10}$$

$$= -\frac{1}{n-1}\sum_{i=1}^{n}\frac{(\partial^i)^2\phi\,\partial^n\phi - \partial^i\phi\,\partial^i\partial^n\phi}{(\partial^n\phi)^2} \ .$$

Moreover

$$\nabla\cdot\left(\frac{\nabla\phi}{|\nabla\phi|}\right) = \sum_{i=1}^{n}\partial^{i}\left(\frac{\partial^{i}\phi}{|\nabla\phi|}\right) = \sum_{i=1}^{n}\frac{(\partial^{i})^{2}\,|\nabla\phi| - \partial^{i}\phi\,\partial^{i}\,|\nabla\phi|}{|\nabla\phi|^{2}}\,. \qquad (9.11)$$

Since $\nabla\gamma(\hat{\mathbf{x}}) = 0$ and $\Omega = \mathrm{level}_{0}(\phi)$ it follows from (9.9) that

$$-\partial^{n}\phi = |\nabla\phi|\,. \qquad (9.12)$$

Using (9.12) the assertion follows from (9.10) and (9.11).   □

Green's Formula

Theorem 9.31 (Gauss–Green). *Let $\Omega \subset \mathbb{R}^{n}$ be bocL. Denote by $\mathbf{n}$ the outward unit normal to Ω on the boundary $\partial\Omega$. Then*

$$\int_{\Omega}\nabla\cdot(\boldsymbol{\phi}) = \int_{\partial\Omega}\mathbf{n}\cdot\boldsymbol{\phi}\,d\mathcal{H}^{n-1}\,, \qquad \boldsymbol{\phi}:\mathbb{R}^{n}\to\mathbb{R}^{n}\,\, Lipschitz\,.$$

Proof. See [159, 4.5.6, 4.5.11, 4.5.12].   □

Corollary 9.32. *Let $\Omega \subset \mathbb{R}^{n}$ be bocL, and let $\boldsymbol{\phi}:\mathbb{R}^{n}\to\mathbb{R}^{n}$ and $u:\mathbb{R}^{n}\to\mathbb{R}$ be Lipschitz. Then*

$$\int_{\Omega}u\,\nabla\cdot(\boldsymbol{\phi}) + \int_{\Omega}\boldsymbol{\phi}\cdot\nabla u = \int_{\partial\Omega}u\,\mathbf{n}\cdot\boldsymbol{\phi}\,d\mathcal{H}^{n-1}\,. \qquad (9.13)$$

Proof. This follows from Theorem 9.31 and the product rule

$$\nabla\cdot(u\,\boldsymbol{\phi}) = u\,\nabla\cdot(\boldsymbol{\phi}) + \boldsymbol{\phi}\cdot\nabla u\,.$$

□

9.4 Sobolev Spaces

Definition 9.33. *Let $\Omega \subset \mathbb{R}^{n}$ be open, $u \in L_{\mathrm{loc}}^{1}(\Omega)$, and $1 \leq i \leq n$. Denote $g_{i} = \partial^{i}u$ the distributional derivative of u with respect to x_{i}. If $g_{i} \in L_{\mathrm{loc}}^{1}(\Omega)$ (via the identification of locally summable functions with distributions), then g_{i} is called the* weak partial derivative *of u with respect to x_{i}.*

In other words, a weak derivative is a distributional derivative, which can be represented by a locally summable function.

If all weak partial derivatives $\partial^{i}u$, $1 \leq i \leq n$, exist, we define the *weak gradient* of u as

$$\nabla u := \left(\partial^{1}u, \ldots, \partial^{n}u\right)\,.$$

In the sequel we do not notationally distinguish between derivatives and weak derivatives of functions, and distributional derivatives.

Definition 9.34. *Let $1 \le p \le \infty$ and Ω an open subset of $\mathbb{R}^n$.*

1. *The function u belongs to the Sobolev space $W^{1,p}(\Omega)$, if $u \in L^p(\Omega)$ and the weak gradient ∇u exists and belongs to $L^p(\Omega; \mathbb{R}^n)$.*
2. *The function u belongs to $W^{1,p}_{\mathrm{loc}}(\Omega)$ if $u|_V \in W^{1,p}(V)$ for each open set $V \subset\subset \Omega$.*

For $1 \le p < \infty$ and $u \in W^{1,p}(\Omega)$, we define

$$\|u\|_{1,p} := \left(\int_\Omega |u|^p + |\nabla u|^p \right)^{1/p} .$$

Moreover,

$$\|u\|_{1,\infty} := \max\left\{ \|u\|_\infty , \|\,|\nabla u|\,\|_\infty \right\} .$$

The space $W^{1,p}(\Omega)$, $1 \le p \le \infty$, with the norm $\|\cdot\|_{1,p}$ is a Banach space. If $1 < p < \infty$, then $W^{1,p}(\Omega)$ is reflexive. Moreover, $W^{1,2}(\Omega)$ is a Hilbert space with the inner product

$$\langle u, v \rangle := \int_\Omega u\,v + \sum_i \int_\Omega \partial^i u\, \partial^i v .$$

Higher Order Sobolev Spaces

Definition 9.35. *Let $\Omega \subset \mathbb{R}^n$ be open, $u \in L^1_{\mathrm{loc}}(\Omega)$, $l \in \mathbb{N}$, and $1 \le p \le \infty$.*

1. *We say that $u \in W^{l,p}(\Omega)$, if $u \in L^p(\Omega)$, and for all multi-indices γ with $|\gamma| \le l$ the distributional derivative $\partial^\gamma u$ belongs to $L^p(\Omega)$.*
2. *We say that $u \in W^{l,p}_{\mathrm{loc}}(\Omega)$, if for all open sets $V \subset\subset \Omega$ we have $u|_V \in W^{l,p}(V)$.*
   The elements of $W^{l,p}_{\mathrm{loc}}(\Omega)$ (and thus in particular the elements of $W^{l,p}(\Omega)$) are called Sobolev functions.

If $u \in W^{l,p}(\Omega)$ and $0 \le k \le l$ we define

$$\nabla^k u = (\partial^\gamma u)_{|\gamma|=k}$$

as the vector of all k-th order weak partial derivatives of u. In particular, $\nabla^0 u := u$. From the definition of $W^{l,p}(\Omega)$ it follows that $\nabla^k u \in L^p(\Omega; \mathbb{R}^{\mathcal{N}(k)})$ for all $0 \le k \le l$, where $\mathcal{N}(k)$ is as defined in (8.4).

For $1 \le p < \infty$ a norm on $W^{l,p}(\Omega)$ is defined by

$$\|u\|_{l,p} := \left(\sum_{k=0}^l \|\nabla^k u\|_p^p \right)^{1/p}, \qquad u \in W^{l,p}(\Omega) .$$

In the case $p = \infty$ we define

$$\|u\|_{l,\infty} := \max_{0 \le k \le l} \|\nabla^k u\|_\infty , \qquad u \in W^{l,\infty}(\Omega) .$$

We need the following subspaces of $W^{l,p}(\Omega)$:

1. For $l \in \mathbb{N}$ and $1 \leq p < \infty$,

$$W_0^{l,p}(\Omega) := \overline{C_0^\infty(\Omega)},$$

where the closure is taken with respect to $\|\cdot\|_{l,p}$. The space $W_0^{l,p}(\Omega)$ is called homogeneous Sobolev space of l-th order.

2. For $l \in \mathbb{N}$,

$$W_0^{l,\infty}(\Omega) := \left\{ u \in W^{l,\infty}(\Omega) \cap C_B^{l-1}(\Omega) : u = 0 \text{ on } \partial\Omega \right\}.$$

Note that by virtue of Theorem 9.38 below it follows that $W^{l,\infty}(\Omega) \subset C_B^{l-1}(\Omega)$ in case $\partial\Omega$ is Lipschitz.

3. Let $\Omega \subset \mathbb{R}^n$ be bounded. For $1 \leq p \leq \infty$ and $l \in \mathbb{N}$,

$$W_\diamond^{l,p}(\Omega) := \left\{ u \in W^{l,p}(\Omega) : \int_\Omega \partial^\gamma u = 0 \text{ for all } |\gamma| \leq l - 1 \right\}.$$

We call $W_\diamond^{l,p}(\Omega)$ the space of Sobolev functions of l-th order with vanishing moments.

4. For $l \in \mathbb{N}$ and $1 \leq p \leq \infty$ we define the periodic Sobolev space

$$W_0^{l,p}(S^1 \times \Omega) := \overline{C_{\mathrm{per},0}^\infty\big((0, 2\pi) \times \Omega\big)}.$$

Again, the closure is taken with respect to $\|\cdot\|_{l,p}$ on $W^{l,p}\big((0, 2\pi) \times \Omega\big)$. Here $S^1 := \{\mathbf{x} \in \mathbb{R}^2 : |\mathbf{x}| = 1\}$ denotes the unit circle in $\mathbb{R}^2$.

Theorem 9.36. *Let $l \in \mathbb{N}$. The spaces $W^{l,p}(\Omega)$, $W_0^{l,p}(\Omega)$, $W_\diamond^{l,p}(\Omega)$, and $W_0^{l,p}(S^1 \times \Omega)$ are Banach spaces when equipped with the norm $\|\cdot\|_{l,p}$. If $1 \leq p < \infty$ then all above spaces are separable, and if $1 < p < \infty$, they are reflexive. If $p = 2$, they are Hilbert spaces.*

Proof. From [3, Thm. 3.2, Thm. 3.5] it follows that $W^{l,p}(\Omega)$ is a Banach space, separable if $1 \leq p < \infty$, reflexive if $1 < p < \infty$, and a Hilbert space, if $p = 2$. Following Lemma 8.12 it is thus enough to show that $W_0^{l,p}(\Omega)$, $W_\diamond^{l,p}(\Omega)$, and $W_0^{l,p}(S^1 \times \Omega)$ are closed.

The spaces $W_0^{l,p}(\Omega)$ and $W_0^{l,p}(S^1 \times \Omega)$, $1 \leq p \leq \infty$, are closed by definition. Moreover, $W_\diamond^{l,p}(\Omega)$ is the intersection of the kernels of the bounded linear operators $u \mapsto \int_\Omega \partial^\gamma u$, for $|\gamma| \leq l - 1$. This shows that $W_\diamond^{l,p}(\Omega)$ is closed, too. $\qquad\square$

Theorem 9.37. *Let $l \in \mathbb{N}_0$. Then the following hold:*

1. *If $1 \leq p \leq \infty$, then $W^{0,p}(\Omega) = L^p(\Omega)$.*
2. *If $1 \leq p < \infty$, then $W_0^{0,p}(\Omega) = L^p(\Omega)$.*
3. *If $1 \leq p < \infty$, then $W^{l,p}(\Omega) \cap C^\infty(\Omega)$ is dense in $W^{l,p}(\Omega)$.*
4. *If $1 \leq p < \infty$ and $\partial\Omega$ is Lipschitz, then $\{u|_\Omega : u \in C_0^\infty(\mathbb{R}^n)\}$ is dense in $W^{l,p}(\Omega)$. In particular this applies to the case $\Omega = \mathbb{R}^n$, which shows that $W^{l,p}(\mathbb{R}^n) = W_0^{l,p}(\mathbb{R}^n)$.*

5. If $\Omega \subset \mathbb{R}^n$ is bocL and $1 \leq p \leq q \leq \infty$, then $W^{l,q}(\Omega)$ is a dense subset of $W^{l,p}(\Omega)$.

Proof. The first two Items are stated in [3, p. 45], Item 3 follows from [3, Thm. 3.16], Item 4 from [3, Thm. 3.17], and Item 5 follows from Item 4 together with Lemma 9.12 and the fact that $C^\infty(\bar{\Omega}) \subset W^{1,\infty}(\Omega)$.   □

Embedding Theorems

In the following we summarize *Sobolev's embedding* theorems. The results are collected from [3, Chap. V].

Theorem 9.38 (Sobolev embedding). *Assume that $\Omega \subset \mathbb{R}^n$ is an open set with Lipschitz boundary. Let $j, l \in \mathbb{N} \cup \{0\}$, and $1 \leq p < \infty$.*

1. If

$$lp < n \quad and \quad p \leq q \leq \frac{np}{n-lp},$$

then the embedding

$$i: W^{j+l,p}(\Omega) \to W^{j,q}(\Omega), \qquad j \in \mathbb{N} \cup \{0\},$$

is bounded. In particular, the embedding

$$i: W^{l,p}(\Omega) \to L^q(\Omega)$$

is bounded.

2. If

$$lp = n \quad and \quad p \leq q < \infty,$$

then the embedding

$$i: W^{j+l,p}(\Omega) \to W^{j,q}(\Omega), \qquad j \in \mathbb{N} \cup \{0\},$$

is bounded. In particular the embedding

$$i: W^{l,p}(\Omega) \to L^q(\Omega)$$

is bounded.

3. If

$$lp > n,$$

then the embedding

$$i: W^{j+l,p}(\Omega) \to C_B^j(\Omega), \qquad j \in \mathbb{N} \cup \{0\},$$

is bounded.

Proof. See [3, Thm. 5.4].   □

Compact embeddings are usually referred to as *Rellich–Kondrašov embedding* theorems.

Theorem 9.39 (Rellich–Kondrašov). *Let $\Omega \subset \mathbb{R}^n$ be an open set with Lipschitz boundary, and let $\Omega_0 \subset \Omega$ be a* bounded *subdomain. For $j \in \mathbb{N} \cup \{0\}$, $l \in \mathbb{N}$, and $1 \leq p < \infty$ the following embeddings are compact:*

1. *For $lp < n$ and $1 \leq q < np/(n-lp)$ the embedding*

$$i : W^{j+l,p}(\Omega) \to W^{j,q}(\Omega_0) .$$

2. *For $lp = n$ and $1 \leq q < \infty$ the embedding*

$$i : W^{j+l,p}(\Omega) \to W^{j,q}(\Omega_0) .$$

3. *For $lp > n$ the embedding*

$$i : W^{j+l,p}(\Omega) \to C^j(\bar{\Omega}_0) .$$

Proof. See [3, Thm. 6.2]. $\qquad\qquad\qquad\qquad\qquad\qquad\qquad\qquad\qquad\quad$ □

Remark 9.40. The compactness of an embedding $i : W^{j+l,p}(\Omega) \to W^{j,q}(\Omega_0)$ in particular implies that whenever $(u_k) \subset W^{j+l,p}(\Omega)$ weakly converges to u, then $\big(i(u_k)\big)$ strongly converges to $i(u)$ (that is, i is weak-strong sequentially continuous).

Indeed, if $(u_k) \rightharpoonup u$, then the sequence is bounded. Therefore the compactness of i implies that $i(u_k)$ has a strongly convergent subsequence converging to some $v \in W^{j,q}(\Omega_0)$. Since $i(u_k)$ weakly converges to $i(u)$, it follows that $v = i(u)$. Thus the strong convergence of $\big(i(u_k)\big)$ follows from Lemma 8.2. $\quad\Diamond$

Equivalent Norms on $W_0^{l,p}(\Omega)$ and $W_\diamond^{l,p}(\Omega)$

For $u \in W^{l,p}(\Omega)$, $l \in \mathbb{N}$, $1 \leq p \leq \infty$, define the Sobolev semi-norm

$$|u|_{l,p} := \big\|\nabla^l u\big\|_p .$$

Theorem 9.41. *Let $\Omega \subset \mathbb{R}^n$ be bounded. Then there exists a constant $C(\Omega, l, p)$ such that*

$$|u|_{l,p} \leq \|u\|_{l,p} \leq C(\Omega, l, p) |u|_{l,p} , \qquad u \in W_0^{l,p}(\Omega) .$$

In particular, $|\cdot|_{l,p}$ and $\|\cdot\|_{l,p}$ are equivalent norms on $W_0^{l,p}(\Omega)$.

Proof. See [3, Thm. 6.28]. $\qquad\qquad\qquad\qquad\qquad\qquad\qquad\qquad\qquad\qquad\quad$ □

Theorem 9.42. *Let $\Omega \subset \mathbb{R}^n$ be bocL. There exists a constant $C(\Omega, l, p)$ such that*

$$|u|_{l,p} \leq \|u\|_{l,p} \leq C(\Omega, l, p) |u|_{l,p} , \qquad u \in W_\diamond^{l,p}(\Omega) .$$

In particular, $|\cdot|_{l,p}$ and $\|\cdot\|_{l,p}$ are equivalent norms on $W_\diamond^{l,p}(\Omega)$.

Proof. See [405, Thm. 4.4.2]. □

Lemma 9.43. *The semi-norm* $|\cdot|_{l,p}$ *is a norm on* $C_0^\infty(\Omega)$.

Proof. Assume that $u \in C_0^\infty(\Omega)$ with $|u|_{l,p} = 0$.

Let $\Omega_0 \subset \Omega$ be a connected component of Ω. Then in particular $\nabla^l u = 0$ on Ω_0. Since u is arbitrarily differentiable, it follows that $u|_{\Omega_0}$ is a polynomial of degree at most $l - 1$. Since $u \in C_0^\infty(\Omega)$, it follows that $K := \mathrm{supp}(u|_{\Omega_0})$ is compactly contained in Ω_0. In particular, $\Omega_0 \setminus K$ is a non-empty open set, and $u = 0$ on $\Omega_0 \setminus K$. Since $u|_{\Omega_0}$ is a polynomial, this shows that $u = 0$ on Ω_0.

Since this argument applies to every connected component of Ω, this proves that $u = 0$. Consequently, $|\cdot|_{l,p}$ is a norm on $C_0^\infty(\Omega)$. □

If Ω is an unbounded set, then in general the semi-norm $|u|_{l,p}$ is not equivalent to the norm $\|u\|_{l,p}$. We therefore define

$$\widehat{W}^{l,p}(\Omega) := \overline{\{u \in C_0^\infty(\Omega)\}}, \qquad (9.14)$$

the completion of $C_0^\infty(\Omega)$ with respect to $|\cdot|_{l,p}$.

Lemma 9.44. *Assume that* $\Omega \subset \mathbb{R}^n$ *is open and bounded. Then* $\widehat{W}^{l,p}(\Omega) = W_0^{l,p}(\Omega)$.

Proof. From the definition of the completion of a normed linear space in Lemma 8.9 it follows that it is enough to show that $C_0^\infty(\Omega)$ is dense in $W_0^{l,p}(\Omega)$ with respect to the topology induced by $|\cdot|_{l,p}$. From Theorem 9.41 it follows that $|\cdot|_{l,p}$ and $\|\cdot\|_{l,p}$ are equivalent, which shows that they induce the same topologies on $W_0^{l,p}(\Omega)$. Thus the claim follows from the definition of $W_0^{l,p}(\Omega)$. □

Duals of Sobolev Spaces

In the following we characterize bounded linear functionals on Sobolev spaces:

Theorem 9.45. *Assume that* $1 \le p < \infty$ *and* $l \in \mathbb{N}_0$. *For every* $L \in \left(W^{l,p}(\Omega)\right)^*$ *there exists* $\mathbf{v} \in L^{p_*}(\Omega; \mathbb{R}^{\mathcal{N}(l)})$ *such that*

$$\langle L, u \rangle = \sum_{|\gamma| \le l} \int_\Omega v_\gamma \, \partial^\gamma u, \qquad u \in W^{l,p}(\Omega). \qquad (9.15)$$

Moreover,

$$\|L\|_{(W^{l,p}(\Omega))^*} = \min\{\|\mathbf{v}\|_{p_*} : \mathbf{v} \in L^{p_*}(\Omega; \mathbb{R}^{\mathcal{N}(l)}) \text{ satisfies } (9.15)\}.$$

Proof. See [3, Thm. 3.8]. □

Theorem 9.46. *Assume that Ω is bocL, $1 \leq p < \infty$, and $l \in \mathbb{N}_0$. For every $L \in \left(W_\diamond^{l,p}(\Omega)\right)^*$ there exists $\mathbf{v} \in L^{p_*}(\Omega; \mathbb{R}^{\mathcal{N}(l)})$ such that*

$$\langle L, u \rangle = \langle \mathbf{v}, \nabla^l u \rangle_{p,p_*} = \sum_{|\gamma|=l} \int_\Omega v_\gamma \, \partial^\gamma u \,, \qquad u \in W_\diamond^{l,p}(\Omega) \,. \tag{9.16}$$

Moreover,

$$\|L\|_{(W_\diamond^{l,p}(\Omega))^*} = \min\{\|\mathbf{v}\|_{p_*} : \mathbf{v} \in L^{p_*}(\Omega; \mathbb{R}^{\mathcal{N}(l)}) \text{ satisfies } (9.16)\} \,. \tag{9.17}$$

Proof. Let $L \in \left(W_\diamond^{l,p}(\Omega)\right)^*$ and denote $X := L^p(\Omega; \mathbb{R}^{\mathcal{N}(l)})$. From the definition of $|\cdot|_{l,p}$ it follows that the operator $P := \nabla^l : W_\diamond^{l,p}(\Omega) \to X$ is a linear isometry from $W_\diamond^{l,p}(\Omega)$ into a linear subspace G of X. In particular, ∇^l is injective. Thus a linear functional $\tilde{L}$ on G is defined by

$$\tilde{L}(Pu) := L(u) \,, \qquad u \in W_\diamond^{l,p}(\Omega) \,.$$

Since P is an isometry, it follows that

$$\sup\{\tilde{L}(Pu) : \|Pu\|_p = 1\} = \sup\{L(u) : |u|_{l,p} = 1\} = \|L\|_{(W_\diamond^{l,p}(\Omega))^*} \,.$$

In particular, $\tilde{L} : G \to \mathbb{R}$ is bounded. From the Hahn–Banach Theorem 8.20 it follows that there exists an extension $\hat{L} : X \to \mathbb{R}$ such that $\|\hat{L}\|_{X^*} = \|L\|_{(W_\diamond^{l,p}(\Omega))^*}$. Since X^* can be identified with $L^{p_*}(\Omega; \mathbb{R}^{\mathcal{N}(l)})$ (see Lemma 9.11), there exists $\mathbf{v} \in L^{p_*}(\Omega; \mathbb{R}^{\mathcal{N}(l)})$ such that $\|\mathbf{v}\|_{p_*} = \|\hat{L}\|_{X^*}$ and

$$\hat{L}(Pu) = \sum_{|\gamma|=l} \int_\Omega v_\gamma \, \partial^\gamma u \,.$$

This shows (9.16).

Now let $\mathbf{w} \in L^{p_*}(\Omega; \mathbb{R}^{\mathcal{N}(l)})$ be another function satisfying (9.16). Then

$$\|\mathbf{w}\|_{p_*} \geq \sup\left\{\sum_{|\gamma|=l} \int_\Omega w_\gamma \, \partial^\gamma u : |u|_{l,p} \leq 1\right\} = \|L\|_{(W^{l,p}(\Omega))^*} \,.$$

Since on the other hand $\|\mathbf{v}\|_{p_*} = \|L\|_{(W_\diamond^{l,p}(\Omega))^*}$, equation (9.17) follows. $\quad\square$

Theorem 9.47. *Assume that $1 \leq p < \infty$ and $l \in \mathbb{N}_0$. For every $L \in \left(\widehat{W}^{l,p}(\Omega)\right)^*$ there exists $\mathbf{v} \in L^{p_*}(\Omega; \mathbb{R}^{\mathcal{N}(l)})$ such that*

$$\langle L, u \rangle = \langle \mathbf{v}, \nabla^l u \rangle_{p,p_*} = \sum_{|\gamma|=l} \int_\Omega v_\gamma \, \partial^\gamma u \,, \qquad u \in \widehat{W}^{l,p}(\Omega) \,. \tag{9.18}$$

Moreover,

$$\|L\|_{(\widehat{W}^{l,p}(\Omega))^*} = \min\{\|\mathbf{v}\|_{p_*} : \mathbf{v} \in L^{p_*}(\Omega; \mathbb{R}^{\mathcal{N}(l)}) \text{ satisfies } (9.18)\} \,.$$

Proof. This can be shown similarly as Theorem 9.46. $\quad\square$

9.5 Convolution

We recall the definition of the convolution and its properties. We refer to [11] for an overview and [7, 2.12–2.14] for details including proofs.

Definition 9.48 (Convolution). *We define the* convolution $u * v$ *of two functions u, $v \in L^1_{\text{loc}}(\mathbb{R}^n)$ as*

$$(u * v)(\mathbf{x}) := \int_{\mathbb{R}^n} u(\mathbf{y})\, v(\mathbf{x} - \mathbf{y})\, d\mathbf{y}$$

whenever the integral makes sense for almost every $\mathbf{x} \in \mathbb{R}^n$.

Lemma 9.49. *Assume that $u \in L^1(\mathbb{R}^n)$ and $v \in L^p(\mathbb{R}^n)$, $1 \le p \le \infty$. Then $u * v \in L^p(\mathbb{R}^n)$, and $\|u * v\|_p \le \|u\|_1 \|v\|_p$. Moreover, $u * v = v * u$ almost everywhere.*

Theorem 9.50. *Assume that $u \in L^1_{\text{loc}}(\mathbb{R}^n)$ and $v \in C^\infty_0(\mathbb{R}^n)$. Then $u * v = v * u \in C^\infty(\mathbb{R}^n)$, and*

$$\partial^\gamma(u * v) = u * (\partial^\gamma v)$$

for every multi-index γ.

In particular, in the two cases above the convolution is well-defined.

Definition 9.51. *A function $\rho \in C^\infty(\mathbb{R}^n)$ is a* mollifier, *if $\rho(\mathbf{x}) \ge 0$ for all $\mathbf{x}$, $\text{supp}(\rho) \subset \overline{B_1(0)}$, and $\int_{\mathbb{R}^n} \rho = \|\rho\|_1 = 1$.*

If ρ is a mollifier and $\varepsilon > 0$, we define the rescaled functions $\rho_\varepsilon \in C^\infty_0(\mathbb{R}^n)$ setting

$$\rho_\varepsilon(\mathbf{x}) := \varepsilon^{-n} \rho(\mathbf{x}/\varepsilon)\ .$$

The functions ρ_ε, $\varepsilon > 0$, satisfy $\rho_\varepsilon \in C^\infty_0(\mathbb{R}^n)$, $\text{supp}(\rho) \subset \overline{B_\varepsilon(0)}$, and $\|\rho_\varepsilon\|_1 = 1$.

Lemma 9.52. *Let $u \in L^1(\mathbb{R}^n)$ and ρ be a mollifier. Then*

$$\text{supp}(u * \rho_\varepsilon) \subset \overline{\{\mathbf{x} + \mathbf{y} : \mathbf{x} \in \text{supp}(u),\ |\mathbf{y}| < \varepsilon\}}\ .$$

One example of a mollifier is the function

$$\rho(\mathbf{x}) = \begin{cases} C \exp\left(-1/\left(1 - |\mathbf{x}|^2\right)^2\right), & \text{if } |\mathbf{x}| < 1, \\ 0, & \text{if } |\mathbf{x}| \ge 1, \end{cases} \tag{9.19}$$

where C is chosen in such a way that $\int_{\mathbb{R}^n} \rho = 1$.

Lemma 9.53. *Let ρ be a mollifier and $u \in L^p_{\text{loc}}(\mathbb{R}^n)$. Then $u_\varepsilon := \rho_\varepsilon * u$ converges to u in $L^p_{\text{loc}}(\mathbb{R}^n)$ as $\varepsilon \to 0$, that is, $\|u_\varepsilon - u\|_{L^p(V)} \to 0$ for every open set $V \subset\subset \mathbb{R}^n$.*

Similarly, if $u \in W^{l,p}_{\text{loc}}(\mathbb{R}^n)$ for some $l \in \mathbb{N}_0$, then $\partial^\gamma u_\varepsilon \to \partial^\gamma u$ in $L^p_{\text{loc}}(\mathbb{R}^n)$ for every multi-index γ with $|\gamma| \le l$.

If $u \in W^{l,p}(\mathbb{R}^n)$, then $\|u_\varepsilon - u\|_{l,p} \to 0$.

Lemma 9.54. *Let ρ be a mollifier and $u \in C(\mathbb{R}^n)$. Then $u_\varepsilon := \rho_\varepsilon * u$ converges to u locally uniformly, that is, for every $\mathbf{x} \in \mathbb{R}^n$ there exists $r > 0$ such that u_ε uniformly converges to u in $B_r(\mathbf{x})$.*

Example 9.55. Convolving a function with a kernel $\rho \in C^\infty(\mathbb{R}^n)$ is a method for smoothing data $f \in L^1_{\text{loc}}(\mathbb{R}^n)$. Consider for instance the Gaussian kernel K_ε, $\varepsilon > 0$, given by

$$K_\varepsilon(\mathbf{x}) := \left(\frac{1}{\varepsilon\sqrt{2\pi}}\right)^n \exp\left(-\frac{|\mathbf{x}|^2}{2\varepsilon^2}\right).$$

Then $f_\varepsilon := f * K_\varepsilon \in C^\infty(\mathbb{R}^n)$, and $f_\varepsilon \to f$ as $\varepsilon \to 0$. Note moreover that f_ε is a solution of the heat equation (cf. Example 6.35)

$$\partial_t u - \Delta u = 0,$$
$$u(0) = f,$$

at time $t = \sqrt{\varepsilon^2/2}$.

In applications in imaging, the function f is often defined on a rectangle $\Omega \subset \mathbb{R}^2$. Since the convolution requires values on $\mathbb{R}^2$, it is convenient to define an extension $\tilde{f}$ of f to $\mathbb{R}^2$ by mirroring f at $\partial\Omega$. Then the convolution $\tilde{f} * K_\varepsilon$ is computed (see for instance [9]).   ◇

9.6 Sobolev Spaces of Fractional Order

Sobolev spaces of fractional order are often required to characterize the smoothness of the exact solution of an operator equation, for instance in the case of the circular Radon transform. In the following we will introduce the spaces $W^{s,2}(\Omega)$, where $s \geq 0$ and $\Omega \subset \mathbb{R}^n$ is bocL. We essentially follow the method presented in [259, Chap. 1, Sect. 2.1, Sect. 9.1].

Let X and Y be separable Hilbert spaces. Assume that X is dense in Y with respect to the topology on Y, and that the inclusion $i : X \to Y$, $i(x) = x$, is continuous and compact with respect to the topologies on X and Y.

From Theorem 8.39 it follows that i has an SVD (u_k, v_k, σ_k), that is,

$$x = i(x) = \sum_k \sigma_k \langle u_k, x\rangle_X v_k, \qquad x \in X.$$

For $0 \leq \theta \leq 1$, we define $\Lambda^\theta : \mathcal{D}(\Lambda^\theta) \subset Y \to Y$ by

$$\Lambda^\theta y := \sum_k \sigma_k^{-\theta} \langle v_k, y\rangle_Y v_k, \qquad y \in \mathcal{D}(\Lambda^\theta),$$

$$\mathcal{D}(\Lambda^\theta) := \left\{y \in Y : \sum_k \left|\sigma_k^{-\theta} \langle v_k, y\rangle_Y\right| < \infty\right\}.$$

In particular, $\mathcal{D}(\Lambda^0) = Y$ and $\mathcal{D}(\Lambda^1) = i(X) = X$.

We define the *interpolation space* $[X, Y]_\theta := \mathcal{D}(\Lambda^{1-\theta})$, which becomes a Hilbert space with the inner product

$$\langle x, y \rangle_{[X,Y]_\theta} := \langle x, y \rangle_Y + \langle \Lambda^{1-\theta} x, \Lambda^{1-\theta} y \rangle_Y \tag{9.20}$$

and the associated norm $\|x\|_{[X,Y]_\theta} := \left(\langle x, x \rangle_{[X,Y]_\theta} \right)^{1/2}$.

Definition 9.56. *Let* $l \in \mathbb{N}$, $s \in (l, l+1)$ *and* $\Omega \subset \mathbb{R}^n$ *be bocL. The Hilbert space* $W^{s,2}(\Omega)$ *is defined as the interpolation space*

$$W^{s,2}(\Omega) := \left[W^{l+1,2}(\Omega), W^{l,2}(\Omega) \right]_{1+l-s}.$$

The inner product and the norm on $W^{s,2}(\Omega)$ *defined by* (9.20) *are denoted by* $\langle \cdot, \cdot \rangle_{s,2}$ *and* $\|\cdot\|_{s,2}$, *respectively.*

Let $s \in (l, l+1)$. The Sobolev space $W^{l+1,2}(\Omega)$ is dense in $W^{s,2}(\Omega)$ (see [259, Chap. 1, Rem. 2.6]). In particular, this implies that $\{u|_\Omega : u \in C_0^\infty(\mathbb{R}^n)\}$ is dense in $W^{s,2}(\Omega)$, see Theorem 9.37.

Definition 9.57. *Let* $s \geq 0$ *be a non-negative real number and* $\Omega \subset \mathbb{R}^n$ *be bocL. We define*

$$W_0^{s,2}(\Omega) := \overline{C_0^\infty(\Omega)}, \quad W_0^{s,2}(S^1 \times \Omega) := \overline{C_{\mathrm{per},0}^\infty((0, 2\pi) \times \Omega)},$$

where the closures are taken with respect to the topology induced by $\|\cdot\|_{s,2}$. *The dual space of* $W_0^{s,2}(\Omega)$ *is denoted by* $W_0^{-s,2}(\Omega) := \left(W_0^{s,2}(\Omega) \right)^*$.

The spaces $W_0^{s,2}(\Omega)$ and $W_0^{s,2}(S^1 \times \Omega)$ are closed subspaces of $W^{s,2}(\Omega)$ and $W^{s,2}(S^1 \times \Omega)$, respectively.

9.7 Bochner Spaces

Bochner spaces are generalizations of function spaces to mappings defined on arbitrary measure spaces and taking on values in a Banach space. We present the results on Bochner spaces that are needed in this book. More details can be found in [156, Sect. 5.9.2] or [392, §§24–25].

In the following, X always denotes a Banach space with corresponding norm $\|\cdot\|_X$, $I \subset \mathbb{R}_{\geq 0}$ denotes a (possibly unbounded) interval on the positive real line, and $1 \leq p \leq \infty$.

Definition 9.58 (L^p Bochner spaces). *The Bochner space* $L^p(I; X)$ *is the space of measurable functions* $u : I \to X$ *such that*

$$\|u\|_{L^p(I;X)} := \left(\int_I \|u(s)\|_X^p \right)^{1/p} < \infty.$$

For $p = \infty$ *we set*

$$\|u\|_{L^\infty(I;X)} := \operatorname{ess\,sup}_{s \in I} \|u(s)\|_X.$$

Definition 9.59 (*l*-times differentiable Bochner spaces). *The space* $C^l(I; X)$ *is the space of l-times continuously differentiable mappings from I to X satisfying*

$$\|u\|_{C^l(I;X)} := \sum_{m=0}^{l} \sup_{s \in I} \|\partial^m u(s)\|_X < \infty .$$

Definition 9.60. *A function* $u : I \to X$ *is* simple *if there exist a finite number of disjoint Lebesgue measurable sets* $E_i \subset I$, $1 \le i \le m$, *and* $c_i \in X$ *such that*

$$u(s) = \sum_{i=1}^{m} \chi_{E_i}(s) c_i , \qquad a.e.\ s \in I .$$

If u is simple we define its integral by

$$\int_I u := \sum_{i=1}^{m} \mathcal{L}^1(E_i) c_i \in X .$$

A function $u : I \to X$ *is* strongly measurable *if there exists a sequence of simple functions* (u_k) *such that*

$$\lim_k \int_I \|u - u_k\|_X = 0 . \tag{9.21}$$

If u is strongly measurable, then its integral $\int_I u$ *is defined as*

$$\int_I u := \lim_k \int_I u_k , \tag{9.22}$$

where we consider any sequence (u_k) *of simple functions satisfying* (9.21).

Theorem 9.61. *A function* $u : I \to X$ *is strongly measurable if and only if* $u \in L^1(I; X)$. *In this case the integral* $\int_I u$ *defined in* (9.22) *does not depend on the choice of the approximating sequence* (u_k).

Proof. See [401, Sect. V.5].   □

Definition 9.62 (Sobolev Bochner spaces). *Let* $u \in L^1(I; X)$. *If there exists a function* $g \in L^1(I; X)$ *such that*

$$\int_I \phi' u = - \int_I \phi g , \qquad \phi \in C_0^\infty(I) , \tag{9.23}$$

then g is called the weak derivative *of u. In this case we denote* $u' := g$. *Note that the integral in* (9.23) *is the Bochner integral introduced in Definition 9.60.*

The space $W^{1,p}(I; X)$ *is defined as the space of all functions* $u \in L^p(I; X)$ *such that* $u' \in L^p(I; X)$. *The norm on* $W^{1,p}(I; X)$ *is defined as*

$$\|u\|_{W^{1,p}(I;X)} := \begin{cases} \left(\int_I \left(\|u\|_X^p + \|u'\|_X^p\right)\right)^{1/p}, & \text{if } 1 \le p < \infty, \\ \operatorname{ess\,sup}_{s \in I}\left(\|u(s)\|_X + \|u'(s)\|_X\right), & \text{if } p = \infty. \end{cases}$$

A mapping u belongs to $W_{\mathrm{loc}}^{1,p}(I;X)$, the Bochner space of weakly differentiable, locally p-integrable functions with values in the Banach space X if $u|_V \in W^{1,p}(V;X)$ for all open $V \subset\subset I$.

9.8 Functions of Bounded Variation

We review some basic properties of functions of bounded variation, which are mainly collected from [11, 157].

Definition 9.63. *Let $\Omega \subset \mathbb{R}^n$ be open. The space of functions of bounded variation $BV(\Omega)$ on $\Omega \subset \mathbb{R}^n$ consists of those functions $u \in L^1(\Omega)$ such that for every $1 \le i \le n$ the weak derivative $D_i u := \partial^i u$ is a finite Radon measure on Ω. We denote by*

$$Du := (D_1 u, \ldots, D_n u)$$

the vector valued Radon measure of weak partial derivatives of u.

From the definition of the weak derivative it follows that for every $u \in BV(\Omega)$ we have

$$\int_\Omega u\, \partial^i \phi = -\int_\Omega \phi \, \mathrm{d}D_i u, \qquad \phi \in C_0^\infty(\Omega), \quad i = 1, \ldots, n.$$

Definition 9.64. *Let $\Omega \subset \mathbb{R}^n$ be open. We define the total variation (or BV semi-norm) $\mathcal{R}_1(u) \in [0, \infty]$ of $u \in L_{\mathrm{loc}}^1(\Omega)$ as*

$$\mathcal{R}_1(u) := \sup\left\{\int_\Omega u\, \nabla\!\cdot\!(\phi) : \phi \in C_0^\infty(\Omega; \mathbb{R}^n),\ |\phi| \le 1\right\}.$$

Theorem 9.65. *Let $\Omega \subset \mathbb{R}^n$ be open and $u \in L^1(\Omega)$. Then $u \in BV(\Omega)$, if and only if $\mathcal{R}_1(u) < \infty$.*

Proof. See [11, Prop. 3.6]. □

Remark 9.66. Let $u \in BV(\Omega)$. Then $\mathcal{R}_1(u) = |Du|\,(\Omega)$, where $|Du|\,(\Omega)$ denotes the total variation of the Radon measure Du, evaluated on Ω (cf. Theorem 9.18). ◇

Theorem 9.67. *The space $BV(\Omega)$ becomes a Banach space with the norm*

$$\|u\|_{BV} := \|u\|_1 + \mathcal{R}_1(u).$$

The space $BV(\Omega)$ is the dual of a normed linear space. If the set Ω has Lipschitz boundary, this space can be characterized directly from the definition of $BV(\Omega)$. Denote by $\bar{Y}$ the closure of the set

$$Y := \left\{ \phi = (\phi_0, \phi_1, \dots, \phi_n) : (\phi_1, \dots, \phi_n) \in C_0^\infty(\Omega; \mathbb{R}^n), \sum_{i=1}^n \frac{\partial \phi_i}{\partial x_i} = \phi_0 \right\}$$

with respect to $\|\cdot\|_\infty$. It can be shown that $BV(\Omega)$ can be identified with the dual of the quotient space $C_0(\Omega; \mathbb{R}^{n+1})/\bar{Y}$ (see [11, Rem. 3.12]).

The weak* convergence on $BV(\Omega)$ can be characterized as follows:

Lemma 9.68. *A sequence (u_k) in $BV(\Omega)$ weakly* converges to a function $u \in BV(\Omega)$, if and only if $\lim_k \|u_k - u\|_1 = 0$ and $\sup_k \mathcal{R}_1(u_k) < \infty$.*

Proof. See [11, Prop. 3.13]. □

Since $BV(\Omega)$ is the dual of a separable Banach space, it follows that bounded sets are weakly* pre-compact:

Lemma 9.69. *Let $\Omega \subset \mathbb{R}^n$ be bocL. Every sequence (u_k) in $BV(\Omega)$ satisfying*

$$\sup_k \{ \|u_k\|_1 + \mathcal{R}_1(u_k) \} < \infty$$

has a subsequence weakly converging to some function $u \in BV(\Omega)$.*

Proof. See [11, Thm. 3.23]. □

Definition 9.70. *A sequence (u_k) strictly converges to $u \in BV(\Omega)$, if and only if $\lim_k \|u_k - u\|_1 = 0$ and $\lim_k \mathcal{R}_1(u_k) = \mathcal{R}_1(u)$.*

Theorem 9.71. *Let $\Omega \subset \mathbb{R}^n$ be open and $u \in BV(\Omega)$. There exists a sequence $(u_k) \subset C^\infty(\Omega) \cap BV(\Omega)$ strictly converging to u.*

Proof. See [11, Thm. 3.9]. □

Lemma 9.72. *Let $u \in BV(\Omega)$. Then for $\mathcal{H}^{n-1}$-a.e. $\mathbf{x} \in \Omega$ the approximate upper and lower limits*

$$u_+(\mathbf{x}) := \inf \left\{ t \in \mathbb{R} : \lim_{r \to 0} \frac{\mathcal{L}^n\left(\mathrm{level}_t(u) \cap B_r(\mathbf{x}) \right)}{\mathcal{L}^n\left(B_r(\mathbf{x}) \right)} = 1 \right\},$$

$$u_-(\mathbf{x}) := \sup \left\{ t \in \mathbb{R} : \lim_{r \to 0} \frac{\mathcal{L}^n\left(\mathrm{level}_t(u) \cap B_r(\mathbf{x}) \right)}{\mathcal{L}^n\left(B_r(\mathbf{x}) \right)} = 0 \right\},$$

exist. Define

$$\Sigma(u) := \left\{ \mathbf{x} \in \Omega : u_+(\mathbf{x}) > u_-(\mathbf{x}) \right\}.$$

Then $\Sigma(u)$ is σ-finite with respect to $\mathcal{H}^{n-1} \llcorner \Sigma(u)$, and $D^j u := Du \llcorner \Sigma(u) = (u_+ - u_-)\mathcal{H}^{n-1} \llcorner \Sigma(u)$. The set $\Sigma(u)$ is called the jump set of u, and $D^j u$ the jump part of Du.

Proof. This is a consequence of the much stronger statements presented in [11, Thms. 3.76, 3.78, Prop. 3.65]. □

Definition 9.73. *Let* $u \in BV(\Omega)$. *Denote by* ∇u *the Radon–Nikodým derivative of* Du *with respect to* $\mathcal{L}^n$ *and by* $D^s u$ *the singular part. Define moreover* $D^c u := D^s u - D^j u$ *the Cantor part of* Du. *Then we have the decomposition*

$$Du = \nabla u \, \mathcal{L}^n + D^s u = \nabla u \, \mathcal{L}^n + (u_+ - u_-) \, \mathcal{H}^{n-1} \, \llcorner \, \Sigma(u) + D^c u$$

into three mutually singular measures.

If $D^s u = 0$, i.e., $Du = \nabla u \, \mathcal{L}^n$, the function u is contained in the Sobolev space $W^{1,1}(\Omega)$, and the weak derivative of u equals ∇u. More precisely, we have the equality of spaces

$$W^{1,1}(\Omega) = \{u \in BV(\Omega) : D^s u = 0\} \ .$$

Definition 9.74. *Let* $\Omega \subset \mathbb{R}^n$ *be open, and let* $E \subset \Omega$ *be measurable with* $\mathcal{L}^n(E) < \infty$. *The perimeter* $\mathrm{Per}(E; \Omega)$ *of* E *in* Ω *is defined as*

$$\mathrm{Per}(E; \Omega) := \mathcal{R}_1(\chi_E) \ .$$

If $\mathrm{Per}(E; \Omega) < \infty$ *we say that* E *is a* set of finite perimeter *in* Ω.

Theorem 9.75 (Coarea formula). *Let* $\Omega \subset \mathbb{R}^n$ *be open and bounded, and* $u \in L^1_{\mathrm{loc}}(\Omega)$. *Then* $u \in BV(\Omega)$, *if and only if*

$$\int_{-\infty}^{+\infty} \mathrm{Per}(\{u > t\}; \Omega) \, \mathrm{d}t = c < \infty \ .$$

In this case, $c = \mathcal{R}_1(u)$. *In particular, if* $u \in BV(\Omega)$, *then for almost every* t *the set* $\{u > t\}$ *has finite perimeter.*

Proof. See [11, Thm. 3.40]. □

Definition 9.76. *Let* $\Omega \subset \mathbb{R}^n$ *be open and bounded. The space* $BV_\diamond(\Omega)$ *consists of all functions of bounded variation with zero mean, that is,*

$$BV_\diamond(\Omega) = BV(\Omega) \cap L^1_\diamond(\Omega) \ .$$

Note that the function $u \mapsto \int_\Omega u$ is continuous with respect to the weak* topology on $BV(\Omega)$. Thus $BV_\diamond(\Omega)$ is the kernel of a weakly* continuous functional, and thus a weakly* closed subspace of $BV(\Omega)$.

Theorem 9.77. *Let* $\Omega \subset \mathbb{R}^n$ *be bocL. There exists a constant* $C(\Omega)$ *such that*

$$\mathcal{R}_1(u) \leq \|u\|_{BV} \leq C(\Omega)\mathcal{R}_1(u) \,, \qquad u \in BV_\diamond(\Omega) \ .$$

In particular, $\mathcal{R}_1(u)$ *is a norm on* $BV_\diamond(\Omega)$ *that is equivalent to* $\|\cdot\|_{BV}$.

Proof. See [11, Thm. 3.44]. □

Theorem 9.78. *Let $\Omega \subset \mathbb{R}^n$ be bocL. Then the embedding*

$$i : BV(\Omega) \to L^q(\Omega)$$

is continuous for every $1 \le q \le n/(n-1)$. Moreover, it is compact for $1 \le q < n/(n-1)$.

Proof. See [11, Cor. 3.49]. □

Theorem 9.79. *Let $n \ge 2$. There exists a constant $C(n)$ such that*

$$\|u\|_{n/(n-1)} \le C(n)\mathcal{R}_1(u), \qquad u \in BV(\mathbb{R}^n).$$

In particular, $BV(\mathbb{R}^n)$ is continuously embedded in $L^{n/(n-1)}(\mathbb{R}^n)$. Moreover, $\mathcal{R}_1(u)$ is a norm on $BV(\mathbb{R}^n)$.

Moreover, there exists a constant $C(1)$ such that

$$\|u\|_\infty \le C(1)\mathcal{R}_1(u), \qquad u \in BV(\mathbb{R}),$$

which implies that $BV(\mathbb{R})$ is continuously embedded in $L^\infty(\mathbb{R})$ and that $\mathcal{R}_1(u)$ is a norm on $BV(\mathbb{R})$.

Proof. See [11, Thm. 3.47]. □

Definition 9.80. *We define*

$$\widehat{BV}(\mathbb{R}^n) := \overline{BV(\mathbb{R}^n)},$$

where the completion is taken with respect to the norm $\mathcal{R}_1(u)$. From Theorem 9.77 it follows that $\widehat{BV}(\mathbb{R}^n) \subset L^{n/(n-1)}(\mathbb{R}^n)$.

Functions of Bounded Higher Order Variation

Definition 9.81. *Let $\Omega \subset \mathbb{R}^n$ be open, and $l \in \mathbb{N}$. The space $BV^l(\Omega)$ of functions of bounded l-th order variation consists of those functions $u \in L^1(\Omega)$ such that $\partial^\gamma u \in L^1(\Omega)$ for all multi-indices γ with $|\gamma| < l$, and $\partial^\gamma u$ is a finite Radon measure for all multi-indices γ with $|\gamma| = l$.*

If $u \in BV^l(\Omega)$ we denote by

$$D^l u := (\partial^\gamma u)_{|\gamma|=l}$$

the vector valued Radon measure of l-th order derivatives of u.

Lemma 9.82. *Let $\Omega \subset \mathbb{R}^n$ be open. Then $u \in BV^l(\Omega)$, if and only if $u \in W^{l-1,1}(\Omega)$, and $\partial^\gamma u \in BV(\Omega)$ for all multi-indices γ with $|\gamma| = l - 1$.*

Proof. This follows from the definition of $BV^l(\Omega)$ and the fact that the distributional derivative satisfies $\partial^{\gamma+\sigma} u = \partial^\gamma \partial^\sigma u$ whenever γ and σ are multi-indices. $\qquad \square$

We define for $u \in L^1_{\mathrm{loc}}(\Omega)$ the *l-th order total variation* (or *l-th order BV semi-norm*)

$$\mathcal{R}_l(u) := \sup \left\{ \int_\Omega u \, (\nabla^l \cdot \phi) : \phi \in C^\infty_0(\Omega; \mathbb{R}^{\mathcal{N}(l)}), \; |\phi| \le 1 \right\}. \qquad (9.24)$$

Note that there exists $C \ge 1$ only depending on n and l such that

$$C^{-1} \mathcal{R}_l(u) \le \sum_{|\gamma|=l-1} \mathcal{R}_1(\partial^\gamma u) \le C \mathcal{R}_l(u), \qquad u \in L^1_{\mathrm{loc}}(\Omega).$$

Consequently it follows as in the case of functions of bounded variation, that $u \in BV^l(\Omega)$ if and only if $u \in L^1(\Omega)$ and $\mathcal{R}_l(u) < \infty$.

On $BV^l(\Omega)$ we define the norm

$$\|u\|_{BV^l} := \|u\|_{l-1,1} + \mathcal{R}_l(u).$$

The space $BV^l(\Omega)$ with $\|\cdot\|_{BV^l}$ is a Banach space.

We say that a sequence $(u_k) \subset BV^l(\Omega)$ *weakly* converges* to $u \in BV^l(\Omega)$, if $\|u_k - u\|_{l-1,1} \to 0$, and $\sup_k \mathcal{R}_l(u_k) < \infty$.

Theorem 9.83. *Let $(u_k) \subset BV^l(\Omega)$ be a sequence satisfying $\sup_k \|u_k\|_{BV^l} < \infty$. Then there exists a subsequence $(u_{k'})$ weakly* converging to a function $u \in BV^l(\Omega)$.*

Proof. For every multi-index γ with $|\gamma| \le l-1$ we have $\partial^\gamma u_k \in BV(\Omega)$, $k \in \mathbb{N}$, and $\sup_k \|u_k\|_{BV} < \infty$. Consequently, it follows from Lemma 9.69 applied to the sequences $(\partial^\gamma u_k)$, $|\gamma| \le l-1$, that there exists a subsequence $(u_{k'})$ such that $\|\partial^\gamma u_{k'} - \partial^\gamma u\|_1 \to 0$ and $\sup_{k'} \mathcal{R}_1(\partial^\gamma u_{k'}) < \infty$ for all $|\gamma| \le l-1$. This subsequence has the properties required in the assertion. $\qquad \square$

Definition 9.84. *Let $\Omega \subset \mathbb{R}^n$ be bounded and $l \in \mathbb{N}$. We define*

$$BV^l_\diamond(\Omega) := BV^l(\Omega) \cap W^{l-1,1}_\diamond(\Omega).$$

The space $BV^l_\diamond(\Omega)$ is a closed subspace of $BV^l(\Omega)$, and thus a Banach space.

Lemma 9.85. *The space $BV^l_\diamond(\Omega)$ is weakly* sequentially closed. That is, whenever $(u_k) \subset BV^l_\diamond(\Omega)$ weakly* converges to a function $u \in BV^l(\Omega)$, then $u \in BV^l_\diamond(\Omega)$.*

Proof. From the definition of the weak* convergence on $BV^l(\Omega)$, it follows that (u_k) strongly converges to u in $W^{l-1,1}(\Omega)$. Since $W^{l-1,1}_\diamond(\Omega)$ is a (strongly) closed subspace of $W^{l-1,1}(\Omega)$, we obtain that $u \in W^{l-1,1}_\diamond(\Omega)$, which proves the claim. $\qquad \square$

Theorem 9.86. *Let $\Omega \subset \mathbb{R}^n$ be bocL. There exists a constant $C(\Omega, l)$ such that*
$$\mathcal{R}_l(u) \leq \|u\|_{BV^l} \leq C(\Omega, l)\mathcal{R}_l(u), \qquad u \in BV^l_\diamond(\Omega) \,.$$

Proof. This is a consequence of Theorems 9.42 and 9.77.   □

Lemma 9.87. *The l-th order total variation $\mathcal{R}_l(u)$ is a norm on $BV^l(\mathbb{R}^n)$.*

Proof. Assume that $\mathcal{R}_l(u) = 0$. Applying Theorem 9.79 to the derivatives $\partial^\gamma u$, $|\gamma| = l - 1$, it follows that $\partial^\gamma u = 0$ for all $|\gamma| = l - 1$, which shows that $\mathcal{R}_{l-1}(u) = 0$. Iterative application of Theorem 9.79 thus shows that $u = 0$.   □

Definition 9.88. *Let $l \in \mathbb{N}$. We define*
$$\widehat{BV}^l(\mathbb{R}^n) := \overline{BV^l(\mathbb{R}^n)} \,,$$

where the completion is formed with respect to the norm $\mathcal{R}_l(u)$.

One-dimensional Functions of Bounded Variation

We now consider the one-dimensional case $\Omega \subset \mathbb{R}$. In this case it can be shown that functions of bounded variation are fairly regular.

For the following results we first need some notation. We define for $x_0 \in \Omega$ and $u \in L^1_{\mathrm{loc}}(\Omega)$ the one-sided essential lower and upper limits

$$\operatorname*{ess\,lim\,inf}_{x \to x_0^+} u(x) := \sup_{\varepsilon > 0} \operatorname{ess\,inf}\{u(x) : x \in (x_0, x_0 + \varepsilon)\} \,,$$

$$\operatorname*{ess\,lim\,sup}_{x \to x_0^+} u(x) := \inf_{\varepsilon > 0} \operatorname{ess\,sup}\{u(x) : x \in (x_0, x_0 + \varepsilon)\} \,,$$

$$\operatorname*{ess\,lim\,inf}_{x \to x_0^-} u(x) := \sup_{\varepsilon > 0} \operatorname{ess\,inf}\{u(x) : x \in (x_0 - \varepsilon, x_0)\} \,,$$

$$\operatorname*{ess\,lim\,sup}_{x \to x_0^-} u(x) := \inf_{\varepsilon > 0} \operatorname{ess\,sup}\{u(x) : x \in (x_0 - \varepsilon, x_0)\} \,.$$

In case $\operatorname{ess\,lim\,inf}_{x \to x_0^\pm} u(x)$ and $\operatorname{ess\,lim\,sup}_{x \to x_0^\pm} u(x)$ coincide, we define

$$u^{(l)}(x_0) := \operatorname*{ess\,lim\,inf}_{x \to x_0^-} u(x) = \operatorname*{ess\,lim\,sup}_{x \to x_0^-} u(x) \,,$$

$$u^{(r)}(x_0) := \operatorname*{ess\,lim\,inf}_{x \to x_0^+} u(x) = \operatorname*{ess\,lim\,sup}_{x \to x_0^+} u(x) \,.$$

Theorem 9.89. *Let $u \in BV(\Omega)$ with $\Omega = (a, b) \subset \mathbb{R}$. For every $x \in \Omega$ there exist $u^{(l)}(x)$ and $u^{(r)}(x)$, and they are equal outside of $\Sigma(u)$. In particular, u almost everywhere equals the function $\tilde{u}(x) := \big(u^{(l)}(x) + u^{(r)}(x)\big)/2$.*

Moreover, there exist $u^{(r)}(a)$ and $u^{(l)}(b)$. In particular, for every $\Omega \subset\subset \tilde{\Omega} \subset\subset \mathbb{R}$ the function

$$\tilde{u}(x) := \begin{cases} u^{(l)}(b), & x \geq b, \\ u(x), & x \in \Omega, \\ u^{(r)}(a), & x \leq a, \end{cases}$$

is in $BV(\tilde{\Omega})$.

Proof. See [11, Thm. 3.28]. □

In this book we will always identify u with the *good representative* $\tilde{u}$ defined in Theorem 9.89. Using this identification it follows that $u^{(l)}(x)$ and $u^{(r)}(x)$ exist for every $x \in \Omega$, and $u^{(l)}(x) = u^{(r)}(x) = u(x)$ for $x \notin \Sigma(u)$.

If additionally $u \in W^{1,1}(\Omega)$, then u is continuous on Ω.

The following result shows the relation between u and its derivative Du:

Lemma 9.90. *Let* $u \in BV(\Omega)$ *and* $x_0 \in \Omega$. *Then*

$$\begin{aligned} u^{(l)}(x) &= u^{(l)}(x_0) + Du([x_0, x)) = u^{(r)}(x_0) + Du((x_0, x)), \\ u^{(r)}(x) &= u^{(l)}(x_0) + Du([x_0, x]) = u^{(r)}(x_0) + Du((x_0, x]), \end{aligned} \qquad x \geq x_0 .$$

In particular, u is non-decreasing in $[x_0, x]$ if and only if $Du \llcorner [x_0, x]$ is a positive Radon measure.

Proof. See [11, Thm. 3.28]. □

Corollary 9.91. *The function* $u \in BV(\Omega)$ *is non-decreasing, if and only if*

$$\int_\Omega u\,\phi' \leq 0, \qquad \phi \in C_0^\infty(\Omega), \ \phi \geq 0 .$$

Proof. From Lemma 9.90 it follows that u is non-decreasing if and only Du is a positive Radon measure. Thus the assertion follows from the definition of Du and the characterization of positive Radon measures in Theorem 9.18. □

Lemma 9.92. *Let* $\Omega = (a, b) \subset \mathbb{R}$ *be an open and bounded interval. For every* $u \in BV^l(\Omega)$ *with* $l \in \mathbb{N}$ *there exists a sequence* $(u_k) \subset C^\infty(\bar{\Omega})$ *with* $\|u - u_k\|_1 \to 0$ *and* $\mathcal{R}_l(u_k) \to \mathcal{R}_l(u)$.

Proof. We prove the assertion by induction on l.

First let $l = 1$. From Theorem 9.89 it follows that we can continue u by a function $\tilde{u} \in BV(a - 1, b + 1)$ by setting $\tilde{u}(x) = u^{(r)}(a)$ for $x < a$, and $\tilde{u}(x) = u^{(l)}(b)$ for $x > b$. From Theorem 9.71 it follows that there exists a sequence (u_k) in $BV(a - 1, b + 1)$ such that $\|u_k - u\|_1 \to 0$ and $\mathcal{R}_1(u_k) \to \mathcal{R}_1(\tilde{u}) = \mathcal{R}_1(u)$. Thus, the sequence $(u_k|_\Omega)$ has the desired properties.

Now assume that the assertion holds for $l - 1$. Since $u' \in BV^{l-1}(\Omega)$, it follows that there exists a sequence $(\tilde{u}_k)$ in $BV^{l-1}(\Omega)$ with $\|\tilde{u}_k - u'\|_1 \to 0$, and $\mathcal{R}_{l-1}(\tilde{u}_k) \to \mathcal{R}_{l-1}(u') = \mathcal{R}_l(u)$. Define

$$u_k(x) := (u')^{(r)}(a) + \int_a^x \tilde{u}_k .$$

Then $\mathcal{R}_l(u_k) = \mathcal{R}_{l-1}(u_k') = \mathcal{R}_{l-1}(\tilde{u}_k) \to \mathcal{R}_l(u)$, and

$$\|u_k - u\|_1 = \int_a^b |u_k - u| \le \int_a^b \int_a^x |\tilde{u}_k - u'| \le (b-a) \|\tilde{u}_k - u'\|_1 \to 0 .$$

Thus the assertion follows. $\square$

10

Convex Analysis and Calculus of Variations

In the following, we review some basic concepts of convex analysis (see, for instance, [27, 143, 144]).

Definition 10.1. *Let U be a linear space, and $K \subset U$. The set K is convex, if*

$$\lambda u + (1 - \lambda)v \in K, \qquad u, v \in K, \ \lambda \in (0,1).$$

If $E \subset U$, we denote by

$$\mathrm{conv}(E) := \bigcap \{K : E \subset K, \ K \ convex\},$$

the convex hull of E.

Definition 10.2. *Let U be a linear space and $\mathcal{S} : U \to \mathbb{R} \cup \{\infty\}$ a functional.*

1. *The domain of $\mathcal{S}$ is the set*

$$\mathcal{D}(\mathcal{S}) := \{u \in U : \mathcal{S}(u) \neq \infty\}.$$

2. *The functional $\mathcal{S}$ is proper, if $\mathcal{D}(\mathcal{S}) \neq \emptyset$.*
3. *The functional $\mathcal{S}$ is convex, if it satisfies*

$$\mathcal{S}(\lambda u + (1-\lambda)v) \leq \lambda \mathcal{S}(u) + (1-\lambda)\mathcal{S}(v), \quad u, v \in U, \quad \lambda \in (0,1). \quad (10.1)$$

   Here we use the convention that $\infty \leq \infty$, $\infty + \infty = \infty$, and $t \cdot \infty = \infty$ for $t > 0$.
4. *The functional $\mathcal{S}$ is strictly convex, if the inequality (10.1) is strict whenever $u \neq v \in \mathcal{D}(\mathcal{S})$.*

Remark 10.3. Note that the definition of convexity implies that a functional $\mathcal{S} : U \to \mathbb{R} \cup \{\infty\}$ is convex, if and only if the restriction of $\mathcal{S}$ to every line $\{u + tv : t \in \mathbb{R}\}$ with $u, v \in U$ is a convex function. ◇

O. Scherzer et al., *Variational Methods in Imaging*,
© Springer Science+Business Media, LLC 2009

10.1 Convex and Lower Semi-continuous Functionals

We recall the fundamental relation between lower semi-continuity of S and properties of its epigraph.

Theorem 10.4. *Let U be a locally convex space and $S : U \to \mathbb{R} \cup \{\infty\}$. The following conditions are equivalent:*

1. *S is lower semi-continuous.*
2. *The epigraph*

$$\mathrm{epi}(S) := \big\{(u, \alpha) \in U \times \mathbb{R} : S(u) \leq \alpha \big\}$$

   of S is closed.

The following conditions are equivalent:

1. *S is convex.*
2. *$\mathrm{epi}(S)$ is convex.*

Moreover, if S is convex, then $\mathrm{level}_\alpha(S)$ is convex for every α.

Proof. See [144, Chap. I, Prop. 2.1, Prop. 2.3].   □

Note, however, that the convexity of every level set of S does not imply the convexity of S. This can be seen by considering the non-convex function $S : \mathbb{R} \to \mathbb{R}$, $S(t) = \sqrt{|t|}$.

Lemma 10.5. *Let U be a locally convex space and (S_i) be a family of functionals on U with values in $\mathbb{R} \cup \{\infty\}$. Denote by $S := \sup_i S_i$ their pointwise supremum.*

- *If every functional S_i is convex, then S is convex.*
- *If every functional S_i is lower semi-continuous, then S is lower semi-continuous.*

Proof. See [144, Chap. I, Prop. 2.2] for the first part of the assertion.

For the second part of the assertion, note that $\mathrm{epi}\, S = \bigcap_i \mathrm{epi}\, S_i$. Thus the assertion follows from Theorem 10.4, as the intersection of closed sets is closed.   □

Lemma 10.6. *Every lower semi-continuous and convex functional S on the locally convex space U is weakly lower semi-continuous.*

Proof. See [144, Chap. I, Cor. 2.2].   □

In particular, Lemma 10.6 applies to the norm on a Banach space U.

Proposition 10.7. *Let* $1 \leq p < \infty$, $\Omega \subset \mathbb{R}^n$ *be open and let* $U := L^p(\Omega)$ *be associated with the* L^p *norm. For every* $1 < s < \infty$ *and* $1 \leq l < \infty$, *define* $\mathcal{S} : U \to \mathbb{R} \cup \{\infty\}$ *by*

$$\mathcal{S}(u) := \left\| \nabla^l u \right\|_s = \left(\int_\Omega |\nabla^l u|^s \right)^{1/s}$$

whenever defined, and $\mathcal{S}(u) := \infty$, *if* u *is not* l-*times weakly differentiable or* $\nabla^l u \notin L^s(\Omega)$. *Then* $\mathcal{S}$ *is convex and lower semi-continuous.*

Proof. Let L_u be the distribution defined by u (see Example 9.22). Recall that the distributional l-th order gradient of u is the linear functional on $C_0^\infty(\Omega; \mathbb{R}^{\mathcal{N}(l)})$ defined by

$$(\nabla^l L_u)\phi = (-1)^l \int_\Omega u \left(\nabla^l \cdot \phi \right), \qquad \phi \in C_0^\infty(\Omega; \mathbb{R}^{\mathcal{N}(l)}).$$

Now note that $C_0^\infty(\Omega; \mathbb{R}^{\mathcal{N}(l)}) \subset L^{s*}(\Omega; \mathbb{R}^{\mathcal{N}(l)})$, which implies that $\nabla^l L_u$ can be regarded as linear functional on a subspace of $L^{s*}(\Omega; \mathbb{R}^{\mathcal{N}(l)})$. Moreover, $\nabla^l L_u$ is bounded, if and only if

$$\left\| \nabla^l L_u \right\|_{(L^{s*})^*} = \sup \left\{ (\nabla^l L_u)\phi : \phi \in C_0^\infty(\Omega; \mathbb{R}^{\mathcal{N}(l)}), \ \|\phi\|_{s*} \leq 1 \right\} < \infty.$$

Because $C_0^\infty(\Omega; \mathbb{R}^{\mathcal{N}(l)})$ is dense in $L^{s*}(\Omega; \mathbb{R}^{\mathcal{N}(l)})$, it follows that in this (and only this) case, the operator $\nabla^l L_u$ can be extended in a unique way to an operator $\hat{L}_u \in \left(L^{s*}(\Omega; \mathbb{R}^{\mathcal{N}(l)}) \right)^*$. From the definition of the weak gradient and the identification of $\left(L^{s*}(\Omega; \mathbb{R}^{\mathcal{N}(l)}) \right)^*$ with $L^s(\Omega; \mathbb{R}^{\mathcal{N}(l)})$ via the isomorphism $\Im_{s*}$, it follows that $\nabla^l u = \Im_{s*} \hat{L}_u$ and $\left\| \nabla^l u \right\|_s = \left\| \nabla^l L_u \right\|_{(L^{s*})^*}$. This shows that

$$\mathcal{S}(u) = \sup \left\{ (-1)^l \int_\Omega u \left(\nabla^l \cdot \phi \right) : \phi \in C_0^\infty(\Omega; \mathbb{R}^{\mathcal{N}(l)}), \ \|\phi\|_{s*} \leq 1 \right\}.$$

Thus, $\mathcal{S}$ is the pointwise supremum of the bounded linear functionals $u \mapsto (-1)^l \int_\Omega u \left(\nabla^l \cdot \phi \right)$. Consequently, it follows from Lemma 10.5 that $\mathcal{S}$ is convex and lower semi-continuous. $\square$

Proposition 10.8. *Let* $\Omega \subset \mathbb{R}^n$ *be open and bounded,* $l \in \mathbb{N}$, *and* $1 \leq p < \infty$. *Define* $\mathcal{S} : L^p(\Omega) \to \mathbb{R} \cup \{\infty\}$ *by* $\mathcal{S}(u) := \mathcal{R}_l(u)$ *if* $u \in BV^l(\Omega)$ *and* ∞ *otherwise. Then* $\mathcal{S}$ *is convex and lower semi-continuous.*

Proof. Note that

$$\mathcal{S}(u) = \sup \left\{ \mathcal{F}_\phi(u) : \phi \in C_0^\infty(\Omega; \mathbb{R}^{\mathcal{N}(l)}), \ \|\phi\|_\infty \leq 1 \right\},$$

where $\mathcal{F}_\phi(u) := (-1)^l \int_\Omega u \left(\nabla^l \cdot \phi \right)$. As in the proof of Proposition 10.7, it follows that $\mathcal{F}_\phi$ is convex and lower semi-continuous. Taking into account Lemma 10.5, this implies that $\mathcal{S}$ is convex and lower semi-continuous. $\square$

10.2 Fenchel Duality and Subdifferentiability

Definition 10.9. *Assume that U is a locally convex space. The* dual, *also called the* polar, *of the proper functional $S : U \to \mathbb{R} \cup \{\infty\}$ is defined as*

$$S^* : U^* \to \mathbb{R} \cup \{\infty\}, \quad u^* \mapsto S^*(u^*) := \sup_{u \in U} (\langle u^*, u \rangle - S(u)),$$

where $\langle \cdot, \cdot \rangle$ denotes the dual pairing with respect to U^* and U.

For a definition of the dual in a finite dimensional space setting, we refer to [334], and for the infinite dimensional setting, we refer to [27, 144].

The next result summarizes some basic properties of dual functionals:

Theorem 10.10. *Let $S : U \to \mathbb{R} \cup \{\infty\}$ be proper. The following assertions hold:*

1. *The functional S^* is weakly* lower semi-continuous and convex.*
2. *For every $\alpha > 0$,*

$$(\alpha S)^*(u^*) = \alpha S^*(u^*/\alpha).$$

3. *For every $t \in \mathbb{R}$,*

$$(S + t)^*(u^*) = S^*(u^*) - t.$$

4. *Let*

$$T(u) = S(u - u_0)$$

for some $u_0 \in U$. Then

$$T^*(u^*) = S^*(u^*) + \langle u^*, u_0 \rangle.$$

Proof. See [144, Sect. I.4].   □

Convention 10.11 *If $1 \le p < \infty$ and $U = L^p(\Omega)$, we regard the dual of $S : U \to \mathbb{R} \cup \{\infty\}$ as a functional on $L^{p*}(\Omega)$. More precisely, we identify $S^* : \big(L^p(\Omega)\big)^* \to \mathbb{R} \cup \{\infty\}$ with the functional $S^* \circ \Im_p^{-1} : L^{p*}(\Omega) \to \mathbb{R} \cup \{\infty\}$.*

Lemma 10.12. *Assume that U is a Banach space and that $\phi : \mathbb{R} \to \mathbb{R} \cup \{\infty\}$ is a lower semi-continuous, convex, and proper function satisfying $\phi(-t) = \phi(t)$ for all $t \in \mathbb{R}$. Define*

$$S : U \to \mathbb{R} \cup \{\infty\}, \qquad S(u) := \phi(\|u\|_U).$$

The dual of S is

$$S^* : U^* \to \mathbb{R} \cup \{\infty\}, \qquad S^*(u^*) = \phi^*(\|u^*\|_{U*}),$$

where $\phi^* : \mathbb{R} \to \mathbb{R} \cup \{\infty\}$ is the dual of ϕ.

Proof. See [144, Chap. I, Prop. 4.2].   □

We use Theorem 10.10 and Lemma 10.12 to compute the dual in one simple but important case:

Example 10.13. Let $1 \leq p < \infty$ and p_* be the conjugate of p. Let $\Omega \subset \mathbb{R}^n$ be open, and $u^\delta \in L^p(\Omega)$.

We compute the dual of the functional

$$S_p(u) = \frac{1}{p} \|u - u^\delta\|_p^p =: T(u - u^\delta) .$$

From Theorem 10.10, it follows that

$$(S_p)^*(u^*) = T^*(u^*) + \langle u^*, u^\delta \rangle .$$

Let $\phi : \mathbb{R} \to \mathbb{R}$, $\phi(t) := \frac{1}{p} |t|^p$, then from Lemma 10.12 it follows that

$$T^*(u^*) = \phi^*(\|u^*\|_{p_*}) .$$

The dual of ϕ is

$$\phi^*(t^*) = \sup_{t \in \mathbb{R}} \left(tt^* - \frac{1}{p} |t|^p \right) .$$

The supremum is attained at $t \in \mathbb{R}$ satisfying $t^* = |t|^{p-1} \operatorname{sgn}(t)$.

In the case $p > 1$, this shows that $\phi^*(t^*) = \frac{1}{p_*} |t^*|^{p_*}$, which implies that

$$(S_p)^*(u^*) = \frac{1}{p_*} \int_\Omega |u^*|^{p_*} + \int_\Omega u^* u^\delta .$$

In the case $p = 1$, we obtain that

$$(S_1)^*(u^*) = \begin{cases} \infty, & \text{if } \|u^*\|_\infty > 1, \\ \int_\Omega u^* u^\delta, & \text{else .} \end{cases}$$

$\diamondsuit$

Definition 10.14. *Let U be a locally convex space and $S : U \to \mathbb{R} \cup \{\infty\}$ be convex. The subdifferential $\partial S(u) \subset U^*$ of S at $u \in U$ is defined as the set of all $u^* \in U^*$ satisfying*

$$S(v) - S(u) - \langle u^*, v - u \rangle \geq 0, \qquad v \in U .$$

Similarly, we define the subdifferential $\partial S^*(u^*)$ of S^* at $u^* \in U^*$ as the set of all $u \in U$ satisfying

$$S^*(v^*) - S^*(u^*) - \langle v^* - u^*, u \rangle \geq 0, \qquad v^* \in U^* .$$

If $\partial S(u)$ contains only a single element, we always identify this element with the set $\partial S(u) \in 2^{U^*}$.

The subdifferential of $\mathcal{S}$ at $u \in U$ is a (possibly empty) weakly* closed and convex subset of U^* (see [144, Chap. I, Cor. 5.1]).

Lemma 10.15. *Let $\mathcal{S} : U \to \mathbb{R} \cup \{\infty\}$ be convex. Then $u \in U$ is a minimizer of $\mathcal{S}$, if and only if $0 \in \partial\mathcal{S}(u)$.*

Proof. The definition of $\partial\mathcal{S}(u)$ implies that $0 \in \partial\mathcal{S}(u)$ if and only if $\mathcal{S}(u) \leq \mathcal{S}(v)$ for all $v \in U$, which is equivalent to stating that u minimizes $\mathcal{S}$.   □

The next result collects some important properties of the subdifferential.

Lemma 10.16. *Let $\mathcal{S} : U \to \mathbb{R} \cup \{\infty\}$ be convex and $\lambda > 0$. Then*

$$\partial(\lambda\mathcal{S})(u) = \lambda\,\partial\mathcal{S}(u)\,, \qquad u \in U\,.$$

Let $\mathcal{S}$, $\mathcal{R} : U \to \mathbb{R} \cup \{\infty\}$ be convex and assume that there exists $v \in \mathcal{D}(\mathcal{R}) \cap \mathcal{D}(\mathcal{S})$ such that $\mathcal{S}$ is continuous in v. Then

$$\partial(\mathcal{S} + \mathcal{R})(u) = \partial\mathcal{S}(u) + \partial\mathcal{R}(u)\,, \qquad u \in U\,.$$

Let U and V be locally convex spaces, $L \in L(U, V)$, and $\mathcal{S} : V \to \mathbb{R} \cup \{\infty\}$ convex. Assume that there exists $v \in V$ such that $\mathcal{S}(v) < \infty$ and $\mathcal{S}$ is continuous in v. Then

$$\partial(\mathcal{S} \circ L)(u) = L^{\#}\big(\partial\mathcal{S}(Lu)\big)\,, \qquad u \in U\,.$$

Here $L^{\#} : V^* \to U^*$ is the dual-adjoint of L (see Proposition 8.18).

Proof. See [143, Chap. I, Prop. 5.6, Prop. 5.7].   □

Convention 10.17 *As in the case of the dual space, we consider for $U = L^p(\Omega)$, $1 \leq p < \infty$, the subdifferential of $\mathcal{S} : L^p(\Omega) \to \mathbb{R} \cup \{\infty\}$ as a subset of $L^{p*}(\Omega)$. More precisely, we identify $\partial\mathcal{S}(u)$ with the set $\Im_p\big(\partial\mathcal{S}(u)\big)$.*

The following result relates the subdifferential of $\mathcal{S}$ with the dual functional $\mathcal{S}^*$.

Theorem 10.18. *Assume that U is a locally convex space and $\mathcal{S} : U \to \mathbb{R} \cup \{\infty\}$ is convex and proper. Then, from $u^* \in \partial\mathcal{S}(u)$, it follows that $u \in \partial\mathcal{S}^*(u^*)$. If $\mathcal{S}$ additionally is lower semi-continuous, then also the converse implication holds.*

Moreover, we have the characterization $u^* \in \partial\mathcal{S}(u)$ if and only if

$$\mathcal{S}(u) + \mathcal{S}^*(u^*) = \langle u^*, u \rangle\,.$$

Proof. See [144, Chap. I, Prop. 5.1, Cor. 5.2].   □

Definition 10.19. *Let U be locally convex and let*

$$\mathcal{T}(u) := \mathcal{S}(u) + \mathcal{R}(u) , \qquad u \in U ,$$

where $\mathcal{S}$, $\mathcal{R} : U \to \mathbb{R} \cup \{\infty\}$ are convex. The Fenchel transform $\mathcal{T}^* : U^* \to \mathbb{R} \cup \{\infty\}$ is defined as

$$\mathcal{T}^*(u^*) := \mathcal{S}^*(u^*) + \mathcal{R}^*(-u^*) , \qquad u^* \in U^* .$$

Remark 10.20. Note that the Fenchel transform strongly depends on the choice of the decomposition of $\mathcal{T}$ in two convex functionals $\mathcal{S}$ and $\mathcal{R}$. ◇

Theorem 10.21. *Let U be locally convex and $\mathcal{S}$, $\mathcal{R} : U \to \mathbb{R} \cup \{\infty\}$ be convex, lower semi-continuous, and proper.*
If $u^\dagger$ minimizes $\mathcal{T} := \mathcal{S} + \mathcal{R}$, that is,

$$u^\dagger = \arg \min \big(\mathcal{S}(u) + \mathcal{R}(u) \big) , \tag{10.2}$$

$u^{\dagger *}$ minimizes the Fenchel transform of $\mathcal{T}$, that is,

$$u^{\dagger *} = \arg \min \big(\mathcal{S}^*(u^*) + \mathcal{R}^*(-u^*) \big) , \tag{10.3}$$

and

$$\inf_{u \in U} \big(\mathcal{S}(u) + \mathcal{R}(u) \big) = - \inf_{u^* \in U^*} \big(\mathcal{S}^*(u^*) + \mathcal{R}^*(-u^*) \big) < \infty , \tag{10.4}$$

then

$$\mathcal{S}(u^\dagger) + \mathcal{R}(u^\dagger) + \mathcal{S}^*(u^{\dagger *}) + \mathcal{R}^*(-u^{\dagger *}) = 0 . \tag{10.5}$$

Conversely, if $u \in U$ and $u^* \in U^*$ satisfy (10.5), then u, u^* satisfy (10.2), (10.3), and (10.4), respectively.

Moreover, the extremality condition (10.5) is equivalent to either of the Kuhn–Tucker conditions

$$\boxed{u^{\dagger *} \in \partial \mathcal{S}(u^\dagger) \qquad and \qquad -u^{\dagger *} \in \partial \mathcal{R}(u^\dagger) ,}$$

or

$$\boxed{u^\dagger \in \partial \mathcal{S}^*(u^{\dagger *}) \qquad and \qquad u^\dagger \in \partial \mathcal{R}^*(-u^{\dagger *}) .}$$

Proof. This follows from [144, Chap. III, Prop. 2.4, Prop. 4.1, Rem. 4.2]. ☐

Theorem 10.22. *Let U be locally convex and $\mathcal{S}$, $\mathcal{R} : U \to \mathbb{R} \cup \{\infty\}$ be convex, lower semi-continuous, and proper. Moreover, assume that one of the functionals $\mathcal{S}$ or $\mathcal{R}$ is continuous in one point and that there exists $v \in U$ with $\mathcal{S}(v) + \mathcal{R}(v) < \infty$. Then (10.4) holds.*

Proof. See [144, Chap. III, Thm. 4.1]. ☐

10.3 Duality Mappings

Definition 10.23. *Let U be a Banach space.*

1. *A continuous and strictly increasing function $\phi : [0, \infty) \to [0, \infty)$ satisfying $\phi(0) = 0$ and $\lim_{t \to \infty} \phi(t) = \infty$ is called* weight function.
2. *The* duality mapping *according to the weight function ϕ is the set-valued mapping $\mathcal{J} : U \to 2^{U^*}$ defined by*

$$\mathcal{J}(u) = \left\{ u^* \in U^* : \langle u^*, u \rangle_{U^*, U} = \|u^*\|_{U^*} \|u\|_U , \ \|u^*\|_{U^*} = \phi(\|u\|_U) \right\} .$$

3. *In the case $\phi(t) = t$, which implies that $\|u\|_U = \|u^*\|_{U^*}$ for every $u^* \in \mathcal{J}(u)$, the mapping $\mathcal{J}$ is called* normalized *duality mapping.*

It can be shown that the set $\mathcal{J}(u)$ is non-empty for every $u \in U$.

Remark 10.24. Let ϕ be a weight function, then its primitive $\Phi(t) = \int_0^t \phi(s) \, \mathrm{d}s$ is convex. $\Diamond$

Theorem 10.25 (Asplund's theorem). *Let U be a Banach space and Φ the primitive of a weight function on $[0, \infty)$. Then*

$$\mathcal{J}(u) = \partial\Phi(\|u\|_U) , \qquad u \in U .$$

In particular, the normalized duality mapping $\mathcal{J}$ is the subdifferential of the mapping $u \mapsto \frac{1}{2} \|u\|_U^2$.

Proof. See [108, Chap. 1, Thm. 4.4]. $\square$

Lemma 10.26. *Let U be a reflexive Banach space and ϕ a weight function with corresponding duality mapping $\mathcal{J} : U \to 2^{U^*}$. Denote by $\mathcal{J}_* : U^* \to 2^{U^{**}}$ the duality mapping on U^* with respect to ϕ^{-1}. Then $\mathcal{J}_* = i\mathcal{J}^{-1}$, where $i : U \to U^{**}$ is the isomorphism between the reflexive space U and its bi-dual U^{**} (see (8.1)).*

Proof. See [108, Chap. 2, Cor. 3.5]. $\square$

The mapping $\mathcal{J}_*$ is called the *adjoint duality mapping*.

Note that in Lemma 10.26, the inverse $\mathcal{J}^{-1}$ has to be understood set valued in the sense that

$$\mathcal{J}^{-1}(u^*) = \left\{ u \in U : u^* \in \mathcal{J}(u) \right\} .$$

Example 10.27. We present two examples of duality mappings:

1. On $L^p(\Omega)$, the duality mapping with respect to the weight $\phi(t) = t^{p-1}$ is given by

$$\mathcal{J}_{L^p}(u) = (\Im_p)^{-1} \circ \mathcal{J}_p(u) , \quad u \in L^p(\Omega) ,$$

   where

$$\mathcal{J}_p : L^p(\Omega) \to L^{p^*}(\Omega) ,$$
$$u \mapsto |u|^{p-2} u . \tag{10.6}$$

$\mathcal{J}_p$ is called the *p-duality mapping*. The *p*-duality mapping satisfies:
a)

$$\int_\Omega \mathcal{J}_p(u)\, u = \|u\|_{L^p}^p = \|\mathcal{J}_p(u)\|_{L^{p*}}^{p*} \,.$$

b) $(\mathcal{J}_p)^{-1} = \mathcal{J}_{p*}$ and $\mathcal{J}_2 = \mathrm{Id}$.

c) $(\mathfrak{I}_p)^{-1} \circ \mathcal{J}_p(u)$ is an element of the subdifferential of the functional $v \mapsto \|v\|_{L^p}^p$ for $u \in L^p(\Omega)$.

2. We consider the spaces $W_\diamond^{1,p}(\Omega)$ and $W_0^{1,p}(\Omega)$ associated with the norm $\left(\int_\Omega |\nabla u|^p\right)^{1/p}$. Then the duality mappings with respect to the weight $\phi(t) = t^{p-1}$ are given by

$$\mathcal{J}_{W_\diamond^{1,p}} : W_\diamond^{1,p}(\Omega) \to \left(W_\diamond^{1,p}(\Omega)\right)^* ,$$

$$u \mapsto -\nabla \cdot \left(|\nabla u|^{p-2} \nabla u\right) ,$$

and

$$\mathcal{J}_{W_0^{1,p}} : W_0^{1,p}(\Omega) \to \left(W_0^{1,p}(\Omega)\right)^* ,$$

$$u \mapsto -\nabla \cdot \left(|\nabla u|^{p-2} \nabla u\right) .$$

Proof. The duality mappings for the norms on $L^p(\Omega)$ and $W_0^{1,p}(\Omega)$ have been computed in [108, Chap. 2, Prop. 4.9, Prop. 4.12]. The computation for $W_0^{1,p}(\Omega)$, however, remains valid in the space $W_\diamond^{1,p}(\Omega)$. $\quad\square$

Remark 10.28. If U is a Hilbert space, then the Riesz Representation Theorem 8.25 implies the existence of a linear isometric isomorphism $\mathcal{J}_U : U \to U^*$. Let moreover $\mathcal{J} : U \to 2^{U^*}$ be the normalized duality mapping on U. Then $\mathcal{J} = \mathcal{J}_U$ in the sense that $\mathcal{J}(u) = \{\mathcal{J}_U(u)\}$, $u \in U$. $\quad\diamond$

For more background on duality mappings, we refer to [108, Chaps. I–II].

10.4 Differentiability of Functionals and Operators

We recall the definitions of directional derivatives of functionals $\mathcal{F}$ and operators F. For a survey on various concepts of differentiability, we refer to [109].

Definition 10.29. *A Banach space X has a* Fréchet differentiable norm, *if* $\lim_{t\to 0}(\|x + ty\| - \|x\|)/t$ *exists for all $x \in S = \{z \in X : \|z\| = 1\}$, and the convergence is uniform for all $y \in S$.*

Definition 10.30. *Let $F : U \to V$ be an operator between normed spaces U and V.*

1. *The operator F admits a one-sided directional derivative $F'(u; h) \in V$ at $u \in U$ in direction $h \in U$, if*

$$F'(u; h) = \lim_{t\to 0^+} \frac{F(u + th) - F(u)}{t} \,. \tag{10.7}$$

2. Let $u \in U$, and assume that $F'(u; h)$ exists for all $h \in U$. If there exists a bounded linear operator $F'(u) \in L(U, V)$ such that

$$F'(u; h) = F'(u)h, \qquad h \in U,$$

then F is Gâteaux differentiable, and $F'(u)$ is called the Gâteaux derivative of F at u.

3. The operator F is Fréchet differentiable at u, if it is Gâteaux differentiable and the convergence in (10.7) is uniform with respect to $h \in B_\rho(0)$ for some $\rho > 0$.

If $\mathcal{F} : U \to \mathbb{R} \cup \{\infty\}$ is an extended real valued functional, we use a different terminology for one-sided directional derivatives, as it is necessary to include the possibility that they become $\pm\infty$.

Definition 10.31. Let U be a linear space and $\mathcal{F} : U \to \mathbb{R} \cup \{\infty\}$ a functional. The one-sided directional derivative of $\mathcal{F}$ at $u \in \mathcal{D}(\mathcal{F})$ is defined as

$$\mathcal{F}'(u; h) := \limsup_{t \to 0^+} \frac{\mathcal{F}(u + th) - \mathcal{F}(u)}{t}, \qquad h \in U.$$

Note that $\mathcal{F}'(u; h)$ exists for every $u \in \mathcal{D}(\mathcal{F})$ and $h \in U$, but may take the values $\pm\infty$.

In case $\mathcal{F}$ is a convex functional, the subdifferential and the Gâteaux derivative are related as follows:

Lemma 10.32. Let U be locally convex, let $\mathcal{F} : U \to \mathbb{R} \cup \{\infty\}$ be convex, and $u \in U$. If $\mathcal{F}$ is Gâteaux differentiable in u, then $\partial\mathcal{F}(u)$ consists of a single element again denoted by $\partial\mathcal{F}(u) \in U^*$, and $\mathcal{F}'(u) = \partial\mathcal{F}(u)$.

Conversely, if $\mathcal{F}$ is continuous and finite in a neighborhood of u, and if $\partial\mathcal{F}(u)$ consists of a single element, then $\mathcal{F}$ is Gâteaux differentiable in u and $\mathcal{F}'(u) = \partial\mathcal{F}(u)$.

If $U = \mathbb{R}^n$ is finite-dimensional, then $\mathcal{F}$ is differentiable almost everywhere in the interior of its domain.

Proof. See [144, Chap. I, Prop. 5.3] for the differentiability of convex functionals on general locally convex spaces and [334, Thm. 25.5] for the finite-dimensional case. $\qquad\square$

Remark 10.33. Let U be a linear space and $\mathcal{F} : U \to \mathbb{R} \cup \{\infty\}$. If $u \in U$ is a minimizer of $\mathcal{F}$, then by definition

$$\mathcal{F}(u + th) - \mathcal{F}(u) \geq 0, \qquad h \in U, \, t > 0.$$

Consequently,

$$\mathcal{F}'(u; h) \geq 0, \qquad h \in U. \tag{10.8}$$

If $\mathcal{F} : U \to \mathbb{R}$ is Gâteaux differentiable, then (10.8) is equivalent to

$$\mathcal{F}'(u) = 0 \ . \qquad\qquad (10.9)$$

The conditions (10.8) and (10.9) are called *(first order) optimality conditions* for a minimizer of $\mathcal{F}$. $\qquad\qquad\qquad\qquad\qquad\qquad\qquad\qquad\qquad\diamond$

Theorem 10.34 (Chain rule). *Let U, V, and W be Banach spaces, and let $F : U \to V$ and $G : V \to W$ be Fréchet differentiable. Then $G \circ F : U \to W$ is Fréchet differentiable and*

$$(G \circ F)'(u) = G'\big(F(u)\big) \circ F'(u) \ , \qquad u \in U \ .$$

Proof. See [390, Satz III.5.4]. $\qquad\qquad\qquad\qquad\qquad\qquad\qquad\qquad\qquad\square$

Example 10.35. We consider quadratic Tikhonov regularization in a Hilbert space U, where we have to minimize a functional

$$\mathcal{T}_{\alpha,v}(u) = \|F(u) - v\|_V^2 + \alpha \|u - u_0\|_U^2 \ .$$

Here $F : U \to V$ is assumed to be Fréchet differentiable, $v^\delta \in V$, $u_0 \in U$, and $\alpha > 0$. Following Remark 10.33 and Theorem 10.34, a minimizer u_α satisfies the equation $\mathcal{T}'_{\alpha,v}(u)h = 0$ for all $h \in U$, that is,

$$2 \langle F(u_\alpha) - v, F'(u_\alpha)h\rangle_V + 2\alpha \langle u_\alpha - u_0, h\rangle_U = 0 \ , \qquad h \in U \ ,$$

or equivalently,

$$F'(u_\alpha)^* \big(F(u_\alpha) - v\big) + \alpha(u_\alpha - u_0) = 0 \ .$$

More generally, let U and V be Banach spaces and let Φ and G be primitives of weight functions ϕ and g, respectively. Moreover, let $F : U \to V$ be Fréchet differentiable, $v^\delta \in V$, $u_0 \in U$, and $\alpha > 0$. Let $\mathcal{J}_\phi : V \to 2^{V^*}$ and $\mathcal{J}_g : U \to 2^{U^*}$ be the duality mappings with respect to ϕ and g, respectively. Then the optimality condition for a minimizer of

$$\mathcal{T}_{\alpha,v^\delta}(u) = G\big(\big\|F(u) - v^\delta\big\|_V\big) + \alpha\Phi(\|u - u_0\|_U)$$

reads as

$$\big\langle \mathcal{J}_g(F(u) - v^\delta), F'(u)h\big\rangle_{V^*,V} + \alpha \big\langle \mathcal{J}_\phi(u - u_0), h\big\rangle_{U^*,U} \ni 0 \ , \qquad h \in U \ ,$$

or equivalently

$$F'(u)^\# \mathcal{J}_g(F(u) - v^\delta) + \alpha\mathcal{J}_\phi(u - u_0) \ni 0 \ .$$

Note the difference of the adjoints appearing in the optimality conditions in Banach and Hilbert spaces. $\qquad\qquad\qquad\qquad\qquad\qquad\qquad\qquad\qquad\diamond$

10.5 Derivatives of Integral Functionals on $L^p(\Omega)$

In the following, we review some results for characterizing subdifferentials of functionals

$$\mathcal{F} : L^p(\Omega; \mathbb{R}^m) \to \mathbb{R} \cup \{\infty\}, \qquad \mathbf{v} \mapsto \int_\Omega f(\mathbf{x}, \mathbf{v}(\mathbf{x})) . \tag{10.10}$$

For arbitrary measurable functions f, the integral in (10.10) may not be well-defined, as the composition of two measurable functions need not be measurable anymore. Therefore, we have to impose a regularity condition on the integrand f.

Definition 10.36. Let $f : \Omega \times \mathbb{R}^m \to \mathbb{R} \cup \{\infty\}$.

1. *We call f normal, if*
   - *$f(\mathbf{x}, \cdot)$ is lower semi-continuous for almost every $\mathbf{x} \in \Omega$,*
   - *there exists a Borel function $\tilde{f} : \Omega \times \mathbb{R}^m \to \mathbb{R} \cup \{\infty\}$ such that for almost every $\mathbf{x} \in \Omega$*

$$\tilde{f}(\mathbf{x}, \mathbf{s}) = f(\mathbf{x}, \mathbf{s}), \qquad \mathbf{s} \in \mathbb{R}^m .$$

2. *We call f a Carathéodory function, if*
   - *$f(\mathbf{x}, \cdot)$ is continuous for almost every $\mathbf{x} \in \Omega$,*
   - *$f(\cdot, \mathbf{s})$ is measurable for every $\mathbf{s} \in \mathbb{R}^m$.*

Lemma 10.37. *Let $f : \Omega \times \mathbb{R}^m \to \mathbb{R} \cup \{\infty\}$. The integrand f is Carathéodory (normal), if and only if for every $\varepsilon > 0$, there exists a compact set $K \subset \Omega$ with $\mathcal{L}^n(\Omega \setminus K) < \varepsilon$ such that f is continuous (lower semi-continuous) on $K \times \mathbb{R}^m$.*

Proof. See [335, Thm. 2F]. □

We recall the relations between Carathéodory, normal, and Borel functions:

$$\boxed{\text{f Carathéodory} \implies \text{f normal} \implies \text{f equivalent to a Borel function.}}$$

The first implication follows from Lemma 10.37, the second from the definition of normal functions.

Lemma 10.38. *Assume that $f : \Omega \times \mathbb{R}^m \to \mathbb{R} \cup \{\infty\}$ is normal. Then for every measurable function $\mathbf{v} : \Omega \to \mathbb{R}^m$, the function $\mathbf{x} \mapsto f(\mathbf{x}, \mathbf{v}(\mathbf{x}))$ is measurable.*

Proof. See [335, Sect. 3]. □

In particular, the integral

$$\mathcal{F}(\mathbf{v}) := \int_\Omega f(\mathbf{x}, \mathbf{v}(\mathbf{x}))$$

is well-defined (but may be infinite), if the negative part of the function $\mathbf{x} \mapsto f(\mathbf{x}, \mathbf{v}(\mathbf{x}))$ is summable.

Note that, in the examples used in this book, the function f is mostly assumed to be non-negative. In this case, normality of f already implies that the integral $\mathcal{F}(\mathbf{v})$ is well-defined.

Theorem 10.39. *Let f be a normal integrand on $\Omega \times \mathbb{R}^m$ such that $\mathcal{F}$ is proper. Assume that for almost every $\mathbf{x} \in \Omega$ the function $\mathbf{s} \mapsto f(\mathbf{x}, \mathbf{s})$ is convex. Then*

$$\partial \mathcal{F}(\mathbf{v}) = \left\{ \mathbf{v}^* \in L^{p_*}(\Omega; \mathbb{R}^m) : \mathbf{v}^*(\mathbf{x}) \in \partial f(\mathbf{x}, \mathbf{v}(\mathbf{x})) \ a.e. \right\} . \tag{10.11}$$

Here, the subdifferential of f is understood to be computed only with respect to $\mathbf{v}(\mathbf{x})$.

Proof. See [335, Cor. 3E]. ☐

Example 10.40. Let $1 \le p < \infty$. We consider the functional

$$\mathcal{F} : L^p(\Omega) \to \mathbb{R}, \quad u \to \frac{1}{p} \int_\Omega \left| u - u^\delta \right|^p .$$

Because $\mathcal{F}(u^\delta) = 0$, it follows that $\mathcal{F}$ is proper.

The function $f : \Omega \times \mathbb{R} \to \mathbb{R} \cup \{\infty\}$, $(\mathbf{x}, u) \to \frac{1}{p} \left| u - u^\delta(\mathbf{x}) \right|^p$ is normal and convex with respect to u. Thus we have for $u \in L^p(\Omega)$ that

$$\partial \mathcal{F}(u) = \left\{ \left| u - u^\delta \right|^{p-1} \operatorname{sgn}(u - u^\delta) \right\} .$$

◇

Example 10.41. Consider a function $\mathcal{F} : W_0^{1,2}(\Omega) \to \mathbb{R} \cup \{\infty\}$,

$$\mathcal{F}(u) := \int_\Omega f(\mathbf{x}, u(\mathbf{x}), \nabla u(\mathbf{x})) ,$$

where $f : \Omega \times (\mathbb{R} \times \mathbb{R}^n) \to \mathbb{R} \cup \{\infty\}$ is a normal and convex integrand. In order to minimize $\mathcal{F}$, it is necessary and sufficient to solve the inclusion $0 \in \partial \mathcal{F}(u)$. Now denote $j : W_0^{1,2}(\Omega) \to L^2(\Omega) \times L^2(\Omega; \mathbb{R}^n)$, $u \mapsto (u, \nabla u)$. Then $\mathcal{F} = \mathcal{G} \circ j$, where

$$\mathcal{G}(\tilde{v}, \mathbf{v}) = \int_\Omega f(\mathbf{x}, \tilde{v}(\mathbf{x}), \mathbf{v}(\mathbf{x})) , \qquad (\tilde{v}, \mathbf{v}) \in L^2(\Omega) \times L^2(\Omega; \mathbb{R}^n) .$$

From Lemma 10.16, it follows that

$$\partial \mathcal{F}(u) = j^* \, \partial \mathcal{G}(u, \nabla u) . \tag{10.12}$$

Using Theorem 10.39, we obtain that

$$\partial \mathcal{G}(u, \nabla u) = \left(\partial_u f(\mathbf{x}, u, \nabla u), \partial_{\nabla u} f(\mathbf{x}, u, \nabla u) \right), \qquad (10.13)$$

where the right-hand side is to be understood as in (10.11), and $\partial_u f$ and $\partial_{\nabla u} f$ denote the gradients of $f(\mathbf{x}, u, \nabla u)$ with respect to u and ∇u, respectively.

The adjoint j^* is defined by the equation

$$\langle \nabla u, \nabla j^*(\tilde{v}, \mathbf{v}) \rangle_2 = \langle u, \tilde{v} \rangle_2 + \langle \nabla u, \mathbf{v} \rangle_2 ,$$

where $u \in W_0^{1,2}(\Omega)$, and $(\tilde{v}, \mathbf{v}) \in L^2(\Omega) \times L^2(\Omega; \mathbb{R}^n)$. This shows that $w :=$ $j^*(\tilde{v}, \mathbf{v})$ is a solution of the equation

$$\nabla \cdot (\nabla w - \mathbf{v}) = -\tilde{v}$$

in $W_0^{1,2}(\Omega)$. Formally denoting $j^*(\tilde{v}, \mathbf{v}) := \Delta^{-1}(\nabla \cdot (\mathbf{v}) - \tilde{v})$, we obtain from (10.12) and (10.13) that the optimality condition $0 \in \partial \mathcal{F}(u)$ reads as

$$0 = \Delta^{-1} \left(\partial_u f(\mathbf{x}, u, \nabla u) - \nabla \cdot (\partial_{\nabla u} f(\mathbf{x}, u, \nabla u)) \right),$$

or simplified, as the *Euler–Lagrange* equation

$$\partial_u f(\mathbf{x}, u, \nabla u) = \nabla \cdot \left(\partial_{\nabla u} f(\mathbf{x}, u, \nabla u) \right) .$$

References

1. R. Acar and C. R. Vogel. Analysis of bounded variation penalty methods for ill-posed problems. *Inverse Probl.*, 10(6):1217–1229, 1994.
2. E. Acerbi and N. Fusco. Semicontinuity problems in the calculus of variations. *Arch. Ration. Mech. Anal.*, 86(2):125–145, 1984.
3. R. A. Adams. *Sobolev Spaces*. Academic Press, New York, 1975.
4. M. L. Agranovsky, K. Kuchment, and E. T. Quinto. Range descriptions for the spherical mean Radon transform. *J. Funct. Anal.*, 248(2):344–386, 2007.
5. Y. Alber and I. Ryazantseva. *Nonlinear Ill-posed Problems of Monotone Type*. Springer-Verlag, Dordrecht, 2006.
6. S. Alliney. Digital filters as absolute norm regularizers. *IEEE Trans. Signal Process.*, 40(6):1548–1562, 1992.
7. H. W. Alt. *Lineare Funktionalanalysis*. Springer-Verlag, 3rd edition, 1999.
8. L. Alvarez, F. Guichard, P.-L. Lions, and J.-M. Morel. Axioms and fundamental equations of image processing. *Arch. Ration. Mech. Anal.*, 123(3):199–257, 1993.
9. L. Alvarez, P.-L. Lions, and J.-M. Morel. Image selective smoothing and edge detection by nonlinear diffusion. II. *SIAM J. Numer. Anal.*, 29(3):845–866, 1992.
10. U. Amato and W. Hughes. Maximum entropy regularization of Fredholm integral equations of the first kind. *Inverse Probl.*, 7(6):793–808, 1991.
11. L. Ambrosio, N. Fusco, and D. Pallara. *Functions of Bounded Variation and Free Discontinuity Problems*. Oxford University Press, New York, 2000.
12. L. Ambrosio, N. Gigli, and G. Savaré. *Gradient Flows: In Metric Spaces and in the Space of Probability Measures*. Birkhäuser, Boston, 2005.
13. L. Ambrosio and V. M. Tortorelli. Approximation of functionals depending on jumps by elliptic functionals via Γ-convergence. *Comm. Pure Appl. Math.*, 43(8):999–1036, 1990.
14. L. Ambrosio and V. M. Tortorelli. On the approximation of free discontinuity problems. *Boll. Un. Mat. Ital. B*, 6:105–123, 1992.
15. L. E. Andersson. On the determination of a function from spherical averages. *SIAM J. Math. Anal.*, 19(1):214–232, 1988.
16. V. A. Andreev, A. A. Karabutov, S. V. Solomatin, E. V. Savateeva, V. Aleynikov, Y. V. Zhulina, R. D. Fleming, and A. A. Oraevsky. Opto-acoustic tomography of breast cancer with arc-array transducer. In *[305]*, pages 36–47, 2000.

288   References

17. V. G. Andreev, A. A. Karabutov, and A. A. Oraevsky. Detection of ultrawide-band ultrasound pulses in optoacoustic tomography. *IEEE Trans. Ultrason., Ferroeletr., Freq. Control*, 50(10):1383–1390, 2003.

18. F. Andreu, C. Ballester, V. Caselles, and J. M. Mazón. Minimizing total variation flow. *C. R. Acad. Sci. Paris Sér I Math.*, 331(11):867–872, 2000.

19. F. Andreu, C. Ballester, V. Caselles, and J. M. Mazón. The Dirichlet problem for the total variation flow. *J. Funct. Anal.*, 180(2):347–403, 2001.

20. F. Andreu, C. Ballester, V. Caselles, and J. M. Mazón. Minimizing total variation flow. *Differential Integral Equations*, 14(3):321–360, 2001.

21. F. Andreu, V. Caselles, J. I. Díaz, and J. M. Mazón. Some qualitative properties for the total variation flow. *J. Funct. Anal.*, 188(2):516–547, 2002.

22. F. Andreu-Vaillo, V. Caselles, and J. M. Mazón. *Parabolic Quasilinear Equations Minimizing Linear Growth Functionals*, volume 223 of *Progress in Mathematics*. Birkhäuser Verlag, Basel, 2004.

23. L. Antonuk and M. Yaffe, editors. *Medical Imaging 2002: Physics of Medical Imaging*, volume 4682 of *Proceedings of SPIE*, 2002.

24. G. Aubert and J.-F. Aujol. Modeling very oscillating signals. Application to image processing. *Appl. Math. Optim.*, 51(2):163–182, 2005.

25. G. Aubert and J.-F. Aujol. A variational approach to remove multiplicative noise. *SIAM J. Appl. Math.*, 68(4):925–946, 2008.

26. G. Aubert and P. Kornprobst. *Mathematical Problems in Image Processing*. Springer-Verlag, New York, 2002.

27. J.-P. Aubin. *Mathematical Methods of Game and Economic Theory*, volume 7 of *Studies in Mathematics and its Applications*. North-Holland Publishing Co., Amsterdam, 1979.

28. J.-F. Aujol, G. Aubert, L. Blanc-Féraud, and A. Chambolle. Image decomposition into a bounded variation component and an oscillating component. *J. Math. Imaging Vision*, 22(1):71–88, 2005.

29. J.-F. Aujol and A. Chambolle. Dual norms and image decomposition models. *Int. J. Comput. Vision*, 63(1):85–104, 2005.

30. J.-F. Aujol, G. Gilboa, T. Chan, and S. Osher. Structure-texture decomposition by a TV-Gabor model. In *[318]*, 2005.

31. J.-F. Aujol, G. Gilboa, T. Chan, and S. Osher. Structure-texture image decomposition—modeling, algorithms, and parameter selection. *Int. J. Comput. Vision*, 67(1):111–136, 2006.

32. A. Auslender and M. Teboulle. Interior gradient and proximal methods for convex and conic optimization. *SIAM J. Optim.*, 16(3):697–725, 2006.

33. P. Aviles and Y. Giga. Variational integrals on mappings of bounded variation and their lower semicontinuity. *Arch. Ration. Mech. Anal.*, 115(3):201–255, 1991.

34. A. B. Bakushinskii. Remarks on the choice of regularization parameter from quasioptimality and relation tests. *Zh. Vychisl. Mat. Mat. Fiz.*, 24:1258–1259, 1984.

35. C. Ballester, M. Bertalmio, V. Caselles, G. Sapiro, and J. Verdera. Filling-in by joint interpolation of vector fields and grey levels. *IEEE Trans. Image Process.*, 10(8):1200–1211, 2001.

36. H. P. Baltes, editor. *Inverse scattering problems in optics*, volume 20 of *Topics in Current Physics*. Springer-Verlag, Berlin, 1980.

37. R. L. Barbour, M. J. Carvlin, and M. A. Fiddy, editors. *Computational, Experimental, and Numerical Methods for Solving Ill-Posed Inverse Imaging Problems: Medical and Nonmedical Applications*, volume 3171 of *Proceedings of SPIE*, Washington, 1997.

38. V. Barbu. *Nonlinear Semigroups and Differential Equations in Banach Spaces*. Editura Academiei Republicii Socialiste România, Bucharest, 1976.

39. J. Bardsley. An efficient computational method of total variation-penalized poisson likelihood estimation. *Inverse Probl. Imaging*, vol. 2, issue 2, 2008, pp. 167–185.

40. J. Bardsley and A. Luttman. Total variation-penalized poisson likelihood estimation for ill-posed problems. *Adv. Comput. Math.*, 2008. Special Volume on Mathematical Methods for Image Processing, to appear.

41. G. Barles and P. E. Souganidis. Convergence of approximation schemes for fully nonlinear second order equations. *Asymptot. Anal.*, 4(3):271–283, 1991.

42. A. C. Barroso, G. Bouchitté, G. Buttazzo, and I. Fonseca. Relaxation of bulk and interfacial energies. *Arch. Ration. Mech. Anal.*, 135(2):107–173, 1996.

43. G. Bellettini, V. Caselles, and M. Novaga. The total variation flow in $\mathbb{R}^N$. *J. Differential Equations*, 184(2):475–525, 2002.

44. A. Beltukov and D. Feldman. Operator identities relating sonar and Radon transforms in Euclidean space, 2006. arXiv:math/0607437v1.

45. B. Berkels, M. Burger, M. Droske, O. Nemitz, and M. Rumpf. Cartoon extraction based on anisotropic image classification. In *Vision, Modeling, and Visualization Proceedings*, pages 293–300, 2006.

46. M. Bertalmio, A. Bertozzi, and G. Sapiro. Navier–Stokes, fluid dynamics, and image and video inpainting. In *Proc. IEEE Computer Vision and Pattern Recognition (CVPR)*, 2001.

47. M. Bertalmio, G. Sapiro, V. Caselles, and C. Ballester. Image inpainting. In *[214]*, pages 417–424, 2000.

48. M. Bertero, D. Bindi, P. Boccacci, M. Cattaneo, C. Eva, and V. Lanza. A novel blind-deconvolution method with an application to seismology. *Inverse Probl.*, 14(4):815–833, 1998.

49. M. Bertero and P. Boccacci. *Introduction to Inverse Problems in Imaging*. IOP Publishing, London, 1998.

50. M. Bertero, P. Boccacci, A. Custo, C. De Mol, and M. Robberto. A Fourier-based method for the restoration of chopped and nodded images. *Astronom. and Astrophys.*, 406(2):765–772, 2003.

51. M. Bertero, P. Boccacci, and M. Robberto. Wide field imaging at mid-infrared wavelengths: Reconstruction of chopped and nodded data. *Pub. Astronom. Soc. Pac.*, 112(774):1121–1137, 2000.

52. M. Bertero, P. Boccacci, and M. Robberto. Inversion of second-difference operators with application to infrared astronomy. *Inverse Probl.*, 19(6):1427–1443, 2003.

53. E. C. Bingham. *Fluidity and Plasticity*. McGraw-Hill, New York, 1922.

54. L. Blanc-Féraud, P. Charbonnier, G. Aubert, and M. Barlaud. Nonlinear image processing: modeling and fast algorithm for regularization with edge detection. In *International Conference on Image Processing (ICIP'95)*, volume 1, pages 474–477, 1995.

55. G. Bouchitté, I. Fonseca, and L. Mascarenhas. A global method for relaxation. *Arch. Ration. Mech. Anal.*, 145(1):51–98, 1998.

56. C. Bouman and K. Sauer. A generalized Gaussian image model for edge-preserving MAP estimation. *IEEE Trans. Image Process.*, 2(3):296–310, 1993.

57. N. Bourbaki. *Topological Vector Spaces. Chapters 1–5*. Elements of Mathematics. Springer-Verlag, Berlin, 1987.

58. M. A. Breazeale. Schlieren photography in physics. In *[358]*, pages 41–47, 1998.

59. L. M. Bregman. A relaxation method of finding a common point of convex sets and its application to the solution of problems in convex programming. *Zh. Vychisl. Mat. Mat. Fiz.*, 7:620–631, 1967.

60. H. Brézis. *Operateurs Maximaux Monotones et Semi-Groupes de Contractions dans les Espaces de Hilbert*. North-Holland, Amsterdam, 1973.

61. M. Burger, K. Frick, S. Osher, and O. Scherzer. Inverse total variation flow. *Multiscale Model. Simul.*, 6(2):366–395, 2007.

62. M. Burger, G. Gilboa, S. Osher, and J. Xu. Nonlinear inverse scale space methods for image restoration. *Commun. Math. Sci.*, 4(1):179–212, 2006.

63. M. Burger and S. Osher. Convergence rates of convex variational regularization. *Inverse Probl.*, 20(5):1411–1421, 2004.

64. M. Burger and S. Osher. A survey on level set methods for inverse problems and optimal design. *European J. Appl. Math.*, 16(02):263–301, 2005.

65. M. Burger, E. Resmerita, and L. He. Error estimation for Bregman iterations and inverse scale space methods in image restoration. *Computing*, 81(2–3):109–135, 2007. Special Issue on Industrial Geometry.

66. M. Burger and O. Scherzer. Regularization methods for blind deconvolution and blind source separation problems. *Math. Control Signals Systems*, 14(4):358–383, 2001.

67. P. Burgholzer, J. Bauer-Marschallinger, H. Grün, M. Haltmeier, and G. Paltauf. Temporal back-projection algorithms for photoacoustic tomography with integrating line detectors. *Inverse Probl.*, 23(6):65–80, 2007.

68. P. Burgholzer, C. Hofer, G. Paltauf, M. Haltmeier, and O. Scherzer. Thermoacoustic tomography with integrating area and line detectors. *IEEE Trans. Ultrason., Ferroeletr., Freq. Control*, 52(9):1577–1583, 2005.

69. P. Burgholzer, G. J. Matt, M. Haltmeier, and G. Paltauf. Exact and approximate imaging methods for photoacoustic tomography using an arbitrary detection surface. *Phys. Rev. E*, 75(4):046706, 2007.

70. D. Butnariu, Y. Censor, and S. Reich. Iterative averaging of entropic projections for solving stochastic convex feasibility problems. *Comput. Optim. Appl.*, 8(1):21–39, 1997.

71. D. Butnariu, Y. Censor, and S. Reich, editors. *Inherently Parallel Algorithms in Feasibility and Optimization and their Applications*, volume 8 of *Studies in Computational Mathematics*. North-Holland Publishing Co., Amsterdam, 2001.

72. D. Butnariu and A. N. Iusem. *Totally Convex Functions for Fixed Points Computation and Infinite Dimensional Optimization*, volume 40 of *Applied Optimization*. Kluwer Academic Publishers, Dordrecht, 2000.

73. D. Butnariu and E. Resmerita. Bregman distances, totally convex functions, and a method for solving operator equations in Banach spaces. *Abstr. Appl. Anal.*, 2006. Article ID 84919.

74. G. Buttazzo and G. Dal Maso. Γ-limits of integral functionals. *J. Anal. Math.*, 37(1):145–185, 1980.

75. C. Byrne. Bregman–Legendre multidistance projection algorithms for convex feasibility and optimization. In *[71]*, pages 87–99, 2001.

76. C. Byrne. Sequential unconstrained minimization algorithms for constrained optimization. *Inverse Probl.*, 24(1):015013, 2008.

77. E. J. Candès, J. Romberg, and T. Tao. Robust uncertainty principles: exact signal reconstruction from highly incomplete frequency information. *IEEE Trans. Inf. Theory*, 52(2):489–509, 2006.

78. A. S. Carasso. Direct blind deconvolution. *SIAM J. Appl. Math.*, 61(6):1980–2007 (electronic), 2001.

79. A. S. Carasso. Singular integrals, image smoothness, and the recovery of texture in image deblurring. *SIAM J. Appl. Math.*, 64(5):1749–1774 (electronic), 2004.

80. V. Caselles, F. Catté, T. Coll, and F. Dibos. A geometric model for active contours in image processing. *Numer. Math.*, 66(1):1–31, 1993.

81. V. Caselles, A. Chambolle, and M. Novaga. The discontinuity set of solutions of the TV denoising problem and some extensions. *Multiscale Model. Simul.*, 6(3):879–894, 2007.

82. V. Caselles, R. Kimmel, and G. Sapiro. Geodesic active contours. *Int. J. Comput. Vision*, 22(1):61–79, 1997.

83. V. Caselles, R. Kimmel, G. Sapiro, and C. Sbert. Minimal surfaces: A geometric three dimensional segmentation approach. *Numer. Math.*, 77(4):423–451, 1997.

84. F. Catté, P.-L. Lions, J.-M. Morel, and T. Coll. Image selective smoothing and edge detection by nonlinear diffusion. *SIAM J. Numer. Anal.*, 29(1):182–193, 1992.

85. B. Chalmond. *Modeling and Inverse Problems in Image Analysis*, volume 155 of *Applied Mathematical Sciences*. Springer-Verlag, New York, 2003.

86. A. Chambolle. Finite-differences discretizations of the Mumford–Shah functional. *Math. Model. Numer. Anal.*, 33(2):261–288, 1999.

87. A. Chambolle. An algorithm for total variation minimization and applications. *J. Math. Imaging Vision*, 20(1–2):89–97, 2004.

88. A. Chambolle and G. Dal Maso. Discrete approximation of the Mumford–Shah functional in dimension two. *Math. Model. Numer. Anal.*, 33(4):651–672, 1999.

89. A. Chambolle, R. A. DeVore, N. Lee, and B. J. Lucier. Nonlinear wavelet image processing: variational problems, compression, and noise removal through wavelet shrinkage. *IEEE Trans. Image Process.*, 7(3):319–335, 1998.

90. A. Chambolle and P.-L. Lions. Image recovery via total variation minimization and related problems. *Numer. Math.*, 76(2):167–188, 1997.

91. R. Chan, S. Setzer, and G. Steidl. Inpainting by flexible Haar wavelet shrinkage. Preprint, University of Mannheim, 2008.

92. R. H. Chan, C.-W. Ho, and M. Nikolova. Salt-and-pepper noise removal by median-type noise detectors and detail-preserving regularization. *IEEE Trans. Image Process.*, 14(10):1479–1485, 2005.

93. T. Chan and S. Esedoglu. Aspects of total variation regularized L^1 function approximation. *SIAM J. Appl. Math.*, 65(5):1817–1837, 2005.

94. T. Chan, S. Kang, and J. Shen. Euler's elastica and curvature based inpaintings. *SIAM J. Appl. Math.*, 63(2):564–592, 2002.

95. T. Chan, A. Marquina, and P. Mulet. High-order total variation-based image restoration. *SIAM J. Sci. Comput.*, 22(2):503–516, 2000.

96. T. Chan and J. Shen. Non-texture inpaintings by curvature-driven diffusions. *J. Vis. Commun. Image Represent.*, 12(4):436–449, 2001.

292   References

97. T. Chan and J. Shen. Mathematical models for local nontexture inpaintings. *SIAM J. Appl. Math.*, 62(3):1019–1043, 2002.

98. T. Chan and J. Shen. *Image Processing and Analysis—Variational, PDE, Wavelet, and Stochastic Methods*. SIAM, Philadelphia, 2005.

99. T. Chan, J. Shen, and L. Vese. Variational PDE models in image processing. *Notices Amer. Math. Soc.*, 50(1):14–26, 2003.

100. T. Chan and L. Vese. Active contours without edges. *IEEE Trans. Image Process.*, 10(2):266–277, 2001.

101. T. Chan and C. K. Wong. Total variation blind deconvolution. *IEEE Trans. Image Process.*, 7(3):370–375, 1998.

102. T. Chan and C. K. Wong. Convergence of the alternating minimization algorithm for blind deconvolution. *Linear Algebra Appl.*, 316(1–3):259–285, 2000.

103. P. Charbonnier, L. Blanc-Féraud, G. Aubert, and M. Barlaud. Deterministic edge-preserving regularization in computed imaging. *IEEE Trans. Image Process.*, 6(2):298–311, 1997.

104. T. Charlebois and R. Pelton. Quantitative 2d and 3d schlieren imaging for acoustic power and intensity measurements. *Medical Electronics*, pages 789–792, 1995.

105. G. Chavent and K. Kunisch. Regularization of linear least squares problems by total bounded variation. *ESAIM Control Optim. Calc. Var.*, 2:359–376, 1997.

106. Y. Chen and M. Rao. Minimization problems and associated flows related to weighted p energy and total variation. *SIAM J. Math. Anal.*, 34(5):1084–1104, 2003.

107. W. F. Cheong, S. A. Prahl, and A. J. Welch. A review of the optical properties of biological tissues. *IEEE J. Quantum Electron.*, 26(12):2166–2185, 1990.

108. I. Cioranescu. *Geometry of Banach Spaces, Duality Mappings and Nonlinear Problems*, volume 62 of *Mathematics and its Applications*. Kluwer, Dordrecht, 1990.

109. F. H. Clarke. *Optimization and Nonsmooth Analysis*, volume 5 of *Classics in Applied Mathematics*. SIAM, Philadelphia, PA, second edition, 1990.

110. A. Cohen. *Numerical Analysis of Wavelet Methods*, volume 32 of *Studies in Mathematics and its Applications*. North-Holland Publishing Co., Amsterdam, 2003.

111. D. Colton, H. W. Engl, A. K. Louis, J. R. McLaughlin, and W. Rundell, editors. *Surveys on Solution Methods for Inverse Problems*. Springer-Verlag, Vienna, 2000.

112. D. Colton, R. Ewing, and W. Rundell, editors. *Inverse Problems in Partial Differential Equations*. SIAM, Philadelphia, 1990.

113. D. Colton and R. Kress. *Integral Equation Methods in Scattering Theory*. Wiley, New York, 1983.

114. D. Colton and R. Kress. *Inverse Acoustic and Electromagnetic Scattering Theory*. Springer-Verlag, New York, 1992.

115. P. L. Combettes and V. R. Wajs. Signal recovery by proximal forward-backward splitting. *Multiscale Model. Simul.*, 4(4):1168–1200 (electronic), 2005.

116. R. Cook, editor. *Computer Graphics*. SIGGRAPH Conference Proceedings. ACM SIGGRAPH, 1995.

117. A. M. Cormack. Representation of a function by its line integrals, with some radiological applications. *J. App. Phys.*, 34(9):2722–2727, 1963.

118. M. G. Crandall, H. Ishii, and P.-L. Lions. User's guide to viscosity solutions of second order partial differential equations. *Bull. Amer. Math. Soc.*, 27(1):1–67, 1992.

119. M. G. Crandall and T. M. Liggett. Generation of semi-groups of nonlinear transformations on general Banach spaces. *Amer. J. Math.*, 93(2):265–298, 1971.

120. A. Criminisi, P. Perez, and K. Toyama. Object removal by exemplar-based inpainting. In *IEEE Conference on Computer Vision and Pattern Recognition*, volume 2. IEEE Computer Society, 2003.

121. I. Csiszár. Why least squares and maximum entropy? An axiomatic approach to inference for linear inverse problems. *Ann. Statist.*, 19(4):2032–2066, 1991.

122. B. Dacorogna. *Direct Methods in the Calculus of Variations*, volume 78 of *Applied Mathematical Sciences*. Springer-Verlag, Berlin, 1989.

123. B. Dacorogna and P. Marcellini. *Implicit Partial Differential Equations*. Birkhäuser, Boston, 1999.

124. G. Dal Maso. *An Introduction to Γ-Convergence*, volume 8 of *Progress in Nonlinear Differential Equations and their Applications*. Birkhäuser, Boston, 1993.

125. I. Daubechies. *Ten Lectures on Wavelets*. SIAM, Philadelphia, PA, 1992.

126. I. Daubechies, M. Defrise, and C. De Mol. An iterative thresholding algorithm for linear inverse problems with a sparsity constraint. *Comm. Pure Appl. Math.*, 57(11):1413–1457, 2004.

127. I. Daubechies and G. Teschke. Variational image restoration by means of wavelets: simultaneous decomposition, deblurring, and denoising. *Appl. Comput. Harmon. Anal.*, 19(1):1–16, 2005.

128. P. L. Davies and A. Kovac. Local extremes, runs, strings and multiresolution. *Ann. Statist.*, 29(1):1–65, 2001.

129. M. H. DeGroot and M. J. Schervish. *Probability and Statistics*. Addison Wesley, 3rd edition, 2002.

130. F. Demengel and R. Temam. Convex functions of a measure and applications. *Indiana Univ. Math. J.*, 33(5):673–709, 1984.

131. C. L. DeVito. *Functional Analysis*, volume 81 of *Pure and Applied Mathematics*. Academic Press, New York, 1978.

132. V. Dicken and P. Maass. Wavelet-Galerkin methods for ill-posed problems. *J. Inverse Ill-Posed Probl.*, 4:203–221, 1996.

133. D. C. Dobson and C. R. Vogel. Convergence of an iterative method for total variation denoising. *SIAM J. Numer. Anal.*, 34(5):1779–1791, 1997.

134. A. Dold and B. Eckmann, editors. *Nonlinear Operators and the Calculus of Variations, Bruxelles 1975*. Springer-Verlag, Berlin, Heidelberg, New York, 1976.

135. D. L. Donoho. De-noising by soft-thresholding. *IEEE Trans. Inf. Theory*, 41(3):613–627, 1995.

136. D. L. Donoho. Compressed sensing. *IEEE Trans. Inf. Theory*, 52(4):1289–1306, 2006.

137. D. L. Donoho and I. M. Johnstone. Minimax estimation via wavelet shrinkage. *Ann. Statist.*, 26(3):879–921, 1998.

138. I. Drori, D. Cohen-Or, and H. Yeshurun. Fragment-based image completion. *ACM Trans. Graph.*, 22(3):303–312, 2003.

139. M. Droske and M. Rumpf. A level set formulation for Willmore flow. *Interfaces Free Bound.*, 6(3):361–378, 2004.

140. H. Edelsbrunner. *Geometry and Topology for Mesh Generation*, volume 7 of *Cambridge Monographs on Applied and Computational Mathematics*. Cambridge University Press, Cambridge, 2006. Reprint of the 2001 original.

141. A. A. Efros and T. K. Leung. Texture synthesis by non-parametric sampling. In *IEEE International Conference on Computer Vision*, volume 2, pages 1033–1038, Corfu, Greece, September 1999.

142. P. P. B. Eggermont. Maximum entropy regularization for Fredholm integral equations of the first kind. *SIAM J. Math. Anal.*, 24(6):1557–1576, 1993.

143. I. Ekeland and R. Temam. *Analyse convexe et problèmes variationnels*. Dunod, 1974. Collection Études Mathématiques.

144. I. Ekeland and R. Temam. *Convex Analysis and Variational Problems*. North-Holland, Amsterdam, 1976.

145. M. Elad, J.-L. Starck, P. Querre, and D. L. Donoho. Simultaneous cartoon and texture image inpainting using morphological component analysis (MCA). *Appl. Comput. Harmon. Anal.*, 19(3):340–358, 2005.

146. P. Elbau, M. Grasmair, F. Lenzen, and O. Scherzer. Evolution by non-convex energy functionals. in preparation, 2008.

147. C. M. Elliott and S. A. Smitheman. Analysis of the TV regularization and H^{-1} fidelity model for decomposing an image into cartoon plus texture. *Commun. Pure Appl. Anal.*, 6(4):917–936, 2007.

148. J. P. Emerson. Observing far-infrared and submillimeter continuum emission. In *[327]*, pages 125–156, 1994.

149. R. Engelking. *Outline of General Topology*. North-Holland, Amsterdam, 1968.

150. H. W. Engl and H. Gfrerer. A posteriori parameter choice for general regularization methods for solving linear ill-posed problems. *Appl. Numer. Math.*, 4(5):395–417, 1988.

151. H. W. Engl and W. Grever. Using the L-curve for determining optimal regularization parameters. *Numer. Math.*, 69(1):25–31, 1994.

152. H. W. Engl, M. Hanke, and A. Neubauer. *Regularization of Inverse Problems*. Kluwer Academic Publishers, Dordrecht, 1996.

153. H. W. Engl, K. Kunisch, and A. Neubauer. Convergence rates for Tikhonov regularization of nonlinear ill-posed problems. *Inverse Probl.*, 5(3):523–540, 1989.

154. H. W. Engl and G. Landl. Convergence rates for maximum entropy regularization. *SIAM J. Numer. Anal.*, 30(5):1509–1536, 1993.

155. S. Esedoglu and J. Shen. Digital inpainting based on the Mumford–Shah–Euler image model. *European J. Appl. Math.*, 13:353–370, 2002.

156. L. C. Evans. *Partial Differential Equations*, volume 19 of *Graduate Studies in Mathematics*. American Mathematical Society, Providence, RI, 1998.

157. L. C. Evans and R. F. Gariepy. *Measure Theory and Fine Properties of Functions*. Studies in Advanced Mathematics. CRC Press, Boca Raton, 1992.

158. J. A. Fawcett. Inversion of n-dimensional spherical averages. *SIAM J. Appl. Math.*, 45(2):336–341, 1985.

159. H. Federer. *Geometric Measure Theory*. Die Grundlehren der Mathematischen Wissenschaften, Band 153. Springer-Verlag New York Inc., New York, 1969.

160. W. Feller. *An Introduction to Probability Theory and Its Applications*. Wiley Series in Probability and Mathematical Statistics. Wiley & Sons, Inc., New York, London, Sydney, 1966.

161. A. L. Fetter and J. D. Walecka. *Theoretical Mechanics of Particles and Continua.* McGraw-Hill, New York, 1980. International Series in Pure and Applied Physics.

162. M. Figueiredo, J. Zerubia, and A. Jain, editors. *Energy Minimization Methods in Computer Vision and Pattern Recognition,* volume 2134 of *Lecture Notes in Computer Science.* Springer-Verlag, New York, 2001.

163. D. Finch, M. Haltmeier, and Rakesh. Inversion of spherical means and the wave equation in even dimensions. *SIAM J. Appl. Math.,* 68(2):392–412, 2007.

164. D. Finch, S. Patch, and Rakesh. Determining a function from its mean values over a family of spheres. *SIAM J. Math. Anal.,* 35(5):1213–1240, 2004.

165. D. Finch and Rakesh. The spherical mean value operator with centers on a sphere. *Inverse Probl.,* 23(6):37–49, 2007.

166. D. Finch and Rakesh. Recovering a function from its spherical mean values in two and three dimensions. In *[380],* 2008.

167. I. Fonseca and G. Leoni. Bulk and contact energies: nucleation and relaxation. *SIAM J. Math. Anal.,* 30(1):190–219 (electronic), 1999.

168. I. Fonseca and S. Müller. Quasi-convex integrands and lower semicontinuity in L^1. *SIAM J. Math. Anal.,* 23(5):1081–1098, 1992.

169. I. Fonseca and P. Rybka. Relaxation of multiple integrals in the space $BV(\Omega, \mathbf{R}^p)$. *Proc. Roy. Soc. Edinburgh Sect. A,* 121:321–348, 1992.

170. M. Fornasier. Nonlinear projection recovery in digital inpainting for color image restoration. *J. Math. Imaging Vision,* 24(3):359–373, 2006.

171. K. Frick. *The Augmented Lagrangian Method and Related Evolution Equations.* PhD thesis, University of Innsbruck, Austria, 2008.

172. K. Frick and O. Scherzer. Applications of non-convex BV regularization for image segmentation. In *[368],* pages 211–228, 2007.

173. I. A. Frigaard, G. Ngwa, and O. Scherzer. On effective stopping time selection for visco-plastic nonlinear BV diffusion filters used in image denoising. *SIAM J. Appl. Math.,* 63(6):1911–1934 (electronic), 2003.

174. I. A. Frigaard and O. Scherzer. Herschel–Bulkley diffusion filtering: non-Newtonian fluid mechanics in image processing. *Z. Angew. Math. Mech.,* 86(6):474–494, 2006.

175. F. Frühauf, A. Leitão, and O. Scherzer. Analysis of regularization methods for the solution of ill-posed problems involving discontinuous operators. *SIAM J. Numer. Anal.,* 43(2):767–786, 2005.

176. J. Garnett, T. Le, Y. Meyer, and L. Vese. Image decompositions using bounded variation and generalized homogeneous Besov spaces. *Appl. Comput. Harmon. Anal.,* 23(1):25–56, 2007.

177. D. Geman and G. Reynolds. Constrained restoration and the recovery of discontinuities. *IEEE Trans. Pattern Anal. Mach. Intell.,* 14(3):367–383, 1992.

178. D. Geman and C. Yang. Nonlinear image recovery with half-quadratic regularization. *IEEE Trans. Image Process.,* 4(7):932–946, 1995.

179. S. Geman and D. Geman. Stochastic relaxation, Gibbs distributions, and the Bayesian restoration of images. *IEEE Trans. Pattern Anal. Mach. Intell.,* 6(6):721–741, 1984.

180. S. Geman, D. E. McClure, and G. Geman. A nonlinear filter for film restoration and other problems in image processing. *CVGIP: Graph. Models Image Process.,* 54(4):281–289, 1992.

181. G. Gilboa, N. A. Sochen, and Y. Y. Zeevi. Estimation of the optimal variational parameter via SNR analysis. In *[236],* pages 230–241, 2005.

182. E. Giusti. *Direct Methods in the Calculus of Variations.* World Scientific Publishing, River Edge, NJ, 2003.

183. R. Glowinski. *Numerical Methods for Nonlinear Variational Problems.* Springer-Verlag, Berlin, New York, 1984.

184. R. C. Gonzales and R. E. Woods. *Digital Image Processing.* Pearson, Upper Saddle River, New Jersey, third edition, 2008.

185. R. Gorenflo and S. Vessella. *Abel integral equations,* volume 1461 of *Lecture Notes in Mathematics.* Springer-Verlag, Berlin, 1991. Analysis and applications.

186. Y. Gousseau and J.-M. Morel. Are natural images of bounded variation? *SIAM J. Math. Anal.,* 33(3):634–648, 2001.

187. M. Grasmair. *Relaxation of Nonlocal Integrals with Rational Integrands.* PhD thesis, University of Innsbruck, Austria, 2006.

188. M. Grasmair and A. Obereder. Generalizations of the taut string method. *Numer. Funct. Anal. Optim.,* vol. 29, issue 3–4, pp. 346–361, 2008.

189. P. J. Green. Bayesian reconstructions from emission tomography data using a modified EM algorithm. *IEEE Trans. Med. Imag.,* 9(1):84–93, 1990.

190. J. B. Greer and A. L. Bertozzi. H^1 solutions of a class of fourth order nonlinear equations for image processing. *Discrete Contin. Dynam. Systems,* 10(1–2):349–366, 2004.

191. C. W. Groetsch. *The Theory of Tikhonov Regularization for Fredholm Equations of the First Kind.* Pitman, Boston, 1984.

192. C. W. Groetsch and O. Scherzer. Nonstationary iterated Tikhonov–Morozov method and third order differential equations for the evaluation of unbounded operators. *Math. Methods Appl. Sci.,* 23(15):1287–1300, 2000.

193. H. Grossauer. A combined PDE and texture synthesis approach to inpainting. In *Proc. European Conference on Computer Vision,* volume 3022 of *Lecture Notes in Computer Science,* pages 214–224. Springer, New York, 2004.

194. F. Guichard, J.-M. Morel, and R. Ryan. *Contrast Invariant Image Analysis and PDE's.* preprint, Paris, 2007. work in preparation.

195. W. Hackbusch. *Elliptic Differential Equations,* volume 18 of *Springer Series in Computational Mathematics.* Springer-Verlag, Berlin, 1992.

196. A. Haddad and Y. Meyer. An improvement of Rudin–Osher–Fatemi model. *Appl. Comput. Harmon. Anal.,* 22(3):319–334, 2007.

197. M. Haltmeier and T. Fidler. Frequency domain reconstruction in photo- and thermoacoustic tomography with line detectors. *arXiv:math/0610155v3,* 2007. submitted.

198. M. Haltmeier, O. Scherzer, P. Burgholzer, R. Nuster, and G. Paltauf. Thermoacoustic tomography & the circular Radon transform: Exact inversion formula. *Math. Models Methods Appl. Sci.,* 17(4):635–655, 2007.

199. M. Haltmeier, O. Scherzer, P. Burgholzer, and G. Paltauf. Thermoacoustic imaging with large planar receivers. *Inverse Probl.,* 20(5):1663–1673, 2004.

200. M. Haltmeier, T. Schuster, and O. Scherzer. Filtered backprojection for thermoacoustic computed tomography in spherical geometry. *Math. Methods Appl. Sci.,* 28(16):1919–1937, 2005.

201. A. B. Hamza and H. Krim. A variational approach to maximum a posteriori estimation for image denoising. In *[162],* 2001.

202. A. B. Hamza, H. Krim, and G. B. Unal. Unifying probabilistic and variational estimation. *IEEE Signal Process. Mag.,* 19(5):37–47, 2002.

203. A. Hanafy and C. I. Zanelli. Quantitative real-time pulsed schlieren imaging of ultrasonic waves. *Proc. IEEE Ultrasonics Symposium*, 2:1223–1227, 1991.

204. M. Hanke. *Conjugate Gradient Type Methods for Ill-Posed Problems*, volume 327 of *Pitman Research Notes in Mathematics Series*. Longman Scientific & Technical, Harlow, 1995.

205. M. Hanke and P. C. Hansen. Regularization methods for large-scale problems. *Surveys Math. Indust.*, 3(4):253–315, 1994.

206. M. Hanke and O. Scherzer. Inverse problems light: numerical differentiation. *Amer. Math. Monthly*, 108(6):512–521, 2001.

207. P. C. Hansen. *Rank-Deficient and Discrete Ill-Posed Problems*. SIAM Monographs on Mathematical Modeling and Computation. SIAM, Philadelphia, PA, 1998.

208. D. J. Heeger and J. R. Bergen. Pyramid-based texture analysis/synthesis. In *[116]*, pages 229–238, 1995.

209. S. Helgason. *The Radon Transform*, volume 5 of *Progress in Mathematics*. Birkhäuser, Boston, 1980.

210. E. Hewitt and K. Stromberg. *Real and Abstract Analysis*. Springer-Verlag, New York, 1965.

211. W. Hinterberger, M. Hintermüller, K. Kunisch, M. von Oehsen, and O. Scherzer. Tube methods for BV regularization. *J. Math. Imaging Vision*, 19(3):219–235, 2003.

212. M. Hintermüller and K. Kunisch. Total bounded variation regularization as a bilaterally constrained optimization problem. *SIAM J. Appl. Math.*, 64(4):1311–1333 (electronic), 2004.

213. C. G. A. Hoelen, F. F. M. de Mul, R. Pongers, and A. Dekker. Three-dimensional photoacoustic imaging of blood vessels in tissue. *Opt. Letters*, 23(8):648–650, 1998.

214. S. Hoffmeyer, editor. *Proceedings of the Computer Graphics Conference 2000 (SIGGRAPH-00)*. ACM Press, New York, 2000.

215. B. Hofmann, B. Kaltenbacher, C. Pöschl, and O. Scherzer. A convergence rates result in Banach spaces with non-smooth operators. *Inverse Probl.*, 23(3):987–1010, 2007.

216. T. Hohage. Regularization of exponentially ill-posed problems. *Numer. Funct. Anal. Optim.*, 21(3&4):439–464, 2000.

217. R. A. Horn and C. R. Johnson. *Matrix Analysis*. Cambridge University Press, Cambridge, 1990. Corrected reprint of the 1985 original.

218. G. N. Hounsfield. Computerised transverse axial scanning (tomography). Part 1: Description of system. *Brit. J. Radiology*, 46(552):1016–1022, 1973.

219. P. J. Huber. *Robust Statistics*. John Wiley & Sons Inc., New York, 1981. Wiley Series in Probability and Mathematical Statistics.

220. A. D. Ioffe. On lower semicontinuity of integral functionals. I. *SIAM J. Control Optim.*, 15(4):521–538, 1977.

221. K. Ito and K. Kunisch. An active set strategy based on the augmented Lagrangian formulation for image restoration. *Math. Model. Numer. Anal.*, 33(1):1–21, 1999.

222. A. N. Iusem and M. Teboulle. A regularized dual-based iterative method for a class of image reconstruction problems. *Inverse Probl.*, 9(6):679–696, 1993.

223. B. Jähne. *Digitale Bildverarbeitung*. Springer, Berlin, 5th edition, 2002.

224. J. Jia and C. K. Tang. Image repairing: robust image synthesis by adaptive ND tensor voting. In *Proc. IEEE Conference on Computer Vision and Pattern Recognition*, volume 1, pages 643–650, 2003.

225. L. Jiang, X. Feng, and H. Yin. Variational image restoration and decomposition with curvelet shrinkage. *J. Math. Imaging Vision*, 30(2):125–132, 2008.

226. F. John. *Plane Waves and Spherical Means Applied to Partial Differential Equations*. Wiley, New York, 1955.

227. F. John. *Partial Differential Equations*, volume 1 of *Applied Mathematical Sciences*. Springer-Verlag, New York, fourth edition, 1982.

228. J. Jost. *Postmodern Analysis*. Springer, third edition, 2005.

229. L. Justen and R. Ramlau. A non-iterative regularization approach to blind deconvolution. *Inverse Probl.*, 22(3):771–800, 2006.

230. U. Kaeufl. Observing extended objects with chopping restrictions on 8m class telescopes in the thermal infrared. In *ESO Conf. and Workshop Proc.: Calibrating and Understanding HSR and ESO Instruments*, volume 53, pages 159–163, 1995.

231. J. Kaipio and E. Somersalo. *Statistical and Computational Inverse Problems*, volume 160 of *Applied Mathematical Sciences*. Springer-Verlag, New York, 2005.

232. A. C. Kak and M. Slaney. *Principles of Computerized Tomographic Imaging*, volume 33 of *Classics in Applied Mathematics*. Society for Industrial and Applied Mathematics (SIAM), Philadelphia, PA, 2001. Reprint of the 1988 original.

233. A. Kartsatos, editor. *Theory and Applications of Nonlinear Operators of Accretive and Monotone Type*, volume 178 of *Lecture Notes in Pure and Applied Mathematics*. Marcel Dekker, New York, 1996.

234. J. L. Kelley. *General Topology*. D. Van Nostrand Company, Toronto-New York-London, 1955.

235. R. Kimmel, R. Malladi, and N. A. Sochen. Images as embedded maps and minimal surfaces: movies, colour, texture, and volumetric medical images. *Int. J. Comput. Vision*, 39(2):111–129, 2000.

236. R. Kimmel, N. A. Sochen, and J. Weickert, editors. *Scale Space and PDE Methods in Computer Vision*, volume 3459 of *Lecture Notes in Computer Science*. Springer, New York, 2005.

237. S. Kindermann and A. Neubauer. Identification of discontinuous parameters by regularization for curve representations. *Inverse Probl.*, 15(6):1559–1572, 1999.

238. S. Kindermann and A. Neubauer. Estimation of discontinuous parameters of elliptic partial differential equations by regularization for surface representations. *Inverse Probl.*, 17(4):789–803, 2001.

239. S. Kindermann and A. Neubauer. Regularization for surface representations of discontinuous solutions of linear ill-posed problems. *Numer. Funct. Anal. Optim.*, 22(1&2):79–105, 2001.

240. S. Kindermann and A. Neubauer. Parameter identification by regularization for surface representation via the moving grid approach. *SIAM J. Control Optim.*, 42(4):1416–1430 (electronic), 2003.

241. R. Klette, R. Kozera, L. Noakes, and J. Weickert, editors. *Geometric Properties of Incomplete Data*, volume 31 of *Computational Imaging and Vision*. Springer-Verlag, New York, 2005.

242. R. G. M. Kolkman, E. Hondebrink, W. Steenbergen, and F. F. M. De Mul. In vivo photoacoustic imaging of blood vessels using an extreme-narrow aperture sensor. *IEEE J. Sel. Topics Quantum Electron.*, 9(2):343–346, 2003.

243. J. Kristensen. Lower semicontinuity of quasi-convex integrals in BV. *Calc. Var. Partial Differential Equations*, 7(3):249–261, 1998.

244. R. A. Kruger, W. L. Kiser, D. R. Reinecke, G. A. Kruger, and K. D. Miller. Thermoacoustic molecular imaging of small animals. *Mol. Imaging*, 2(2):113–123, 2003.

245. R. A. Kruger, P. Lui, Y. R. Fang, and R. C. Appledorn. Photoacoustic ultrasound (PAUS)—reconstruction tomography. *Med. Phys.*, 22(10):1605–1609, 1995.

246. R. A. Kruger, K. D. Miller, H. E. Reynolds, W. L. Kiser, D. R. Reinecke, and G. A. Kruger. Breast cancer in vivo: contrast enhancement with thermoacoustic CT at 434 MHz-feasibility study. *Radiology*, 216(1):279–283, 2000.

247. R. A. Kruger, K. M. Stantz, and W. L. Kiser. Thermoacoustic CT of the breast. In *[23]*, pages 521–525, 2002.

248. G. Ku and L. V. Wang. Deeply penetrating photoacoustic tomography in biological tissues enhanced with an optical contrast agent. *Opt. Letters*, 30(5): 507–509, 2005.

249. P. Kuchment and L. A. Kunyansky. Mathematics of thermoacoustic and photoacoustic tomography. *European J. Appl. Math.*, vol. 19, issue 2, 2008, pp. 191–224.

250. H. R. Künsch. Robust priors for smoothing and image restoration. *Ann. Inst. Statist. Math.*, 46(1):1–19, 1994.

251. L. A. Kunyansky. Explicit inversion formulae for the spherical mean Radon transform. *Inverse Probl.*, 23(1):373–383, 2007.

252. P. O. Lagage, J. W. Pel, M. Authier, J. Belorgey, A. Claret, C. Doucet, D. Dubreuil, G. Durand, E. Elswijk, P. Girardot, H. U. Kufl, G. Kroes, M. Lortholary, Y. Lussignol, M. Marchesi, E. Pantin, R. Peletier, J.-F. Pirard, J. Pragt, Y. Rio, T. Schoenmaker, R. Siebenmorgen, A. Silber, A. Smette, M. Sterzik, and C. Veyssiere. Successful commissioning of VISIR: the mid-infrared VLT instrument. *The Messenger*, 117:12–17, 2004.

253. G. Landl and R. S. Anderssen. Non-negative differentially constrained entropy-like regularization. *Inverse Probl.*, 12(1):35–53, 1996.

254. C. J. Larsen. Quasiconvexification in $W^{1,1}$ and optimal jump microstructure in BV relaxation. *SIAM J. Math. Anal.*, 29(4):823–848, 1998.

255. D.R. Larson, P. Massopust, Z. Nashed, M.C. Nguyen, M. Papadakis, and A. Zayed. *Frames and operator theory in analysis and signal processing. AMS-SIAM special session, San Antonio, TX, USA, January 12–15, 2006.* Contemporary Mathematics 451. Providence, RI: American Mathematical Society (AMS), 2008.

256. M. M. Lavrentiev, V. G. Romanov, and V. G. Vasiliev. *Multidimensional Inverse Problems for Differential Equations*, volume 167 of *Lecture Notes in Mathematics*. Springer-Verlag, Berlin, 1970.

257. Y. G. Leclerc. Constructing simple stable descriptions for image partitioning. *Int. J. Comput. Vision*, 3(1):73–102, 1989.

258. J. Lie and J. M. Nordbotten. Inverse scale spaces for nonlinear regularization. *J. Math. Imaging Vision*, 27(1):41–50, 2007.

300   References

259. J.-L. Lions and E. Magenes. *Non-Homogeneous Boundary Value Problems and Applications I*, volume 181 of *Die Grundlehren der Mathematischen Wissenschaften*. Springer-Verlag, New York, 1972.

260. F. Liu and M. Z. Nashed. Convergence of regularized solutions of nonlinear ill-posed problems with monotone operators. In *[269]*, pages 353–361. Marcel Dekker, New York, 1996.

261. F. Liu and M. Z. Nashed. Regularization of nonlinear ill-posed variational inequalities and convergence rates. *Set-Valued Anal.*, 6(4):313–344, 1998.

262. D. Lorenz. Convergence rates and source conditions for Tikhonov regularization with sparsity constraints. *arXiv:0801.1774v1, submitted*, 2008.

263. F. Luk, editor. *Advanced Signal Processing Algorithms*, volume 2563 of *Proceedings of SPIE*, 1995.

264. M. Lysaker, A. Lundervold, and X. Tai. Noise removal using fourth-order partial differential equation with applications to medical magnetic resonance images in space and time. *IEEE Trans. Image Process.*, 12(12):1579–1590, 2003.

265. S. Mallat. *A Wavelet Tour of Signal Processing*. Academic Press, San Diego, CA, second edition, 1999.

266. E. Mammen and S. van de Geer. Locally adaptive regression splines. *Ann. Statist.*, 25(1):387–413, 1997.

267. P. Marcellini. Approximation of quasiconvex functions, and lower semicontinuity of multiple integrals. *Manuscripta Math.*, 51(1–3):1–28, 1985.

268. P. Marcellini and C. Sbordone. On the existence of minima of multiple integrals of the calculus of variations. *J. Math. Pures Appl. (9)*, 62:1–9, 1983.

269. P. Marcellini, G. Talenti, and E. Vesentini, editors. *Partial Differential Equations and Applications : Collected Papers in Honor of Carlo Pucci*, volume 177 of *Lecture Notes in Pure and Applied Mathematics*. Marcel Dekker, New York, 1996.

270. R. March and M. Dozio. A variational method for the recovery of smooth boundaries. *Image Vision Comput.*, 15(9):705–712, 1997.

271. A Marquina. Inverse scale space methods for blind deconvolution. Technical Report 06/36, UCLA, Los Angeles, 2007.

272. S. Masnou. Disocclusion: a variational approach using level lines. *IEEE Trans. Image Process.*, 11(2):68–76, 2002.

273. S. Masnou and J.-M. Morel. Level lines based disocclusion. In *[389]*, pages 259–263, 1998.

274. R. E. Megginson. *An Introduction to Banach Space Theory*, volume 183 of *Graduate Texts in Mathematics*. Springer-Verlag, New York, 1989.

275. Y. Meyer. *Oscillating Patterns in Image Processing and Nonlinear Evolution Equations*, volume 22 of *University Lecture Series*. American Mathematical Society, Providence, RI, 2001.

276. J.-M. Morel and S. Solimini. *Variational Methods in Image Segmentation*, volume 14 of *Progress in Nonlinear Differential Equations and their Applications*. Birkhäuser, Boston, 1995.

277. V. A. Morozov. *Methods for Solving Incorrectly Posed Problems*. Springer Verlag, New York, Berlin, Heidelberg, 1984.

278. V. A. Morozov. *Regularization Methods for Ill-Posed Problems*. CRC Press, Boca Raton, 1993.

279. C. B. Morrey. *Multiple Integrals in the Calculus of Variations*, volume 130 of *Die Grundlehren der Mathematischen Wissenschaften*. Springer-Verlag, New York, 1966.

280. P. P. Mosolov and V. P. Miashikov. On stagnant flow regions of a viscous-plastic medium in pipes. *J. Appl. Math. Mech.*, 30(4):841–854, 1966.

281. P. P. Mosolov and V. P. Miasnikov. Variational methods in the theory of the fluidity of a viscous-plastic medium. *J. Appl. Math. Mech.*, 29(3):545–577, 1965.

282. P. Mrázek and M. Navara. Selection of optimal stopping time for nonlinear diffusion. *Int. J. Comput. Vision*, 52(2–3):189–203, 2003.

283. D. Mumford and J. Shah. Boundary detection by minimizing functionals. In *Proc. IEEE Conference on Computer Vision and Pattern Recognition*, pages 22–26, 1985.

284. D. Mumford and J. Shah. Optimal approximations by piecewise smooth functions and associated variational problems. *Comm. Pure Appl. Math.*, 42(5):577–685, 1989.

285. M. Z. Nashed and F. Liu. On nonlinear ill-posed problems. II. Monotone operator equations and monotone variational inequalities. In *[233]*, pages 223–240. Marcel Dekker, New York, 1996.

286. M. Z. Nashed and O. Scherzer. Least squares and bounded variation regularization with nondifferentiable functional. *Numer. Funct. Anal. Optim.*, 19(7&8):873–901, 1998.

287. M. Z. Nashed and O. Scherzer, editors. *Interactions on Inverse Problems and Imaging*, volume 313 of *Contemporary Mathematics*. AMS, 2002.

288. F. Natterer. *The Mathematics of Computerized Tomography*, volume 32 of *Classics in Applied Mathematics*. SIAM, Philadelphia, 2001.

289. F. Natterer and F. Wübbeling. *Mathematical Methods in Image Reconstruction*, volume 5 of *Monographs on Mathematical Modeling and Computation*. SIAM, Philadelphia, PA, 2001.

290. A. Neubauer. Tikhonov regularization for non-linear ill-posed problems: optimal convergence rates and finite-dimensional approximation. *Inverse Probl.*, 5(4):541–557, 1989.

291. A. Neubauer and O. Scherzer. Reconstruction of discontinuous solutions from blurred data. In *[37]*, pages 34–41, 1997.

292. A. Neubauer and O. Scherzer. Regularization for curve representations: uniform convergence of discontinuous solutions of ill-posed problems. *SIAM J. Appl. Math.*, 58(6):1891–1900, 1998.

293. M. Nikolova. Minimizers of cost-functions involving nonsmooth data-fidelity terms. Application to the processing of outliers. *SIAM J. Numer. Anal.*, 40(3):965–994, 2002.

294. M. Nikolova. A variational approach to remove outliers and impulse noise. *J. Math. Imaging Vision*, 20(1–2):99–120, 2004. Special issue on mathematics and image analysis.

295. M. Nikolova. Analysis of the recovery of edges in images and signals by minimizing nonconvex regularized least-squares. *Multiscale Model. Simul.*, 4(3):960–991, 2005.

296. M. Nikolova. Model distortions in bayesian map reconstruction. *Inverse Probl. Imaging*, 1(2):399–422, 2007.

297. S. Nilsson. *Application of Fast Backprojection Techniques for Some Inverse Problems of Integral Geometry*. PhD thesis, Linköping University, Dept. of Mathematics, 1997.

298. M. Nitzberg, D. Mumford, and T. Shiota. *Filtering, Segmentation and Depth*, volume 662 of *Lecture Notes in Computer Science*. Springer-Verlag, New York, 1993.

299. S. J. Norton. Reconstruction of a two-dimensional reflecting medium over a circular domain: Exact solution. *J. Acoust. Soc. Amer.*, 67(4):1266–1273, 1980.

300. S. J. Norton and M. Linzer. Ultrasonic reflectivity imaging in three dimensions: Exact inverse scattering solutions for plane, cylindrical and spherical apertures. *IEEE Trans. Biomed. Eng.*, 28(2):202–220, 1981.

301. A. Obereder, S. Osher, and O. Scherzer. On the use of dual norms in bounded variation type regularization. In *[241]*, pages 373–390, 2005.

302. A. Obereder, O. Scherzer, and A. Kovac. Bivariate density estimation using BV regularisation. *Comput. Statist. Data Anal.*, 51(12):5622–5634, 2007.

303. C. Olech. Weak lower semicontinuity of integral functionals. *J. Optim. Theory Appl.*, 19(1):3–16, 1976.

304. M. E. Oman and C. Vogel. Fast numerical methods for total variation minimization in image reconstruction. In *[263]*, pages 359–367, 1995.

305. A. Oraevsky, editor. *Biomedical Optoacoustics*, volume 3916 of *Proceedings of SPIE*, 2000.

306. A. Oraevsky and L. V. Wang, editors. *Photons Plus Ultrasound: Imaging and Sensing 2007: The Eighth Conference on Biomedical Thermoacoustics, Optoacoustics, and Acousto-optics*, volume 6437 of *Proceedings of SPIE*, 2007.

307. S. Osher, M. Burger, D. Goldfarb, J. Xu, and W. Yin. An iterative regularization method for total variation based image restoration. *Multiscale Model. Simul.*, 4(2):460–489, 2005.

308. S. Osher and S. Esedoglu. Decomposition of images by the anisotropic Rudin–Osher–Fatemi model. *Comm. Pure Appl. Math.*, 57(12):1609–1626, 2004.

309. S. Osher and N. Paragios, editors. *Geometric Level Set Methods in Imaging, Vision, and Graphics*. Springer-Verlag, New York, 2003.

310. S. Osher and O. Scherzer. G-norm properties of bounded variation regularization. *Commun. Math. Sci.*, 2(2):237–254, 2004.

311. S. Osher and J. A. Sethian. Fronts propagating with curvature-dependent speed: Algorithms based on Hamilton–Jacobi formulations. *J. Comput. Phys.*, 79(1):12–49, 1988.

312. S. Osher, A. Solé, and L. Vese. Image decomposition and restoration using total variation minimization and the H^{-1}-norm. *Multiscale Model. Simul.*, 1(3):349–370, 2003.

313. V. P. Palamodov. Reconstruction from limited data of arc means. *J. Fourier Anal. Appl.*, 6(1):25–42, 2000.

314. V. P. Palamodov. *Reconstructive Integral Geometry*, volume 98 of *Monographs in Mathematics*. Birkhäuser Verlag, Basel, 2004.

315. V. P. Palamodov. Remarks on the general Funk–Radon transform and thermoacoustic tomography. *arXiv*, page math.AP/0701204, 2007.

316. G. Paltauf, R. Nuster, P. Burgholzer, and M. Haltmeier. Three-dimensional photoacoustic tomography using acoustic line detectors. In *[306]*, pages 23–32, 2007.

317. G. Paltauf, R. Nuster, M. Haltmeier, and P. Burgholzer. Experimental evaluation of reconstruction algorithms for limited view photoacoustic tomography with line detectors. *Inverse Probl.*, 23(6):81–94, 2007.

318. N. Paragios, O. Faugeras, T. Chan, and C. Schnörr, editors. *Variational, Geometric, and Level Set Methods in Computer Vision*, volume 3752 of *Lecture Notes in Computer Science*. Springer, New York, 2005.

319. N. H. Pavel. *Nonlinear Evolution Operators and Semigroups*, volume 1260 of *Lecture Notes in Mathematics*. Springer-Verlag, Berlin, 1987.

320. P. Perona and J. Malik. Scale space and edge detection using anisotropic diffusion. *IEEE Trans. Pattern Anal. Mach. Intell.*, 12(7):629–639, 1990.

321. W. R. Pestman. *Mathematical Statistics*. de Gruyter, Berlin, New York, 1998.

322. T. A. Pitts, J. F. Greenleaf, J.-Y. Lu, and R. R. Kinnick. Tomographic schlieren imaging for measurement of beam pressure and intensity. In *Proc. IEEE Ultrasonics Symposium*, pages 1665–1668, 1994.

323. C. Pöschl and O. Scherzer. Characterization of minimizers of convex regularization functionals. In *[255]*, pages 219 – 248, 2008.

324. J. Radon. Über die Bestimmung von Funktionen durch ihre Integralwerte längs gewisser Mannigfaltigkeiten. *Ber. Verh. Kön. Sächs. Ges. Wiss. Leipzig Math. Phys. Kl.*, 69:262–277, 1917.

325. T. Raus. The principle of the residual in the solution of ill-posed problems. *Tartu Riikl. Ül. Toimetised*, (672):16–26, 1984.

326. T. Raus. The principle of the residual in the solution of ill-posed problems with nonselfadjoint operator. *Tartu Riikl. Ül. Toimetised*, (715):12–20, 1985.

327. T. P. Ray and S. V. W. Beckwith, editors. *Star Formation and Techniques in Infrared and mm-Wave Astronomy*, volume 431 of *Lecture Notes in Physics*. Springer, Berlin / Heidelberg, 1994.

328. C. Reinsch. Smoothing by spline functions. *Numer. Math.*, 10(3):177–183, 1967.

329. E. Resmerita. On total convexity, Bregman projections and stability in Banach spaces. *J. Convex Anal.*, 11(1):1–16, 2004.

330. E. Resmerita. Regularization of ill-posed problems in Banach spaces: convergence rates. *Inverse Probl.*, 21(4):1303–1314, 2005.

331. E. Resmerita and R. S. Anderssen. Joint additive Kullback–Leibler residual minimization and regularization for linear inverse problems. *Math. Methods Appl. Sci.*, 30(13):1527–1544, 2007.

332. E. Resmerita and O. Scherzer. Error estimates for non-quadratic regularization and the relation to enhancing. *Inverse Probl.*, 22(3):801–814, 2006.

333. M. Robberto, S. V. W. Beckwith, N. Panagia, S. G. Patel, T. M. Herbst, S. Ligori, A. Custo, P. Boccacci, and M. Bertero. The Orion nebula in the mid-infrared. *Astronom. J.*, 129(3):1534–1563, 2005.

334. R. T. Rockafellar. *Convex Analysis*, volume 28 of *Princeton Mathematical Series*. Princeton University Press, Princeton, 1970.

335. R. T. Rockafellar. Integral functionals, normal integrands and measurable selections. In *[134]*, pages 157–207, 1976.

336. A. Rosenfeld and A. C. Kak. *Digital Picture Processing*, volume 1+2. Academic Press, New York, 2nd edition, 1989.

337. L. I. Rudin, P.-L. Lions, and S. Osher. Multiplicative denoising and deblurring: theory and applications. In *[309]*, pages 103–119, 2003.

338. L. I. Rudin and S. Osher. Total variation based image restoration with free local constraints. In *Proc. IEEE International Conference on Image Processing*, pages 31–35, 1994.

339. L. I. Rudin, S. Osher, and E. Fatemi. Nonlinear total variation based noise removal algorithms. *Phys. D*, 60(1–4):259–268, 1992.

340. W. Rudin. *Functional Analysis*. McGraw-Hill Series in Higher Mathematics. McGraw-Hill Book Co., New York, 1973.

341. F. Santosa. A level-set approach for inverse problems involving obstacles. *ESAIM Control Optim. Calc. Var.*, 1:17–33, 1996.

342. A. Sarti, R. Malladi, and J. A. Sethian. Subjective surfaces: a method for completing missing boundaries. *Proc. Nat. Acad. Sci. U.S.A.*, 97:6258–6263 (electronic), 2000.

343. O. Scherzer. The use of Morozov's discrepancy principle for Tikhonov regularization for solving nonlinear ill-posed problems. *Computing*, 51(1):45–60, 1993.

344. O. Scherzer. Denoising with higher order derivatives of bounded variation and an application to parameter estimation. *Computing*, 60(1):1–27, 1998.

345. O. Scherzer. A posteriori error estimates for nonlinear ill-posed problems. *Nonlinear Anal.*, 45(4):459–481, 2001.

346. O. Scherzer. Explicit versus implicit relative error regularization on the space of functions of bounded variation. In *[287]*, pages 171–198, 2002.

347. O. Scherzer. Scale space methods for denoising and inverse problem. *Adv. Imaging Electron Phys.*, 128:445–530, 2003.

348. O. Scherzer, H. W. Engl, and K. Kunisch. Optimal a posteriori parameter choice for Tikhonov regularization for solving nonlinear ill-posed problems. *SIAM J. Numer. Anal.*, 30(6):1796–1838, 1993.

349. O. Scherzer and J. Weickert. Relations between regularization and diffusion filtering. *J. Math. Imaging Vision*, 12(1):43–63, 2000.

350. O. Scherzer, W. Yin, and S. Osher. Slope and G-set characterization of set-valued functions and applications to non-differentiable optimization problems. *Commun. Math. Sci.*, 3(4):479–492, 2005.

351. I. J. Schoenberg. Spline functions and the problem of graduation. *Proc. Nat. Acad. Sci. U.S.A.*, 52(4):947–950, 1964.

352. I. J. Schoenberg. Spline interpolation and the higher derivatives. *Proc. Nat. Acad. Sci. U.S.A.*, 51(1):24–28, 1964.

353. L. L. Schumaker. *Spline Functions: Basic Theory*. Wiley, New York, 1981.

354. T. I. Seidman and C. R. Vogel. Well posedness and convergence of some regularisation methods for non-linear ill posed problems. *Inverse Probl.*, 5(2):227–238, 1989.

355. J. Shen and S. H. Kang. Quantum TV and applications in image processing. *Inverse Probl. Imaging*, 1(3):557–575, 2007.

356. J. Shi and S. Osher. A nonlinear inverse scale space method for a convex multiplicative noise model. Technical Report 07/10, UCLA, Los Angeles, 2007.

357. R. E. Showalter. *Monotone Operators in Banach Spaces and Nonlinear Partial Differential Equations*, volume 49 of *Mathematical Surveys and Monographs*. American Mathematical Society, Providence, Rhode Island, 1997.

358. A. Sliwinski, B. Linde, and P. Kwiek, editors. *Acousto-Optics and Applications III*, volume 3581 of *Proceedings of SPIE*, 1998.

359. D. L. Snyder, A. M. Hammoud, and R. L. White. Image recovery from data acquired with a charged-coupled-device camera. *J. Opt. Soc. Amer. A*, 10(5):1014–1023, 1993.

360. M. Sonka and J. M. Fitzpatrik. *Handbook of Medical Imaging, Volume 1: Medical Image Processing and Analysis*. SPIE, 2000.

361. L. A. Steen and A. J. Seebach Jr. *Counterexamples in Topology*. Holt, New York, 1970.

362. G. Steidl. A note on the dual treatment of higher-order regularization functionals. *Computing*, 76(1–2):135–148, 2006.

363. G. Steidl, J. Weickert, T. Brox, P. Mrázek, and M. Welk. On the equivalence of soft wavelet shrinkage, total variation diffusion, total variation regularization, and SIDes. *SIAM J. Numer. Anal.*, 42(2):686–713, 2004.

364. D. Strong and T. Chan. Edge-preserving and scale-dependent properties of total variation regularization. *Inverse Probl.*, 19(6):165–187, 2003. Special section on imaging.

365. M. A. Sychev. Attainment and relaxation results in special classes of deformations. *Calc. Var. Partial Differential Equations*, 19(2):183–210, 2004.

366. E. Tadmor, S. Nezzar, and L. Vese. A multiscale image representation using hierarchical (BV, L^2) decompositions. *Multiscale Model. Simul.*, 2(4):554–579 (electronic), 2004.

367. E. Tadmor, S. Nezzar, and L. Vese. Multiscale hierarchical decomposition of images with applications to deblurring, denoising and segmentation. Technical report, University of Maryland, 2007.

368. X. Tai, K. Lie, T. F. Chan, and S. Osher. *Image Processing Based on Partial Differential Equations: Proceedings of the International Conference on PDE-Based Image Processing and Related Inverse Problems*. Mathematics and Visualization. Springer-Verlag, New York, 2007.

369. A. C. Tam. Applications of photoacoustic sensing techniques. *Rev. Modern Phys.*, 58(2):381–431, 1986.

370. U. Tautenhahn. On the asymptotical regularization of nonlinear ill-posed problems. *Inverse Probl.*, 10(6):1405–1418, 1994.

371. A. N. Tikhonov. Regularization of incorrectly posed problems. *Soviet Math. Dokl.*, 4:1624–1627, 1963.

372. A. N. Tikhonov. Solution of incorrectly formulated problems and the regularization methods. *Soviet Math. Dokl.*, 4:1035–1038, 1963.

373. A. N. Tikhonov and V. Y. Arsenin. *Solutions of Ill-Posed Problems*. John Wiley & Sons, Washington, D.C., 1977.

374. M. Unser. Splines: a perfect fit for signal and image processing. *IEEE Signal Process. Mag.*, 16(6):22–38, 1999.

375. M. Unser and T. Blu. Fractional splines and wavelets. *SIAM Rev.*, 42(2):43–67, 2000.

376. L. Vese. A study in the BV space of a denoising-deblurring variational problem. *Appl. Math. Optim.*, 44(2):131–161, 2001.

377. L. Vese and S. Osher. Modeling textures with total variation minimization and oscillating patterns in image processing. *J. Sci. Comput.*, 19(1–3): 553–572, 2003. Special issue in honor of the sixtieth birthday of Stanley Osher.

378. C. R. Vogel. *Computational Methods for Inverse Problems*, volume 23 of *Frontiers in Applied Mathematics*. SIAM, Philadelphia, 2002.

379. G. Wahba. *Spline Models for Observational Data*, volume 59 of *Regional Conference Series in Applied Mathematics*. SIAM, Philadelphia, 1990.

380. L. V. Wang, editor. *Photoacoustic Imaging and Spectroscopy*. Optical Science and Engineering. CRC Press, Boca Raton, 2008.

381. X. D. Wang, G. Pang, Y. J. Ku, X. Y. Xie, G. Stoica, and L. V. Wang. Noninvasive laser-induced photoacoustic tomography for structural and functional *in vivo* imaging of the brain. *Nature Biotech.*, 21(7):803–806, 2003.

382. X. D. Wang, Y. Xu, M. Xu, S. Yokoo, E. S. Fry, and L. V. Wang. Photoacoustic tomography of biological tissues with high cross-section resolution: Reconstruction and experiment. *Med. Phys.*, 29(12):2799–2805, 2002.

383. A. Webb. *Statistical Pattern Recognition*. Wiley, second edition, 2002.

384. L.-Y. Wei and M. Levoy. Fast texture synthesis using tree-structured vector quantization. In *[214]*, pages 479–488, 2000.

385. J. Weickert. *Anisotropic Diffusion in Image Processing*. Teubner, Stuttgart, 1998. European Consortium for Mathematics in Industry.

386. J. Weickert and C. Schnörr. A theoretical framework for convex regularizers in PDE-based computation of image motion. *Int. J. Comput. Vision*, 45(3):245–264, 2001.

387. J. Weidmann. *Linear Operators in Hilbert Spaces*, volume 68 of *Graduate Texts in Mathematics*. Springer, New York, 1980.

388. E. W. Weisstein. *CRC Concise Encyclopedia of Mathematics*. Chapman & Hall/CRC, Boca Raton, 1999.

389. B. Werner, editor. *Proceedings of the 1998 IEEE International Conference on Image Processing (ICIP-98)*, Los Alamitos, 1998. IEEE Computer Society.

390. D. Werner. *Funktionalanalysis*. Springer-Verlag, Berlin, 2002. Revised 4th edition.

391. G. Winkler. *Image Analysis, Random Fields and Markov Chain Monte Carlo Methods*, volume 27 of *Applications of Mathematics*. Springer-Verlag, New York, second edition, 2003.

392. J. Wloka. *Partielle Differentialgleichungen*. Teubner, Stuttgart, 1982.

393. J. Xu and S. Osher. Iterative regularization and nonlinear inverse scale space applied to wavelet-based denoising. *IEEE Trans. Image Process.*, 16(2):534–544, 2007.

394. M. Xu and L. V. Wang. Time-domain reconstruction for thermoacoustic tomography in a spherical geometry. *IEEE Trans. Med. Imag.*, 21(7):814–822, 2002.

395. M. Xu and L. V. Wang. Analytic explanation of spatial resolution related to bandwidth and detector aperture size in thermoacoustic or photoacoustic reconstruction. *Phys. Rev. E*, 67(5):0566051–05660515 (electronic), 2003.

396. M. Xu and L. V. Wang. Universal back-projection algorithm for photoacoustic computed tomography. *Phys. Rev. E*, 71(1):0167061–0167067 (electronic), 2005.

397. M. Xu and L. V. Wang. Photoacoustic imaging in biomedicine. *Rev. Sci. Instruments*, 77(4):041101, 2006.

398. M. Xu, Y. Xu, and L. V. Wang. Time-domain reconstruction algorithms and numerical simulations for thermoacoustic tomography in various geometries. *IEEE Trans. Biomed. Eng.*, 50(9):1086–1099, 2003.

399. Y. Xu and L. V. Wang. Rhesus monkey brain imaging through intact skull with thermoacoustic tomography. *IEEE Trans. Ultrason., Ferroeletr., Freq. Control*, 53(3):542–548, 2006.

400. W Yin, S. Osher, D. Goldfarb, and J. Darbon. Bregman iterative algorithms for l^1-minimization with applications to compressed sensing. *SIAM J. Imaging Sciences*, 1:143168, 2008.

401. K. Yosida. *Functional Analysis*, volume 123 of *Die Grundlehren der Mathematischen Wissenschaften*. Academic Press Inc., New York, 1965.

402. C. I. Zanelli and M. M. Kadri. Measurements of acoustic pressure in the nonlinear range in water using quantitative schlieren. In *Proc. IEEE Ultrasonics Symposium*, volume 3, pages 1765–1768, 1994.

403. E. Zeidler. *Nonlinear Functional Analysis and its Applications III*. Springer-Verlag, New York, 1985.

404. E. Z. Zhang, J. Laufer, and P. Beard. Three-dimensional photoacoustic imaging of vascular anatomy in small animals using an optical detection system. In *[306]*, 2007.

405. W. P. Ziemer. *Weakly Differentiable Functions. Sobolev Spaces and Functions of Bounded Variation*, volume 120 of *Graduate Texts in Mathematics*. Springer-Verlag, Berlin, 1989.

Nomenclature

The nomenclature is structured into sets, function spaces, norms, functions, functionals and operators, and symbols and abbreviations.

Sets

2^X	Power set of X, page 239
A^0	Minimal section of set-valued operator A, page 190
$\bar{A}$	Closure of the set A, page 221
$\overset{\circ}{A}$	Interior of the set A, page 221
$B_\varepsilon(x)$	Open ball, page 225
$\mathcal{B}_p^*(0)$	Unit ball with respect to $\|\cdot\|_*$, page 212
$\mathcal{B}(X)$	Borel σ-algebra of X, page 240
conv E	Convex hull of the set E, page 273
$\mathcal{D}(A)$	Domain of the set-valued operator A, page 190
$\mathcal{D}(\mathcal{R})$	Proper domain, page 60
$\mathcal{D}_B(\mathcal{R})$	Bregman domain of $\mathcal{R}$, page 61
∂A	Boundary of the set A, page 222
$E(\mathbf{n}, d)$	Plane normal to $\mathbf{n}$, page 12
epi$(\mathcal{S})$	Epigraph, page 274
GL^n	Invertible matrices, page 199
$\mathcal{G}(A)$	Graph of the set-valued operator A, page 190
$\mathcal{G}(F)$	Graph of the operator F, page 224
$\mathcal{I}_1$	Set of pixel indices, page 31
$\mathcal{I}_2$	Subset of pixel indices, page 32
$\ker(L)$	Kernel of the linear operator L, page 227
$\mathrm{level}_t(\mathcal{F})$	t-lower level set of $\mathcal{F}$, page 224
$\mathcal{M}_\alpha(M)$	M-level set for a regularization functional with regularization parameter α, page 60
$Q(x, r)$	Rectangle around x, page 250
$\mathrm{Ran}(\Delta)$	Range of the random variable Δ, page 27
$\mathrm{Ran}(A)$	Range of the set-valued operator A, page 190

$\mathrm{Ran}(L)$	Range of the linear operator L, page 227
S^1	Unit circle, page 256
S^2	Unit sphere, page 6
$\Sigma(u)$	Jump set of $u \in BV(\Omega)$, page 266
$S^{n \times n}$	Symmetric matrices, page 198
$\mathrm{supp}(\mathbf{u})$	Support of $\mathbf{u}$, page 238

Function spaces

$BV(\Omega)$	Space of functions of bounded variation, page 265
$\widehat{BV}(\mathbb{R}^n)$	Space of functions of finite total variation, page 268
$\widehat{BV}^l(\mathbb{R}^n)$	Space of functions of finite higher order total variation, page 270
$\mathcal{BV}^l$	Space of functions of finite total variation on Ω bocL or $\Omega = \mathbb{R}^n$, page 121
$c_0(\mathbb{N})$	Space of zero sequences, pre-dual of $l^1(\mathbb{N})$, page 230
$C(\Omega; \mathbb{R}^m)$	Space of continuous functions, page 237
$C^\infty_{\mathrm{per},0}\big((0,T) \times \Omega; \mathbb{R}^m\big)$	Space of arbitrarily differentiable periodic functions with compact support, page 238
$C^\infty_0(\Omega; \mathbb{R}^m)$	Space of arbitrarily differentiable functions with compact support, page 238
$C^\infty_0(\overline{\Omega}; \mathbb{R}^m)$	Space of arbitrarily differentiable functions with zero boundary, page 238
$C^\infty(\Omega; \mathbb{R}^m)$	Space of arbitrarily differentiable functions, page 238
$C^l_0(\Omega; \mathbb{R}^m)$	Space of l-times differentiable functions with compact support, page 238
$C^l(I; X)$	Bochner space of l-times differentiable functions with values in the Banach space X, page 264
$C^l(\Omega; \mathbb{R}^m)$	Space of l-times differentiable functions, page 237
$C^l_B(\Omega; \mathbb{R}^m)$	Space of l-times differentiable bounded functions, page 238
$C^l_B(\overline{\Omega}; \mathbb{R}^m)$	Space of l-times differentiable bounded functions on $\overline{\Omega}$, page 238
$C^l_K(\Omega; \mathbb{R}^m)$	Space of l-times differentiable functions on Ω with compact support in $K \subset \Omega$, page 238
$L^p(I; X)$	Bochner space of p-integrable functions with values in the Banach space X, page 263
$l^p(\mathbb{N})$	Space of p-summable sequences, page 230
$L^1_{\mathrm{loc}}(\Omega; \mu)$	Space of locally integrable functions, page 244
$L^p(\Omega)$	Space of p-integrable functions, page 243
$L^p_\diamond(\Omega)$	Space of p-integrable functions with zero mean, page 246
$L^\infty(\Omega)$	Space of essentially bounded functions, page 243
$L(X, Y)$	Space of bounded linear operators, page 227
$W^{1,p}(I; X)$	Bochner space of weakly differentiable, p-integrable functions with values in the Banach space X, page 264
$W^{1,p}(\Omega)$	Sobolev space, page 255

$W^{1,p}_{\text{loc}}(I;X)$	Bochner space of weakly differentiable, locally p-integrable functions with values in the Banach space X, page 265
$W^{1,p}_{\text{loc}}(\Omega)$	Sobolev space of locally integrable functions, page 255
$W^{l,p}_0(\Omega)$	Homogeneous Sobolev space, page 256
$W^{l,p}_0(S^1 \times \Omega)$	Periodic Sobolev space, page 256
$W^{l,p}(\Omega)$	Higher-order Sobolev space, page 255
$\mathcal{W}^{l,p}$	Sobolev space on Ω bocL or $\Omega = \mathbb{R}^n$, page 121
$W^{l,p}_\diamond(\Omega)$	Sobolev space with vanishing moments, page 256
$\widehat{W}^{l,p}(\Omega)$	Homogeneous Sobolev space, page 259
$W^{l,p}_{\text{loc}}(\Omega)$	Higher-order Sobolev space of locally integrable functions, page 255

Norms

$\lvert\cdot\rvert_\infty$	Maximum norm on $\mathbb{R}^n$, page 225
$\lvert\cdot\rvert_{l,p}$	Sobolev semi-norm, page 258
$\lvert\cdot\rvert_p$	p-norm on $\mathbb{R}^n$, page 225
$\lVert\cdot\rVert_{1,\infty}$	Norm on the Sobolev space $W^{1,\infty}(\Omega)$, page 255
$\lVert\cdot\rVert_{1,p}$	Norm on the Sobolev space $W^{1,p}(\Omega)$, page 255
$\lVert\cdot + G\rVert_{X/G}$	Norm on the factor space X/G, page 236
$\lVert\cdot\rVert_G$	G-norm, page 120
$\lVert\cdot\rVert_\infty$	L^∞-norm, page 243
$\lVert\cdot\rVert_p$	L^p-norm, page 243
$\lVert\cdot\rVert_{l,p}$	Norm on the higher-order Sobolev space $W^{l,p}(\Omega)$, page 255
$\lVert\cdot\rVert_{s,2}$	Norm on the interpolation space $W^{s,2}(\Omega)$, page 263
$\lVert\cdot\rVert_{[X,Y]_\theta}$	Norm on an interpolation space, page 263

Functions

χ_E	Characteristic function of E, page 242
$\operatorname{co} f$	Convexification of the integrand f, page 163
f^∞	Recession function of f, page 168
ρ_ε	Rescaling of a mollifier, page 261
$\mathbf{u}$	Discrete image data, page 31
$\mathbf{u}^\delta$	Discrete image data with noise, page 33
u_+	Approximate upper limit of u, page 266
u_-	Approximate lower limit of u, page 266
u_α	Regularizer for noise-free data, page 54
u^δ_α	Regularizer for noisy data, page 54
$u^{(k)}_\alpha$	Iterative regularizer, page 53
$u^\dagger$	Minimal norm or $\mathcal{R}$-minimizing solution, page 55
$u_{k,N}$	Approximation of the exponential formula, page 188
$u^{(l)}(x)$	Left limit of u at x, page 270
$u^{(r)}(x)$	Right limit of u at x, page 270
u^-	Non-positive part of the function u, page 241
u^+	Non-negative part of the function u, page 241

v	Unperturbed data, page 54
v^δ	Noisy data, page 54

Functionals and Operators

$\partial^0 \mathcal{R}$	Minimal section of the subdifferential $\partial \mathcal{R}$, page 193
$\partial^\gamma L$	Derivative of a distribution, page 249
$\partial^\gamma u$	Derivative of u with multi-index γ, page 237
$\partial^i u$	Weak partial derivative of u, page 254
$\partial \mathcal{S}$	Subdifferential of $\mathcal{S}$, page 277
$\mathrm{dist}(x, A)$	Distance between $x \in X$ and $A \subset X$, page 222
$D_\mathcal{R}$	Directional Bregman distance, page 67
Du	Weak derivative of a function of bounded variation, page 265
D_ξ	Bregman distance, page 61
E	Mean or sample mean, page 29
$\mathcal{F}_c^{(1)}$	Convexified NCBV functional with exponent 1, extended to $BV(\Omega)$, page 175
$\mathcal{F}_c$	Convexification of the functional $\mathcal{F}$, page 164
$\mathcal{F}^{(p)}$	NCBV functional with exponent p, page 172
$\mathcal{F}_c^{(p)}$	Convexified NCBV functional with exponent p, page 174
$F'(u)$	Gâteaux derivative of F, page 282
$\mathcal{F}'(u; h)$	One-sided derivative of the functional $\mathcal{F}$ in direction h, page 282
$F'(u; h)$	One-sided derivative of F in direction h, page 281
Id	Identity mapping, page 223
$\Im_p$	Identification of $(L^p)^*$ and L^{p*}, page 245
i^*	Adjoint of the embedding operator from L^2 to $W^{1,2}$, equals $-\Delta^{-1}$, page 58
$\mathcal{J}$	Duality mapping: $X \to 2^{X^*}$ with Banach space X, page 280
$\mathcal{J}_{W_0^{1,p}}$	$W_0^{1,p}$-duality mapping, page 281
$\mathcal{J}_{W_\diamond^{1,p}}$	$W_\diamond^{1,p}$-duality mapping, page 281
$\mathcal{J}_{1,s}$	Duality mapping $\mathcal{J}_{W_\diamond^{1,s}}$ or $\mathcal{J}_{W_0^{1,s}}$, page 208
$\mathcal{J}_p$	p-duality mapping: $L^p(\Omega) \to L^{p*}(\Omega)$, page 281
$\mathcal{J}_X$	Identification of X and X^* in Hilbert spaces, page 231
J_f	Jacobian of f, page 28
$(\nabla \cdot \mathbf{u})$	Divergence of $\mathbf{u}$, page 237
$(\nabla^l \cdot \mathbf{u})$	Higher-order divergence of $\mathbf{u}$, page 237
$\nabla_h u$	Discrete gradient of u, page 32
$\nabla^k u$	Vector of k-th order weak partial derivatives of u, page 255
∇u	Gradient of u, page 254
$P_{\overline{\mathcal{B}_2^*(0)}}$	Projection operator from $L^2(\Omega)$ onto $\overline{\mathcal{B}_2^*(0)}$, page 212
$\mathcal{R}_{BV}\mathcal{F}$	Relaxation of $\mathcal{F}$ in $BV(\Omega)$, page 167
$\mathrm{R}_{\mathrm{circ}}$	Circular Radon transform, page 21
$\mathcal{R}\mathcal{F}$	Relaxation of the functional $\mathcal{F}$, page 162
$\mathcal{R}_1$	Total variation, page 265

$\mathcal{R}_l(u)$	Higher-order total variation of a locally summable function, page 269
R_{line}	Linear Radon transform, page 12
R_{plane}	Planar Radon transform, page 19
$\mathcal{R}^{\text{SP}}$	L^1 regularization term, page 87
$\mathcal{R}^{\text{sp}}$	l^p regularization term, page 79
R_{sph}	Spherical Radon transform, page 18
S	Schlieren Transform, page 109
S_λ	Soft thresholding function, page 86
$\mathcal{S}_p$	L^p similarity term, page 118
$\mathcal{T}_{\alpha,u^\delta}^{\text{ME}}$	Maximum entropy functional, page 115
$\mathcal{T}_{\alpha,u^\delta}^{p,l}$	Regularization functional with total variation of the l-th derivative and L^p similarity term, page 118
$\mathcal{T}_{\alpha,u^\delta}^{\text{SP}}$	L^1 regularization, page 87
$\mathcal{T}_{\alpha,u^\delta}^{\text{sp}}$	Sparsity regularization, page 79
$\mathcal{T}_{\alpha,v^\delta}$	Regularization functional, page 53
$\mathcal{T}_{\alpha,v^\delta}^{(k)}$	Iterative regularization functional, page 53
$\mathcal{T}^*$	Fenchel transform of $\mathcal{T}$, page 279
Var	Variance or sample variance, page 29

Symbols and Abbreviations

$\langle\cdot,\cdot\rangle = \langle\cdot,\cdot\rangle_X$	Inner product, page 226
$\langle x,y\rangle_{[X,Y]_\theta}$	Inner product on an interpolation space, page 263
$\langle L,x\rangle$	Evaluation of the linear functional $L \in X^*$ at $x \in X$, page 228
1_*	Conjugate of 1, defined as $1_* = \infty$, page 229
$a \sim b$	a and b are of same order, page 58
bocL	Bounded, open, connected, Lipschitz, page 250
$f^\#\Delta$	Push-forward of the random vector Δ, page 28
$\Gamma\text{-}\lim_k \mathcal{T}_k$	Γ-limit of the sequence $(\mathcal{T}_k)$, page 152
$\mathbf{h}$	Chopping throw, page 7
$\mathcal{H}^s$	s-dimensional Hausdorff measure, page 241
$\text{Lip}(u)$	Lipschitz constant of u, page 250
$\mathcal{L}^n$	Lebesgue measure, page 241
$L^\#$	Dual adjoint operator, page 228
L^*	Adjoint of L, page 231
$L_k \xrightarrow{*} L$	Weak* convergence of (L_k) to L, page 235
$\mu \llcorner E$	Restriction of a measure, page 240
$\mu \perp \nu$	The positive Radon measures μ and ν are mutually singular, page 248
$\mathcal{N}(l)$	Number of multi-indices of length l, page 237
$\overline{\mathcal{N}}(l)$	Number of multi-indices of length at most l, page 237
p_*	Conjugate of p, defined by $1/p + 1/p_* = 1$, page 229
$\text{Per}(E;\Omega)$	Perimeter of E in Ω, page 267

P_Δ	Probability distribution of random variable Δ, page 27
$P_{\mathbf{U}\mid\mathbf{U}^\delta}(\cdot\mid\mathbf{u}^\delta)$	Conditional probability, page 43
p_Δ	Probability density of random variable Δ, page 28
$p_{\mathbf{U}\mid\mathbf{U}^\delta}$	Conditional probability density, page 45
$\lvert\tau\rvert_\infty$	Size of the partition τ, page 206
$\tau=(\tau_k)$	Partition of $[0,\infty)$, page 206
$u*v$	Convolution of u and v, page 261
$V\subset\subset\Omega$	V is compactly contained in Ω, page 223
$\mathbf{x}\cdot\mathbf{y}$	Inner product of $\mathbf{x},\mathbf{y}\in\mathbb{R}^n$, page 226
$x_k\rightharpoonup x$	Weak convergence of (x_k) to x, page 235
x_{ij}	Pixel position, page 31

Index